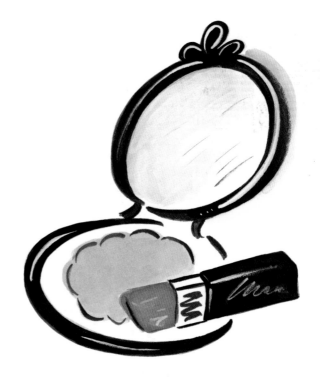

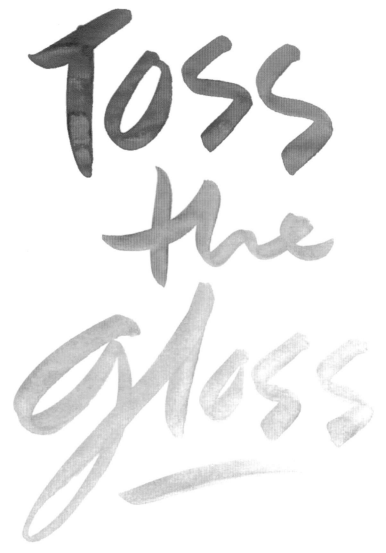

Toss the Gloss

Beauty Tips, Tricks & Truths for Women 50+

ANDREA Q. ROBINSON

SEAL PRESS

Toss the Gloss
Copyright © 2014 Andrea Q. Robinson

Illustrations © Chesley McLaren

Page 4 photo credits: top right © Alex Chatelain, *Vogue France*, October 1969; bottom right © Eric Bowman,
Vogue Australia, November 1993; bottom left © Jennifer Livingston, *Women's Wear Daily*, 2002.

ISBN 978-1-58005-490-4

Library of Congress Cataloging-in-Publication Data

Robinson, Andrea Q.,
Toss the gloss : beauty tips, tricks, and truths for women 50+.
pages cm
ISBN 978-1-58005-490-4
1. Women–Health and hygiene. 2. Middle-aged women–Health and hygiene.
3. Beauty, Personal. I. Title. II. Title: Beauty tips, tricks, and truths
for women 50+.
RA778.R5288 2014
646.7'2–dc23
2013040180

Published by
Seal Press
A Member of the Perseus Books Group
1700 Fourth Street
Berkeley, California
sealpress.com

Cover design by Erin Seaward-Hiatt
Interior design by meganjonesdesign.com
Printed in China
Distributed by Publishers Group West

With love for my mother, the dreamer; my daughter, the naturalist; and my son, the realist. Dazzling inspirations, all of them.

CONTENTS

INTRODUCTION: WHAT'S THAT YOU SAY, MRS. ROBINSON?   1

1   **WABI-SABI:** THE PERFECTION OF IMPERFECTION   11

2   **OUT WITH THE OLD:** CLEAR THE SHELF AND FREE YOURSELF   19

3   **SKINCARE:** GETTING CLEAR ON PRODUCT HELP VS. HYPE   35

4   **ELIMINATE AND ILLUMINATE:** CONCEALER, PRIMER, HIGHLIGHTER   51

5   **FOUNDATION:** THE (NEARLY) NAKED TRUTH   65

6   **BLUSH:** LET'S GET CHEEKY!   85

7   **TANNING:** THE ULTIMATE FAKE BAKE   95

8   **THE EYES HAVE IT:** EYELINER, EYE SHADOW, MASCARA   109

9   **LIPSTICK:** THE MAGIC BULLET   131

10   **HAIR:** HAIR DOS AND HAIR DON'TS   147

11   **THE FORGOTTEN ZONE:** FROM THE NECK DOWN TO THE HANDS UP   169

12   **COSMETIC TWEAKS:** THE NEEDLE, THE KNIFE, THE KNOW-HOW   183

CONCLUSION: SEXY DOESN'T HAVE AN AGE   197

What's that you say, Mrs. Robinson?

INTRODUCTION

HOW MUCH TIME DO YOU HAVE, DEAR READER, BECAUSE I HAVE GOT A LOT TO SAY. WHY LISTEN? BECAUSE I'VE SPENT DECADES RUNNING BEAUTY COMPANIES:

Ultima II, Ralph Lauren, Tom Ford, and Prescriptives, to name just a few. And I'm here to blow the whistle on the beauty industry and give you the real scoop on the business—the good, the bad, and the ugly.

I've tried it all. I've seen it all. I know too much.

Think of me as your personal cosmetics guinea pig. In the name of beauty (and many, many jobs in the beauty industry), I've tried everything out there: lotions, makeup, injections, spas, lasers, you name it. Once I even tried crushed beetle skin on my face, just to test the truth of the Indian legend that extols its youth-preserving magical properties. (As it turned out, it didn't work, but I think you'll agree, that was real commitment!)

After years in the beauty trenches, I've acquired the ultimate beauty industry insider's perspective, and I'm ready to spill it all—even if it means inciting a powder-puff fatwa.

How do I know all these whispered truths? Let's just say it started where all good secrets do: at *Vogue* magazine. Back in the days before The Devil Wore Prada, I was The Beauty Editor Who Wore Revlon . . . and CoverGirl and Lancôme and Maybelline and all the rest. It was my job to try everything, from lipsticks to liposuction, and then report on it. Yes, I tried it all in the name of beauty, and no, you can't see my before and after shots. But thanks to my editor, Grace Mirabella, who reclaimed *Vogue* from a fantasy fashion magazine and made it a bible for real working women who had families and day jobs, I was able to extend her modern point of view on to *Vogue*'s beauty pages and address the needs of real women and their beauty issues.

From my perch at the magazine, I was immersed in the very best the cosmetics industry had to offer, and I spent years testing, comparing, and judging. Then, an unconventional beauty industry executive offered me a job outside *Vogue*'s chic gray walls, and I became president of Ultima II. My job was to reinvent the brand on every level—from product, to packaging, to its image in department stores and in advertising.

How does a girl from an all-women Catholic college, where I practiced pouring tea and holding polite conversation, learn to do battle in the corporate world? I'll tell you how.

The only problem? The male executives in my office. If you think they're a pain in the butt in the boardroom, imagine a group of chauvinistic guys in suits telling you—the only female president in the corporation—that the makeup you've invented won't appeal to women just like you. This was my first business venture (or should I say, adventure), where men, whose only "cosmetic" was deodorant, were telling me what

I wanted in my makeup bag! Well, let's just say they didn't know who they were dealing with. A clash of wit and wills ensued: My instincts took hold and I was determined to deliver to them the non–sugar-coated truth—what we women really want, not what they think we really want. And I did.

How does a girl from an all-women Catholic college, where I practiced pouring tea and holding polite conversation, learn to do battle in the corporate world? I'll tell you how. A friend entered me in *Glamour* magazine's "10 Best Dressed College Girls" contest. I won and that's where my adventure into the "glamorous jungle" began. After graduation, I joined a pool of young college graduates at Condé Nast (the corporation that owns *Vogue*, *Glamour*, and *Vanity Fair*, among many other magazines), assisting editors with whatever they needed. We answered telephones, picked up coffee, ferried clothes to the garment district, scheduled appointments, booked lunch dates at glamorous restaurants, escorted models to the photographer's studio for fashion and beauty shoots, and even typed their children's homework—whatever they needed.

From there, I landed a permanent job working for *Mademoiselle*, where I witnessed the most remarkable explosion of creativity marching through our office each day in the form of artists like Andy Warhol, photographers such as David Bailey, writers like Joyce Carol Oates and Truman Capote, not to mention celebrities, fashion designers, rock stars—The Beatles, Janis Joplin, Grace Slick, Cher (with Sonny), to name a few—and all the top models including Twiggy. Once, I even saw Timothy Leary smoke pot with a very cool editor at the desk next to mine. Edie Locke was the editor-in-chief during that time and turned *Mademoiselle* into the "it" magazine of its time. Nonnie Moore, the legendary editor at *Mademoiselle* magazine and the quintessential modern woman, was my boss and a fabulous mentor who, during the ten years I was there before moving to *Vogue,* not only taught me the basics of editing, but also showed me, by example, how to combine career and family, and in the process also encouraged me to value my own opinions, take chances, break rules when they didn't apply, and tap into my creative talents. That's when I first began to notice the ways in which the cosmetics industry seemed singularly geared to a lack of vision when it came to the basics of addressing the needs and desires of "real women," especially "real women" with real and special needs.

Just in case I'm being too subtle, let me be clear: I believe most men running the major beauty corporations where you undoubtedly have spent a lot of money (even if you're not a cosmetics junkie like me) think you've lost it at fifty. Sure, there are exceptions—men like Ralph Lauren (I was president of his fragrance brand) and Tom Ford (I was president of his beauty company). I'd be a fool to say those men don't understand, explore, and create what real women crave for their vanity table.

> Just in case I'm being too subtle, let me be clear: Most men running the major beauty corporations where you undoubtedly have spent a lot of money think you've lost it at fifty.

But Mr. Lauren and Mr. Ford are geniuses. The fact is that most men in charge of your makeup aren't going to change your world, or even your look. You've "aged out" of their makeup market. The only products they're spending big bucks to market to you are wrinkle creams. Sorry, ladies, but it's true.

But you can't—we can't—listen to them. You, your life, your brain, and—yes, dammit—your looks are at their prime. I know

Pictures from the fashion, beauty, and corporate worlds taken throughout my career, showing the evolution of my style: natural looking makeup and hair.

Clockwise: *Vogue France, Vogue Australia, Women's Wear Daily.*

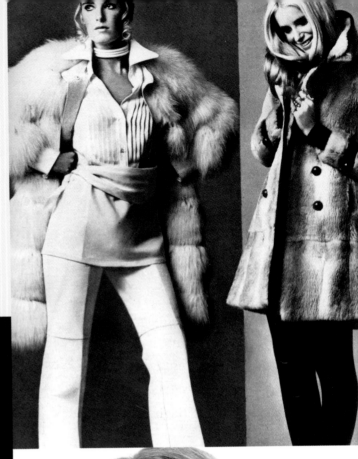

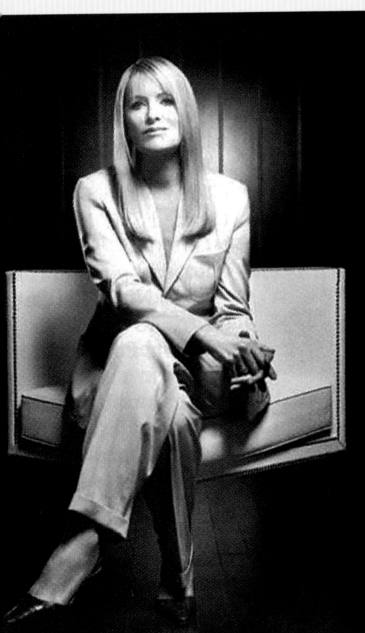

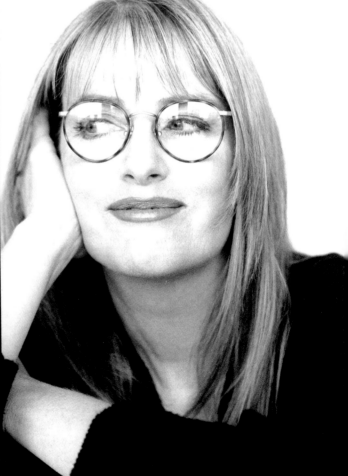

you're just as concerned as ever with looking your best. Want a pair of Manolo Blahnik shoes? How about that sexy little black dress? Who doesn't? So why wouldn't you put your money toward grown-up cosmetics to match?

The depressing, oh-go-to-hell answer for why we don't even have the opportunity to buy cosmetics geared to the color and texture of our menopausal skin is quite simple. Even if there's money to be made, the people running these corporations are afraid to address our specific needs with anything other than antiaging creams because they are worried that they will alienate their younger consumer base, even though we—the fifty+ "real women"—are the largest demographic, with more money to spend. They need to wake up and realize that we're worth their investment.

The disconnect between the industry and us really dawned on me when I accepted a job at Revlon—my first position on the corporate side of the beauty industry. There I relaunched Ultima II with the help of my *Vogue* collaborator, revered photographer Irving Penn. We created a print ad that heralded the start of something new. We set up the shoot so that each letter that spelled out U-L-T-I-M-A got its own makeup item, a visual feast of smeared lipstick, crushed eye shadow, streaked nail polish, and scribbled lip liner. Until then, beauty ads featured either provocative "babes" in overdone makeup or uptight matrons wearing ruffled blouses. The corporate execs didn't get it—frankly, they were shocked, and the ad almost didn't run. But it did, thanks to my persuasive skills with my immediate boss and the company chairman and owner, Ronald Perelman, who overruled the decision that the suits who were running his company made. And soon cash registers were ringing up sales faster than Viagra in a retirement community.

That was just the beginning. Remember "The Nakeds"? It was a groundbreaking line of thirty-eight neutral shades of makeup that predates any of the cosmetic companies that followed, including Bobbi Brown. I created that concept at Revlon. I collaborated on this project with Kevyn Aucoin, the shy, lumbering Texan who helped me with shade selection and would become the biggest makeup artist name in the industry. And I created it because my mission in the beauty business was to help women *look like themselves, only better.* I had to fight the corporate machine to even get the collection on the counters, but, when it arrived in the stores, women loved it, and it sold out everywhere. "Why would a woman want to wear mud on her face?" the suits asked. "Makeup is about

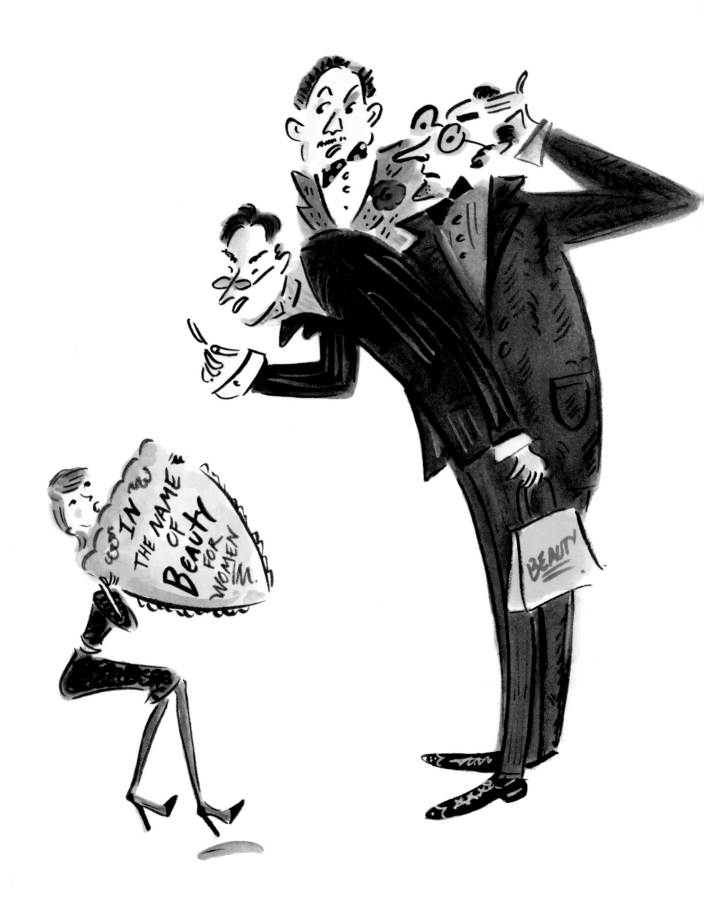

disguise and fantasy." This was 1990, and women had been flooding the workplace with their blue eye shadow, pink lipstick, and orange cheeks—can you imagine? It was war paint for girls (created by men)—for an entire decade. The Nakeds became a cultural statement as well as a fashion statement. Women wholeheartedly embraced the idea of looking like themselves, only better. The concept made millions and catapulted me to the next phase of my career. More important, it catapulted the women of our generation to a new kind of sex appeal, one that relied on who we were instead of a man's fantasy.

The Nakeds were followed by the The Naughty Nakeds, and the first ever long-wearing lipstick (women could go to work and not have to think about reapplying their lipstick all day—remember, it was the '80s. Everyone wore lipstick). After that, I was lured to L'Oreal, where I had the privilege of working with Ralph Lauren and his burgeoning collection of women's fragrances. I helped Ralph create his blockbuster fragrance successes: Romance, Romance Men, Polo Blue, Polo Black, and Ralph. We also worked together on a makeup collection. While I was there, Ralph Lauren Fragrances became the largest fragrance franchise in the world.

I loved those years, but when Estée Lauder came calling again (after a thirty-year courtship on their part to hire me), I signed on. Because the company was founded by a woman, I thought it would further my mis-

> The Nakeds became a cultural statement as well as a fashion statement.

sion to work on a brand that had a built-in audience of fifty+ women who had come of age with the brand. I was named global chief marketing officer for the Estée Lauder brand, and, when Tom Ford created his own brand in the Lauder Corporation, I became its president. My responsibility as president was to help him realize his makeup and fragrance vision. Together, we launched a very successful and unique group of Private Blend fragrances for men and for women, and worked on a makeup collection that would follow later. Ironically, they fired me when I was fifty+. The suit who was running Estée Lauder said he thought it was time for me to retire. *Retire?!* I was just getting started.

WHILE MY LIFE and my career were happening, my own beauty needs were changing. Being married, raising two children, maintaining a full-time career, and supporting a household began to take its toll on my looks, which I had always taken for granted. I noticed the inevitable lines, wrinkles, and shadows under my eyes, and my once fresh-looking skin seemed to have checked out of my face and run for the hills. A visit with my mother crystallized the situation when she gently suggested that I make some time to spend on myself, inferring that I had started to look like I was "letting myself go." She said that I came last on the list when it came to my family. I laughed (probably should have cried) and remarked that I wasn't even on the list! Sound familiar? This was a seminal moment—my mother, who always thought I was beautiful (don't all mothers feel that way?), and this direct conversation prompted me to take immediate action. I was overweight, so I got a membership at the local gym (dropped twenty pounds in four months), and my family went on a healthy diet with me. I went to my dermatologist and started addressing the burgeoning needs of my skin with the Fraxel laser and fillers (more about this later), and I started playing with makeup and treatments to find a regime that would restore that lost youthfulness to my tired little face.

And somewhere between the drama of surgical scaffolding and the myth of miracle skin treatments, I discovered a potent realm of targeted, useful makeup that really works for women over fifty. And thanks to my collaboration with the cosmetic scientists, makeup artists, photographers, actresses, hairdressers, models, dermatologists, cosmetologists, plastic surgeons, witch doctors, rich doctors, and beauty junkies, I knew when and how to apply it. I began to tinker with existing products, mixing and matching formulas, and in the process created new ones geared to my needs.

If your real goal is looking like yourself, only better, this is your go-to book. The surprisingly simple truth I want to share with you, through every chapter, is this: The right makeup, used the right way, is the most powerful weapon in your beauty arsenal. Let this be your first beauty commandment. This book will serve as your guide to recapture the glamorous you. Forget about makeup reclaiming youth. Good makeup reclaims *you*. It's the Chanel in your sample sale, the Splenda in your latte, the fully charged battery in your iPad—it's the sizzle that leads to feeling good and confident; it's instant gratification and major fun, and I'm going to help you get it. Let's go!

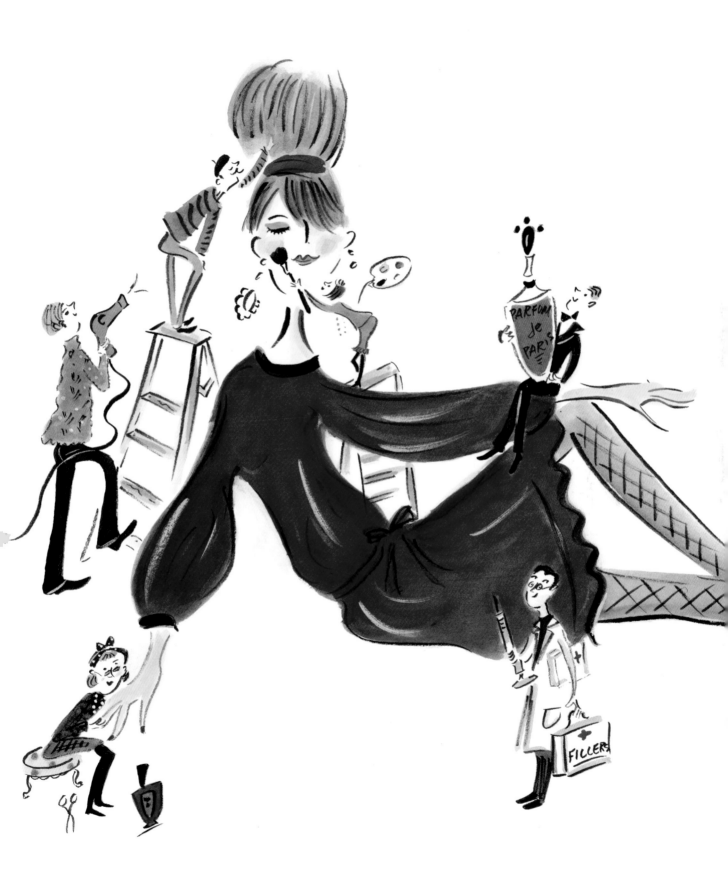

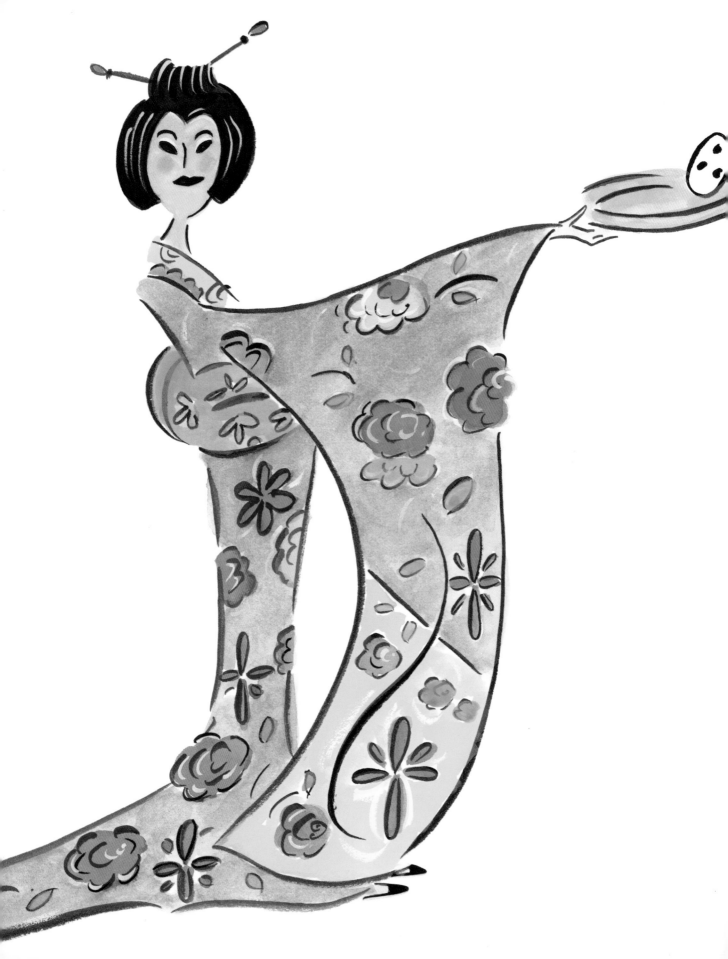

CHAPTER ONE

WABI-SABI

the perfection of imperfection

YEARS AGO, WHEN I WAS TRAVELING THROUGH JAPAN, I MET ISSEY MIYAKE, THE ICONIC JAPANESE DESIGNER KNOWN FOR HIS MODERN FASHION DESIGNS.

Since he was a man of distinctly refined tastes, I jumped at the chance to visit the local spa he recommended. The spa was known for its simple beauty, its organic architectural style (an artful abundance of wood and rock), and its elegant proprietor—a beautiful woman in her fifties. It was here, during a traditional tea ceremony, that she exposed me to the aesthetic of *Wabi-Sabi*, a Japanese concept that celebrates the beauty of imperfection, especially as it relates to the changes experienced with the passage of time. With quiet ritual, she presented a spare bamboo tray laden with an array of irregular-shaped wooden bowls wearing a sheen of time-earned patinas, and old cracked pottery that had been fired with subtle, earth-toned glazes. Together, they presented a beautiful picture of restraint, purity, and color that was a reflection of time's passage. *Wabi-Sabi*, the proprietor explained, was the acknowledgment and respect for imperfection (the

Wabi-Sabi: It is the opposite of trying too hard, and it is understanding the power and seduction of imperfection.

cracks in the pottery), the aesthetic of imperfect beauty (the irregular bowls), and the important notion of honoring time and simplicity (the patinas and glazes). *Wabi-Sabi*: It is the opposite of trying too hard, and it is understanding the power and seduction of imperfection—the beauty of an egg with spots, a seashell with water marks, and, like the beautiful spa owner, a woman with laugh lines. It is the perfection of imperfection, a profound reminder that beauty is best found in its least complex form.

How does this philosophy apply to us? Let me start by sharing an anecdote . . .

When I worked with Ralph Lauren, he told me that the girl he designs for is the one in the convertible with the top down, her hair and clothes blowing in the wind.

I've never forgotten this and I've carried that girl, that image with me, into my womanhood. The French say, "*Elle est bien dans sa peau*"—she is comfortable in her own skin, like the girl in the convertible, not concerned that her hair and makeup look perfect. This is true *Wabi-Sabi*.

We each want to capture that totally natural and carefree girl inside us—the one who is completely at ease with herself and her look at any age. We all know the woman who tries too hard, does too much, and becomes enslaved by the latest trends. She's the woman in the spin class who is so made up that she can't break a sweat, or the woman at the beach with false eyelashes and bright-blue eye shadow, or the woman shopping for groceries wearing lip liner in one color and lipstick in another, or so much lip gloss that she can barely move her mouth when she speaks. She's the woman you don't really ever get to know because her hair, makeup, and clothes enter the room before she does—not a strand of hair, not an eyelash, not a stitch out of place. She has lost that girl.

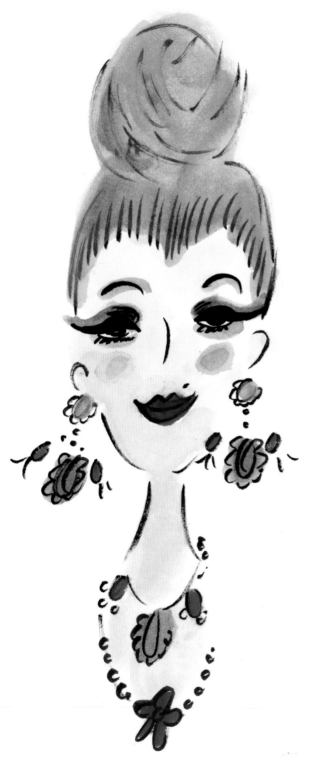

The beautiful older Japanese woman in the spa and the girl in the convertible rule my beauty routine. They are the personification of beauty in its simplest form, not sepa-

She's the woman you don't really ever get to know because her hair, makeup, and clothes enter the room before she does.

rated by age, but joined by their engagement in living and appreciating life as it happens, and the vigorous acceptance of imperfection.

So in light of this, you might ask: How much do I have to worry on the beach, on the ski slope, on a blustery day? How do I strike the balance between not enough and too much control over my appearance? And: Can I still look natural and be fashionable at the same time, young in spirit but not over-the-top trendy? The answer: of course. It's all about *Wabi-Sabi*. And this chapter is about how to make it work for you. Here are the overarching truths:

1 LET GO OF PERFECTION

This is a tough concept, because we've all been brought up to strive for perfection in one way or another. But the truth is that embracing your "flaws" makes you more beautiful, more noticeable, more accessible, more real. How attractive! These are the qualities that come with experience and awareness. Learn to love the bump in your nose, the asymmetry of your eyes, your uneven mouth, your freckles. Learn to love what you consider your flaws.

2 BEWARE OF TRENDS

While I do not subscribe to the rigid rules that many women's magazines like to dictate about how to look good at every age, there certainly are trends you can carry with confidence at age twenty that simply don't work when you're over fifty. Most makeup trends are targeted to women eighteen to forty years old. And that should be your first clue that beauty companies are not thinking about us with the products they market. Furthermore, much of the beauty content we read in fashion magazines is provided by these beauty companies. So beware: What looks good on the model in the magazine may not look good on you. Beware of screaming color. Beware of raccoon eyes. Beware of the latest yellow eye shadow. Beware of heavy eyeliner. Beware of frosted eye and cheek color. Beware of high-gloss lips. Beware of overpenciled, overarched brows. Master the difference between trend "aware" and trend "beware." Just be aware that these looks have been bought and sold by major corporations, but only you can own your personal beauty.

3 DON'T TRY TOO HARD

Let's face it: Wearing heavy makeup when you're over fifty—especially in everyday settings, like the woman at the spin class, the beach, or the supermarket—is as off-putting as seeing short-shorts on jiggly thighs. So the first rule of thumb is to beware of being sold the "short-shorts" of beauty. Remember, department store

cosmetics "experts" get a commission for selling you stuff that you don't need and stuff that is frequently not appropriate. How can you avoid this? First, take a good look at yourself in the mirror and review recent photographs of yourself. Consider what you see. Is your favorite lipstick too harsh? Your eye makeup too heavy? Is that color that the beauty advisor with the ring in her nose at the MAC counter sold you too garish for you? Take an overall assessment: Are you wearing too much powder and paint? Decide what to get rid of. If you're having a hard time with this, pay special attention to Chapter 2 and don't be afraid to consult with a trusted friend whose taste you admire about what works and what doesn't in your makeup kit.

When in doubt, remember what the late Diana Vreeland, the legendary editor of *Vogue* magazine, once said: "Elegance is refusal." And I'll add my own two cents: "Fear of change is for old ladies!" So retire that glittery teal eye shadow. And that matte fuchsia lipstick. Oh, and those colored mascaras, too. Refuse all those inappropriate and cringe-worthy trends of our younger years!

4 HIGH MAINTENANCE HAS TO GO

When it comes to makeup, your routine should be effortless. It shouldn't take more than ten minutes. No, I am not kidding. If it takes much more than that, rethink and re-edit your regimen. This book will help you do that.

And when it comes to cosmetic quick fixes like fillers, please take my advice and don't become a junkie. If Botox is the cocaine of the upper face, then Restylane is the crack of the lower face. Be judicious in what you choose to do. And beware of the Botox/filler parties that closely resemble the Tupperware parties your mother went to. Only now there is a doctor or a nurse with an arsenal of botulism and perhaps some bovine fillers waiting to freeze your face, not the leftovers, at an expense far greater than a set of microwave-safe plastic containers. Just a little reminder: Crow's feet and laugh lines equal a life well lived.

5 SAY "SAYONARA" TO HARSH LINES

And a tough and angry disposition equals a life *not* well lived. And it shows up as scowl lines on your face. And there's nothing pretty about that. The same principle applies to makeup—harsh lines have to go! Check your eyeliner, lip liner, contour lines, and eyebrow pencils. If any of these products are creating sharp lines and hard edges on your face, they should be banished from your makeup case. You need cosmetics that blend, blend, blend. The best look is soft like the wind in the hair of the girl in the convertible. Remember: Makeup is an expression of who you are—not who you were, not who you thought you'd be, and certainly not what the media tells us we should be. Who you are is actually much better. Trust me.

6 DON'T BREAK THE BANK

If you add up all the dough you've ever forked out for beauty products that you either didn't need or didn't use or ended up throwing away, you could probably buy that convertible that inspired Ralph Lauren (or take a trip to that spa in Japan), and you'd still probably have enough money left over for a Birkin bag. To look good, you don't need to spend a lot. It's fine to shell out for certain special "pricey" pieces—but head straight to the drugstore to economize on the rest. You'll find recommendations of how to do this in every chapter.

7 BE PROUD OF WHO YOU REALLY ARE

Do you ever wonder what Dolly Parton looks like under the pounds of makeup and all that blonde, cotton-candy hair? Wouldn't her voice still be as great without it? Wouldn't she still be as funny and clever without it? Wouldn't she still write the most heartfelt and perceptive songs without it? Wouldn't her guitar sound just as good without her long nails? When people say they love her because she's so real I know what they mean, but I always wonder why she needs to pile on the paint, camouflaging her natural beauty. Maybe it's cultural, maybe it's the fans, maybe it's the media. Maybe it's her inner mirror. Does she really *see* herself in all her brilliance? Dolly Parton is not alone. Many other women fall prey to this, despite their innate talent and beauty.

8 LOVE YOUR LINES, YOU'VE EARNED THEM

You're not twenty anymore, and that's a good thing, so I'll say it again: Your lines are what make your face interesting. They are lines of *expression*. Think Diane Keaton in the movie *Something's Gotta Give* (rent it!). She shows us that being beautiful has nothing to do with age or lines or spots. In the end, she, not the younger babe, gets the guy. Remember, you're not twenty anymore and that's a good thing. Accept your laugh lines, laugh about them, and use them to your advantage.

accept your laugh lines . . .

So what does all of this mean? It means appreciating where we are in life, the experiences we've had, and the changes we've made—or those that have been made for us. It's harnessing all of that energy to express the beauty we possess and how to make it work for us in everyday life. In fact, it's understanding that beauty has nothing to do with age and everything to do with a comfort zone the years have provided; that our wisdom, experience, and emotional maturity have coalesced into a beauty that provides a precious platform for our physical appearance. We honor who we are and the abundance of our talents by respecting our physical appearance.

At fifty and beyond, *Wabi-Sabi* teaches us to inhabit the beauty that comes effortlessly with age. It is time for *us* to own our face, not Estée Lauder, not Maybelline, not Revlon, not L'Oreal. It's time to release ourselves from slavish devotion to beauty gimmickry.

At this point in our lives, our beauty routine should be more minimal and effortless, and more strategically focused on the right products and the right procedures in the right places. This is a new day, and we're turning the page to a new beauty chapter for ourselves. And this is where I come in . . . read on.

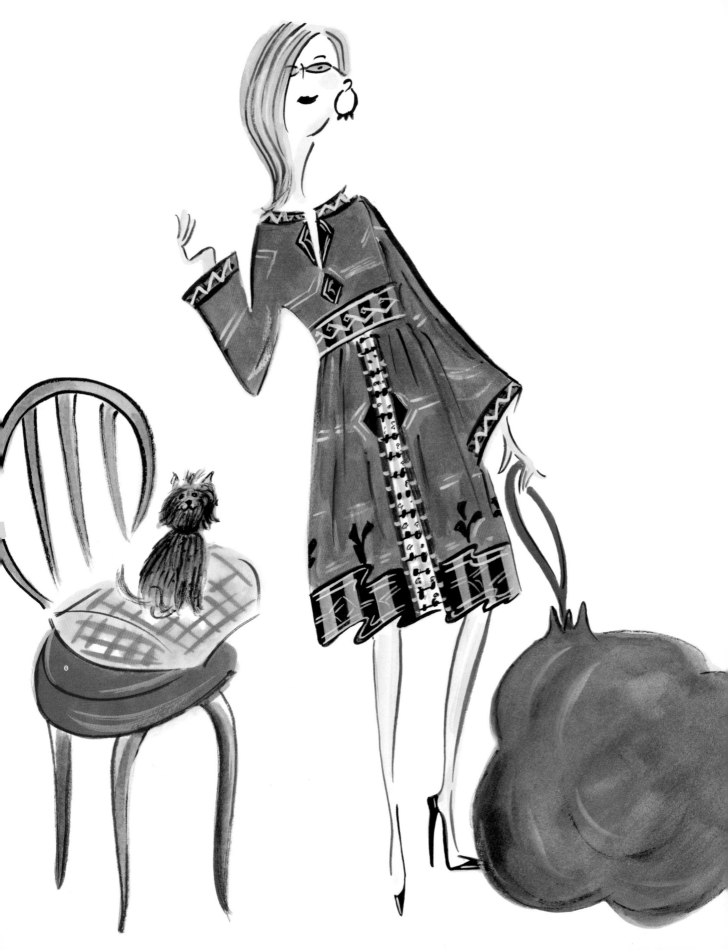

CHAPTER TWO

Out with The Old

clear the shelf and free yourself

BE BRAVE AND TAKE THE FIRST STEP: A FACELIFT. NOW, DON'T GET NERVOUS! IT'S NOT FOR YOU.

It's for your bathroom vanity. By shaving years off your shelves, you'll be left with fresher, healthier beauty products that will enhance your appearance and protect you from the nastier consequences of using old cosmetics. The added beauty of downsizing to the essentials is that you should then be able to tote them easily in a single, well-chosen makeup bag, making storage and retrieval as simple as a one-sided zip.

If you're thinking, *How can I possibly reduce half a dozen drawers and shelves to a single bag?!* I've got news for you. Follow these directions:

1 Get a tall kitchen garbage bag (preferably biodegradable, since the containers you toss will likely be recyclable). If you're at all like me, you will need the big thirty-gallon outdoor garbage bags instead, or maybe even a U-Haul truck!

2 Sweep, dump, or scoop every cosmetic product you've owned longer than one year into that bag. Whatever you do, *don't* stop to debate whether you'll have another chance to wear that sexy red lipstick you bought for New Year's Eve last century, or the shimmery bronzer you bought for your trip to Hawaii three years ago. You won't. *You shouldn't.*

3 Immediately toss the bag(s) into the recycling bin—preferably the one outside—and banish all second thoughts. Congratulations. Now go back inside as fast as you can.

Purging is good. I'm talking about getting rid of all the stuff you don't need—the C-R-A-P that's standing in the way of reclaiming your beauty (and let's face it, your sanity). Chances are, you have a lot of cosmetics that have outlived their expiration date. Keep in mind that the clock starts ticking the moment you open a new tube, wand, bottle, or lipstick, and be aware that natural beauty products have a shorter shelf life because those parabens you've been trying to avoid—the chemicals found in malignant breast tumors that mimic estrogen—were developed to prohibit bacterial growth.

purging is good . . .

Unlike food, cosmetics aren't required to have an expiration date printed on their packaging, so it's up to you to keep track of when you purchased them (see sidebar for specifics about the shelf life of common beauty products). For example, that old tube of opened mascara you've been hoarding for longer than four months is likely laden with bacteria, and there's nothing pretty about a case of pink eye. What about that foundation you've been saving for a rainy day. Is it separating in the bottle? Dump it! Old foundation can clog pores, irritate skin, and cause breakouts. Are your sponges old and torn? Are your powders crumbling? Has that fabulous eye shadow changed color or faded? Do your products look dirty and smell bad? What about all those opened tubes, compacts, and lipsticks that you've had trouble parting with for years?

> "Be brutal" is the operative phrase here.

Think they'll come in handy at some point? *Uh uh,* they've gotta go. If you haven't used a cosmetic in six weeks, it's a pretty safe bet you aren't going to use it any time soon. Get rid of it, all of it.

"Be brutal" is the operative phrase here.

I know this might be difficult, especially if you spend more money at Sephora than you do on your monthly mortgage. But do you really want to risk a bad case of middle-age acne, or, worse, a staph infection? I think not.

Ultimately, you just don't need all those products to begin with. Say buh-bye to all of it and hello to a very important beauty truth:

BEAUTY TRUTH:

Beauty comes from within . . .
a very small makeup bag!

---

the bare necessities

This chapter is about having access to your everyday beauty essentials—not excess; just enough to fill a small and practical makeup pouch, and nothing more. Think of it as a diet program for beauty products—like Weight Watchers for cosmetics, and the following items are the essential "food" groups:

FOUNDATION OR TINTED MOISTURIZER

Because these products give you the color and luminosity that menopause steals. The right one makes you look dewy, fresh, and glowing. The wrong one makes you look like Casper the Friendly Ghost. Choose carefully (see Chapter 5 for more about foundation).

CHEEK COLOR

Because this pick-me-up product takes you from dull to vibrant in five seconds or less. It's like a latte for your face.

LIP LINER

Because it restores fullness and shape to your lips and reins in runaway color that loves to migrate into the vertical lines above your upper lip.

LIPSTICK

Because it restores the creamy texture and volume of youthful lips. (An inconvenient truth: Gooey lip gloss is for Dallas Cowboys cheerleaders and your teenage daughter. Toss it immediately.)

MASCARA

Because the eyes are the most expressive part of the face, which may be why this is the classic "desert island" makeup item of choice (assuming there is someone else on the island and you already have sunscreen).

EYELINER

Because it enhances the natural beauty of the eye. It can even reshape the eye.

Now let's talk about organization, because almost as important as what products you keep on hand is how you organize and store them, what you tote them in when you're on the go, and which cosmetics products you should keep at work for a quick day-to-evening transition without a stop at home.

vital reserves

If your cosmetics storage area is anything like mine, it's so full that you likely have to body-slam the cabinet door shut and hold it for a few seconds before gently letting go, hoping it doesn't burst open and the contents come tumbling out. Yep, I *am* the one who could use a few thirty-gallon garbage bags! So let's do this together.

First, we're only going to save a few pieces from each of the essential "food" groups listed above. For example, assuming their expiration window is still open, keep two foundations or tinted moisturizers (for seasonal changes), two or three blushers to work with seasonal and lipstick changes, three lip liners to match your lipstick colors, three of your favorite lipsticks in a range of colors, two mascaras (one waterproof), and two eyeliners.

Now where do we put all this? Space is the defining factor. Most of us keep our cosmetics in the bathroom medicine cabinet, but this is the worst place to store cosmetics because it is warm and damp, which speeds up the deterioration of the product. Instead, keep your products in a cool dry place removed from moisture and light (for starters, consider a shelf in your clothing or linen closet). To get even more longevity from your products, place your cosmetics

> To get even more longevity from your products, place your cosmetics in a plastic box with a tight lid and store them in the refrigerator.

in a plastic box with a tight lid and store them in the refrigerator. Don't worry, this will not affect the texture or application properties of your cosmetics; just give the products time to warm to room temperature before using.

As for what type of container to store them in, see the list below for some tried-and-true suggestions:

HANGING ORGANIZER WITH CLEAR POCKETS

These affordable organizers can be hung on the back of a closet or bathroom door, and they come in a wide range of sizes and styles. Check out the selection at Bed, Bath and Beyond (www.bedbathandbeyond.com).

STACKABLE STORAGE BOXES

Preferably transparent, with removable drawers. The Container Store (www.containerstore.com) offers a wide range of sizes and styles, including those hard-to-find smaller acrylic organizers and caddies with separators that can be most useful in tight spaces.

TACKLE BOX OR TRAIN CASE

Check out www.target.com for the Soho or Caboodles brand of cosmetic cases. Like tackle boxes, they unfold, revealing several levels of built-in storage cubbies.

DRAWER ORGANIZERS

If you're storing cosmetics in a drawer, try a flatware organizer for simplicity. The Container Store is another great place to look for drawer organizers in various shapes and sizes.

SHOEBOX

Yes, I mean it. In the absence of all of the above, you can go with an old-fashioned sturdy shoebox—or upgrade to a pretty box with a lid. Simply separate the products into clear plastic baggies. Repurposed cups, canisters, and pencil holders also make great receptacles for brushes or eye and lip pencils. Look at it this way—you're saving money *and* reducing your carbon footprint at the same time.

With these few pieces stored in an easily accessible place, there'll be peace in your closet and a feeling of well-being in your soul. Say, *aaah . . .*

say, aaah . . .

office supplies

If you work outside the home, it's always handy to have a stash of the right makeup at the office for impromptu after-work outings or just to freshen up before a staff meeting, client appointment, or power lunch. A little cosmetic pick-me-up during the work day will help boost your confidence and enhance first impressions. Keep in your desk drawer a small, preferably transparent, container or standard makeup pouch—anything that fits neatly at your work station and is accessible—and fill it with the basics and then some. Here are three simple steps to fleshing out your workplace backup kit:

1 Keep on hand cleansing towelettes, a facial moisturizer, a travel-size pack of tissues, and a mini magnifying mirror (if you can find a small one with a suction-cup back, all the better—you can stick it on any flat surface, allowing both hands to be free).

2 Next, choose the lipstick and lip liner that looks best for evening, and buy an extra one of each to go into your office kit. Add an eye shadow for a smidge of drama, and transfer some of your foundation or tinted moisturizer into a travel-size container (available in most chain drugstores). A friend of mine keeps hers in a contact lens case—small enough to fit in a pocket, and it keeps the makeup fresh. (Note: The foundation formula and the plastic container may not be compatible; should the product start to change color or consistency, toss and switch to a small glass container.)

3 Now add your tools. Be sure to keep your sponges, Q-tips, sharpeners, and makeup brushes in a separate container or clean baggie to help limit the buildup of bacteria.

All of this should take up no more than half a desk drawer. A great fashion tip that I learned from my first boss—*Mademoiselle* magazine editor Nonnie Moore, who rarely went home before attending glamorous events and dinners—was to tuck an all-purpose evening clutch in the drawer, in the event of any postwork festivities.

on the go

So now it's time to move on to your handbag, possibly the most important makeup carrier you own. What do you take with you on a daily basis? Do you toss your makeup into your purse alongside your keys, change, and wallet? Or do you keep it in a nice zippered pouch? Your makeup should be kept together in a bag or pouch so you don't have to hunt around the bottom of your purse for your lipstick—or worse, have your makeup leak all over the inside of your bag.

One of the chic-est women I know—a well-respected former *Vogue* magazine editor, Jade Hobson, only uses Ziploc bags to contain her cosmetics because she prefers the ease of seeing the particular product she wants. When the bags get dirty or smudged, she replaces them. If you prefer an actual makeup pouch, look for these important qualities: small and washable, with a dependable closure.

You can find affordable, sturdy, easy-to-clean makeup bags online, or you can often snag higher-end bags at a fraction of the cost at discount department stores like TJ Maxx or Ross, or from vintage resale shops. Check out the following websites for worthy brands that offer quality bags below $100.

www.toryburch.com

www.katespade.com

www.lesportsac.com

www.sephora.com

For those interested in a little splurge (and no doubt you've earned it!), let me introduce you to a few high-end designer makeup bags that will not only stand the test of time and wear but are so well made that each tiny detail conveys their iconic elegance, luxury, and craftsmanship. And, not to be ignored, they pack a lot of purse power (your friends will notice when you take it out of your bag)! Years of experience have shown me that quality really does count, and these three designer classic bags have it in spades:

quality really does count . . .

THE PRADA BLACK NYLON ZIPPERED BAG

Choose the smallest size and make good use of the inner zip pocket. It's lightweight, indestructible, and the zipper is totally reliable. This cosmetic pouch is thoroughly modern and a true favorite of beauty editors.

THE LOUIS VUITTON MONOGRAM MAKEUP TROUSSE

Made of high-quality coated canvas, it's sturdy, rarely shows makeup stains or handbag scuffs, wipes down quickly with a damp cloth, and the monogram design reeks of vintage luxury worthy of nothing less than *Downton Abbey*.

THE HENRI BENDEL POUCH

Made of signature brown and white vinyl-coated cotton twill, its plastic coating makes it impervious to damage, spills, and leaks. This classic makeup carrier is the go-to bag for many makeup artists.

While these designer makeup cases are a big splurge item, investing in them is a great "cost per wear" (CPW) strategy, since they will last you a lifetime and never lose their luxurious presence and appeal.

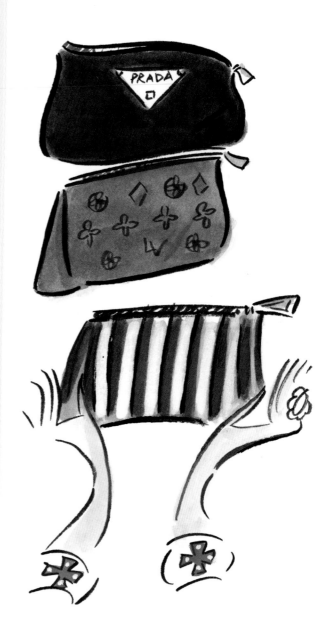

buyer beware

Have you ever fallen prey to the GWP (that's "Gift with Purchase" in makeup speak)? You know, those makeup bags that come "free" when you buy a product from a beauty company? Those little totes brimming with mini makeup products, like mascara, lipsticks, and eye shadows? If you have, don't beat yourself up, we've all been taken in by the Gift with Purchase promotion. Once you read this, you'll think twice about succumbing again. Here's the true scoop on how the

> But the GWP is really not a gift, and it's not free, because you can't get it without making a purchase!

GWPs work: It's the cosmetics company's way of luring you to their counter. You make a purchase, and only then are you rewarded with your Gift with Purchase. You may have intended to purchase only one product, but you'll likely go home with three, since the beauty advisors, who are paid on commission, are trained to not let you escape with less than three products. But the GWP is really not a gift, and it's not free, because

you can't get it without making a purchase! To add insult to injury, the cosmetic pouch is so cheaply made, it can't take a lot of wear and tear (all is not lost—you can use it to store tampons, Q-tips, or cotton balls in your desk drawer). Further, it's filled with tiny product samples with colors and formulas that are often not right for you.

Bottom line, the manufacturers want you to sample and get hooked on these products because they can produce them in huge quantities at a low cost.

Cosmetic companies and retailers spend millions of dollars on full-page newspaper adds, online banner ads, and in-store promotions to advertise these GWPs. Picture the conversation in the marketing department of these companies during a brainstorming session on how to design and sell the GWPs. You know what, never mind—you don't need to imagine the conversation because, as a beauty executive, I've heard hundreds of them. They all go something like this: "The pouch is too expensive! Get rid of the buckle, get rid of the

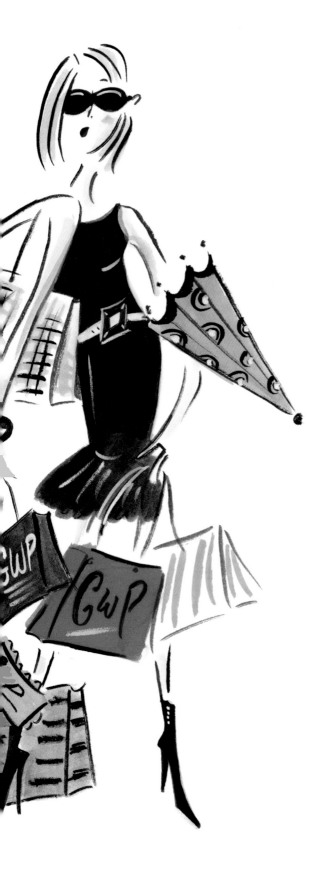

pockets, get rid of the zipper, and use a snap instead. Can't we find a cheaper fabric? Can't we make it in China? How can we produce this pouch for $1.00 instead of $1.10?" It's all about cheap, cheap, cheap.

Still not convinced? Just ask yourself how many of these products and pouches you have actually used, or saved with the intention of regifting them, only to have them take up space in your drawers and cabinets for months, even years, never to see the light of day until you clean out the closet and put them in that thirty-gallon garbage bag.

Bravo to all the hoarders of the world who can bring themselves to take the first step: Toss and make room!

The Gift with Purchase shenanigans were started by Estée Lauder years ago as a sampling vehicle, and much of the cosmetics industry followed that lead because it created enormous sales. That said, beauty companies are increasingly pulling away from these promotions because they are not realizing the same return on investment they once did (too much competition, and loss of interest by the consumer), but nobody's willing to ride out the drop in sales that would come as a result of dropping GWP entirely. So, dear buyer, beware of strangers bearing "gifts" (with purchase).

So here are some questions to ask yourself as you are flinging "gifts" and purchases into the trash bag:

1 How many seasons ago did I buy this product? In other words, is it a "fad" color? (Probably.) Should I be wearing a "fad" color in the first place? (No way.)

2 How many times have I worn this? If the answer is never, time to gift it to someone who can, like the local women's shelter—if the products have never been opened. (Virgin olive oil is great, virgin makeup is wasting valuable counter space.)

3 Am I just hanging onto it because I'm feeling guilty for spending so much? (You might want to ask your wardrobe this one, too.)

4 Am I holding on to an empty bottle thinking I might reuse it? (That's why God invented recycling bins.)

5 Would my daughter wear this? (See also: Would my mother wear this?)

6 Why did I buy this in the first place? Who talked me into it? (If it was one of your friends, maybe you need to toss them, too.)

7 And the key question . . . do I really need all this crap? (No, no, NO!)

Toss and don't look back.

YOU SHOULD KNOW

Face it: It's impossible to mentally keep track of when you purchased which products. Short of creating an Excel spreadsheet, here are some tips to keep you clued in to when your products are out of date:

- Label your products. Stickers are colorful reminders of expiration dates, so you can easily label a specific product by its particular shelf life. You can find waterproof stickers for this purpose at www.beautyalert.biz.

- Download the Beauty Alert! app, which keeps track of your cosmetics. It will notify you when they expire.

- Use a Sharpie pen to write down the purchase date on the product container itself.

- Put a "toss" reminder on your calendar.

Prolong the life of your products and prevent contamination by doing the following:

- Never borrow a product that someone else has used.

- Sharpen lip and eyeliner pencils after each use to remove moisture-causing bacteria, which contaminate the pencil.

- Choose makeup products in sealed pump containers. This allows you to dispense the product without introducing new bacteria.

- Periodically wipe lipsticks with alcohol wipes.

- Do not store makeup in the bathroom if you can help it. Keep it in a cool, dry place to ensure its longevity.

When should you replace your makeup? See the list below for the general rule of thumb on how frequently you should toss and replace standard cosmetics once they've been unsealed. Natural beauty products have a shorter shelf-life since they're free of preservatives, so they should be replaced every six months (except for mascara or unless the product package indicates otherwise).

- **MASCARA:** Every three months

- **LIPSTICK/LIP GLOSS:** Every twelve months

- **EYE SHADOW:** Every twelve months

- **PENCILS FOR EYES AND LIPS:** Every six months

- **LIQUID FOUNDATIONS, CONCEALERS, HIGHLIGHTERS, AND TINTED MOISTURIZERS:** Every six months

- **POWDERED FOUNDATION, BLUSH, HIGHLIGHTERS, AND BRONZERS:** Every twelve months

- **CREAM BLUSH:** Every six months

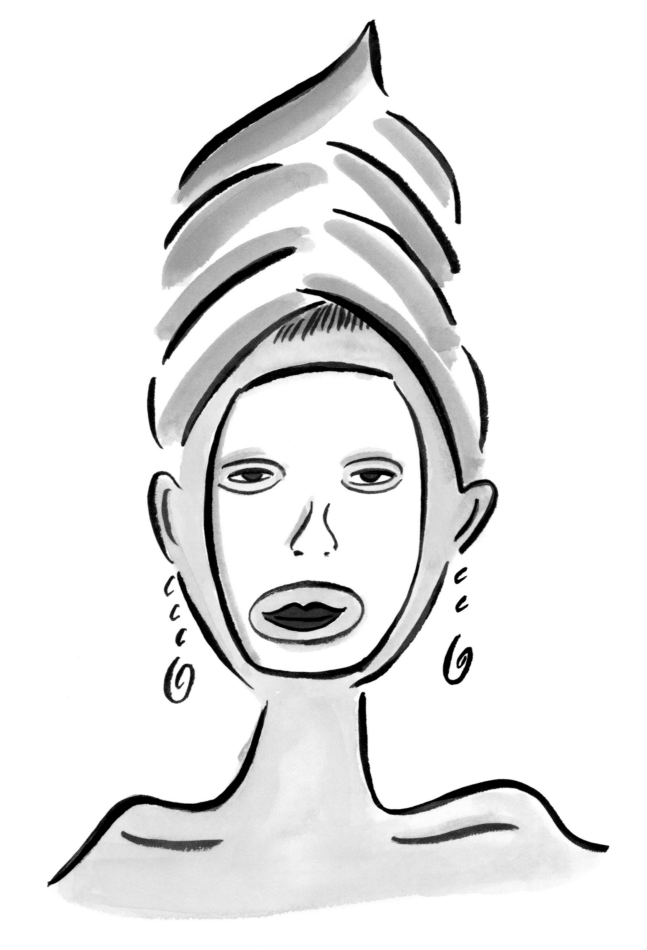

CHAPTER THREE

Skincare

getting clear on product help vs. hype

THERE ARE MORE ANTIAGING PRODUCTS OUT THERE THAN GEORGE CLOONEY HAS EX-GIRLFRIENDS. THE PROBLEM? FEW OF THEM ACTUALLY DELIVER.

The skincare market may be one of the few that has embraced women over fifty with open arms—at least, in theory. The beauty companies are preying on our insecurities about aging rather than acknowledging how damn good we already look. I mean, do we really believe this season's "new" miracle ingredient will make us look ten years younger? (Wait, do you also believe in unicorns?) We might be savvy enough to know when we're getting duped, but even the smartest among us will be surprised at some of the beauty-industry marketing shenanigans. But first a reality check.

BEAUTY TRUTH:

If you're over fifty, you've changed, and so has your skin.

Sure, you've accumulated a few more laugh lines, perhaps even a new age spot or two, but the changes are more than just skin deep. You've also changed *physiologically,* and that means a whole new set of rules for how your skin behaves. That's right, I'm about to invoke the "M" word: menopause. (If you're not quite there yet, you will be, so read on anyway.)

Without getting too technical, I'll just tell you that our skin becomes drier, thinner, and less elastic at menopause because of the natural lowering of estrogen levels (unless you're taking hormone replacement therapy, which has its definite downsides— ask your doctor). The decrease in this key hormone can result in a number of beauty bummers (including less hair on our heads and more on our chinny-chin-chins). For now, however, let's focus on the effect it has on our skin. There is a direct link between lower estrogen levels and reduced collagen

and skin elasticity, thickness, and strength. Gone is the perky plumpness you used to take for granted. Your skin is probably looking and feeling a lot more parched now, and when you pinch the back of your hand, it probably stays pinched for far longer than it used to. Yep, this stinks. But if we're honest and open in talking about it, we can take the necessary steps to deal with these effects and start to get in touch with our new and improved beauty routine instead. The first step is to know the difference between skincare products that help you offset these age-related tempests and skincare products that merely offset your bank account.

brand beware

Beauty counters are brimming with slick-looking moisturizers, serums, peels, oils, masks, eye creams, lotions, and night treatments that promise to combat wrinkles, crow's feet, bags, and sags. The options are seemingly endless and the choices can be overwhelming. And unlike the "beauty consultants" at cosmetics counters who work on commission and are trained to parrot their company's product press releases, I will actually tell you the truth: Smoke and mirrors abound.

Having spent a big chunk of my career in the high-tech research and development laboratories of some of the world's most prominent beauty companies, I can share an industry scoop that most women don't know. Major beauty corporations own or license several brands in a wide range of price points. The Estée Lauder Companies have Bobbi Brown, Clinique, Tom Ford, La Mer, MAC, Estée Lauder, Smashbox, and a myriad of other brands. The L'Oreal Group has Maybelline, L'Oreal Paris, Lancôme, Ralph Lauren, Kiehl's, La Roche-Posay, Redken, Matrix, Essie, and others. Procter and Gamble owns CoverGirl, Max Factor, Olay, SK-II, to name a few. And Coty owns Philosophy, Sally Hansen, Rimmel, and OPI. This information is on the Internet, but it's certainly not broadcast by the individual brands that often compete against each other.

In my career as a beauty editor, I saw the industry's top beauty brands present new skincare offerings every season, and I quickly learned to connect the dots. Basically, one research lab in each corporation fuels the technology development and creates an ingredient that is widely used across many of their brands. They get away with it by using different scientific-sounding names for the ingredient, and they carefully wordsmith the claims for each brand so they don't sound exactly the same. So while L'Oreal Paris would introduce a product with glamorous packaging, a space-age name with ingredient X, and an

> The first step is to know the difference between skincare products that help you offset these age-related tempests and skincare products that merely offset your bank account.

ad campaign featuring a celebrity spokesperson, Lancôme might introduce virtually the same product with ingredient X "respun" with a chic French name, different luxury packaging, and a slightly different claim for essentially the same ingredient. The only real difference? The price. L'Oreal Paris is sold in drugstores and Lancôme is sold in department stores as a higher-end brand. In the end, it's all pretty much the same stuff. For example, a few years ago, Lancôme's big launch of the season was Genifique, a "youth-activating concentrate" stemming from the production of genes. Similarly, a year after this launch, L'Oreal

Paris introduced Youth Code Serum Intense that touts a breakthrough using "gene science"—get the connection?

And even more shocking, did you know that big corporations compete to buy or license a "hot" ingredient or technology very often from the same two or three independent laboratories, and then claim that ingredient as their own creation?

And did you also know that the moment one of these companies creates a new "it" product that garners beauty awards and reaps high retail sales, the rest of these beauty companies waste no time copying it and getting their own version to market, posthaste? All of the above brings us to another . . .

BEAUTY TRUTH:

The tubes from Target will probably work just as well as the bottles from Barneys.

Save your money for a guilty pleasure and invest in skin care the way you would stocks: cautiously, wisely, and well-informed. I'll be your broker.

tricky wordsmithing

When it comes to touting a product's benefits, beauty companies have developed hocus-pocus phrases best left to noncommittal boyfriends to market their promises to unsuspecting consumers.

Do phrases like "may help to diminish" or "results may vary" sound familiar? This is where you need to be extra vigilant. Nontransparent words like "may" express only the *possibility* that the claim may be true. These "promises" or claims are vague for a reason. Companies use the word *may,* as in "may improve" and "may lift" to ensure that they are not caught making false claims about how the product works, which would leave them open to lawsuits based on false advertising. How about promises like, "refill wrinkles in just one hour"—sound tempting? Keep your refills to a glass of Chardonnay! The key word in that phrase is "refill" versus "remove forever," because the reality is, it's temporary and it doesn't say how much your wrinkles will be refilled or that they will go away. You may see some short-term improvement in skin because of hydrating ingredients that soften and "plump" the look of stubborn wrinkles, but the wrinkles will still be there in one hour and tomorrow. This is not necessarily a bad thing, but it's important to be clued in about

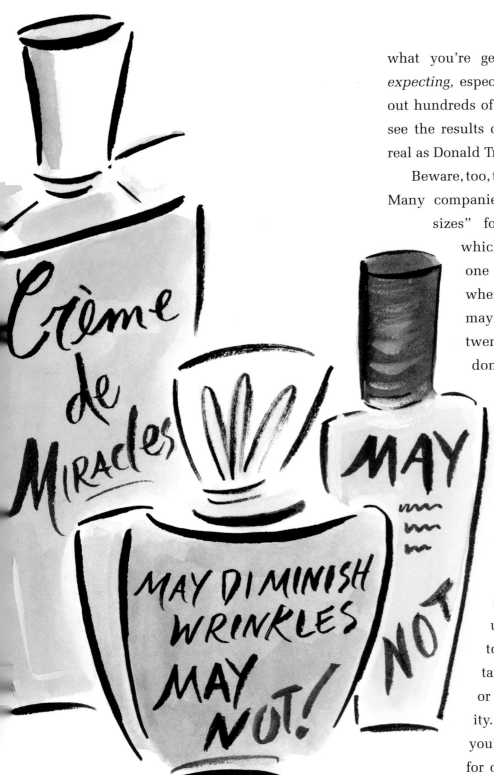

what you're getting versus what you're *expecting,* especially when you're shelling out hundreds of dollars a month hoping to see the results of claims that are about as real as Donald Trump's comb over.

Beware, too, that little asterisk symbol (*). Many companies refer to "small sample sizes" for their research groups, which might suggest that about one hundred women tried it, when in fact the testing group may have only consisted of twenty-five product users. You don't know how the research was conducted, so don't fall prey to this. These claims give the impression that they were conducted using the most rigorous of scientific methods, but often these studies are lacking in real supporting evidence. Beauty companies use this punctuation mark to endorse vague commentary like "in a clinical study" or "instantly improves clarity." Follow the asterisk, and you'll see qualifying statements for claims such as "69 percent clinically measured improvement in overall aging signs after 12 weeks." Sounds promising, right? But read the mice type associated with that asterisk (in the magazine gutter), and you'll read the *context* of that claim: "*12 week clinical test conducted on 32 women aged 26–64." Not a big sample

Brace yourself: Like the promises politicians make during the campaign season, many of these product promises just aren't going to happen.

size, and certainly not a sample size reflective of the target audience. I mean, just how many women were over fifty and how many were dewy-skinned twentysomethings? There is nothing remotely scientific about it. Then why even include it on the packaging? Because this little punctuation mark is intended to protect the company from being accused of misguiding the consumer with unfounded or unsupportable claims, and the company is hedging their bets that you won't bother to read the fine type, and, if you do, that it won't make much of an impression because it still sounds clinical. The same goes for phrases like "dermatologist-tested," which marketers like to use to coax you into thinking a dermatologist hand-picked that product, tested it, and gave it a blessing, when in reality all it means is that a product has reached a certain level of safety in the company that's making the claim, but, since the cosmetics industry regulates itself, there are no industry-wide standards for product testing. And don't be lured in by clinical-sounding language like "Our studies show . . ." Don't get excited that 95 percent of women found positive results. All this means is that 95 percent of the women tested could simply have noticed a difference and liked a product, which isn't the same as 95 percent seeing an improvement that matched the product's claims, like an actual reduction in wrinkles!

Believe me, the research and development labs in these corporations are smart and know how to establish their tests for the appearance of outstanding results. Brace yourself: Like the promises politicians make during the campaign season, many of these product promises just aren't going to happen. But don't be discouraged! Some products actually *do* deliver, and we'll get to that soon.

be wary of endorsements

There are other ways beauty companies mislead consumers in their effort to sell us their products. When it comes to endorsements, for example, beauty editor "favorites" are not always true favorites. Believe me, I know, because I was once the beauty editor for *Vogue*. Here's the scoop: Before I began work on the editorial content for each new issue, I was given a "must list" from my publisher, whose job it was to bring in advertising dollars—which, for the uninitiated, is how all magazines pay for their overhead costs, including staff salaries. As you can imagine, there's a lot of pressure from big advertisers to promote their products, so this list included the products and companies I must mention on the pages of the magazine, based on the number of advertising pages a particular company has bought for the issue or for the year. The silent quid pro quo was basically "no ticket, no laundry," or no editorial mention, no advertising. Sad but true—not all favorites *are* favorites and journalistic integrity is not always exactly pure when it comes to editorial content— let's leave it at that—just be aware that when it comes to "must-have" beauty products, the favorites are often written by editors with fingers crossed behind their backs.

Celebrity endorsements work the same way. The celebrity negotiates a hefty contract (often in the millions of dollars) with a beauty company that requires her to say she uses and loves the product during press events, like product launch parties, store appearances (where it's being sold),

> Just be aware that when it comes to "must-have" beauty products, the favorites are often written by editors with fingers crossed behind their backs.

print advertising, TV commercials, magazine and Internet interviews, and personal appearances on television talk shows. So when you look at Starlet X's skin in the ad and think it's so perfect, remember Photoshop, and, when you hear her praising the product's benefits, remember that she's paid to do so.

And what about skincare brands marketed under the name of a famed dermatologist? Just because a product carries a doctor's name doesn't necessarily mean he created it. Many suppliers (the labs that create and manufacture these formulations) offer "stock" products, similar to a shoe store that has different sizes of the same shoe available in the stock room. Sometimes a scent is changed, a color is adjusted, or an ingredient is added to the base formula, but, basically, the dermatologist often slaps a label on it and calls it his or her own. The products that actually have been developed by doctors usually are aesthetically pleasing and offer a new ingredient, but the truth is that, even with those, nothing new has been added to the equation. Remember that although doctors (derms) are involved with patients' skin issues, they are not scientists (the people who have made the breakthroughs). In most cases, he/she'll sell these products to patients as a follow-up measure to "enhance" or "help prolong" the benefits of the treatment she's just received, and their products are a profit center for them.

But despite all this skincare strife, there are things you can do, buy, and use (and *not* use) that really will enhance the appearance of your skin. Here's some real advice about what works and what tanks, and what I consider to be the most effective, investment-worthy skincare ingredients and products available to you.

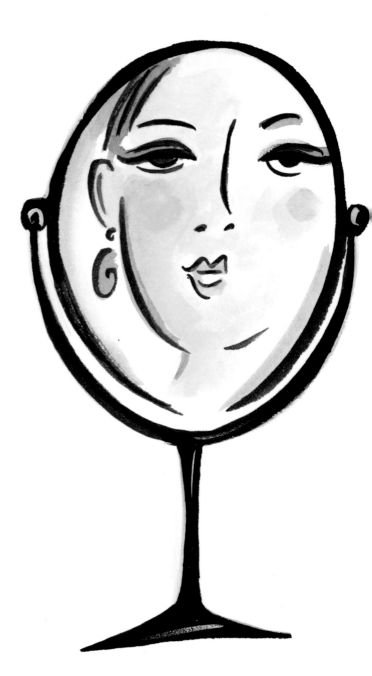

SLEEP

FACT: OUR SKIN CELLS REGENERATE WHILE WE SLEEP!

Get that "beauty" sleep (seven or eight hours nightly does it for most of us) whenever you can for healthy-looking skin. A good night's sleep does make a difference to our skin, as it repairs and restores itself while we rest. Lack of sleep makes the skin appear dull and lifeless and accentuates dark circles under the eyes. The Debbie Downer fact is that menopause is often accompanied by restless nights (sorry to report this) and those sweet dreams can be interrupted by hot flashes and night sweats. But the good news is that we can do something about promoting more restful nights.

It took me a while to get the hang of it, but here are a few tips I've learned for all you sleeping beauties:

- No caffeine for six hours before bedtime
- Eating a light and early dinner regularly
- Going to bed at the same time every night
- Limit alcohol intake to one glass of wine daily
- Regular exercise

Forget sleep aids. I gave those up when a friend emailed me back with question marks in response to an incomprehensible email I'd sent him in the middle of the night, which I had no recollection of doing! No thank you to those little devils. They went into the thirty-gallon bags with my expired cosmetics.

EXERCISE

FACT: INCREASED BLOOD FLOW AND CIRCULATION NOURISHES SKIN CELLS.

It will also chase away those nasty free radicals (see the following page) that damage good healthy skin. Exercise eases stress and therefore we can often fall asleep more easily—one big happy circle of health that feeds into the heart, lungs, and SKIN. Make it a regular routine four or five times weekly, alternating disciplines of aerobic, muscle, and stretching. I also am a great believer in squeezing it in when it presents itself to me (e.g., a flight or two of stairs or a fast walk to a destination—when alone I always walk fast).

SUNSCREENS

FACT: SUN DAMAGE IS THE #1 CAUSE OF WRINKLES.

There is no advice I can offer you that is more important than this: Use a sunscreen! It is the lion at the gate of healthy, even-toned, beautiful skin. Do not leave home without it. Rain, sleet, snow, or hale—not just when you're on the beach—use a sunscreen *every day*, everywhere. Be sure it's "broad-spectrum" (titanium dioxide, zinc oxide, or Parsol 1789), which blocks the wrinkle-causing UVA rays and the burn- and cancer-causing UVB rays. Use at least an SPF 30, but don't waste your money on anything higher than an SPF 50, since there's little evidence that higher SPFs provide more protective benefits. This is a skincare item that can be purchased quite inexpensively just about anywhere, from drugstores to sporting good stores.

Here are a few **Best Bets:**

- Neutrogena Ultra Sheer Sunscreen
- Aveeno Continuous Protection Sunblock Lotion for the Face
- La Roche-Posay Anthelios Face Ultra Light

ANTIOXIDANTS

FACT: FREE RADICALS ATTACK HEALTHY SKIN CELLS AND BREAK DOWN COLLAGEN, CAUSING DULL SKIN AND WRINKLES.

Antioxidants do battle with these nasty molecules, which are produced by pollution, stress, alcohol, cigarettes, and sun. Antioxidants are found in berries, pomegranates, grapes, and foods rich in Vitamin C and E, green tea and even chocolate(!), to give a few examples. Additionally, topical use of antioxidants in the form of an oil, serum, or cream has proven effective relating to natural and synthetic light damage.

Some **Best Bets** worth considering:

- SkinCeuticals CE Ferulic
- Elizabeth Arden Prevage Face Advanced Anti-Aging Serum
- Neutrogena Ageless Intensives Anti-Wrinkle Serum

RETINOIDS

FACT: THE ONLY PROVEN ANTIAGING COMPOUND THAT REDUCES LINES AND WRINKLES.

Retinoids increase cell turnover and stimulate collagen renewal, which is the support structure that gives skin a firmer look—exactly what our fifty+ skin needs. The most powerful punch comes from prescription strength retinoids, but over-the-counter products will still yield impressive results. Retinoids should only be used at night, as sunlight can inactivate them and there are risks or side effects, like redness and flakiness from exfoliating skin with prescription strength that your doctor can help you manage.

A few **Best Bets** to try:
- RoC Retinol Correxion Deep Wrinkle Serum
- Vichy LiftActiv Retinol HA Night Total Wrinkle Plumping Care
- SkinCeuticals Retinol 1.0 Maximum Strength Refining Night Cream
- Philosophy Miracle Worker

ALPHA HYDROXY ACIDS

FACT: ALPHA HYDROXY ACIDS REMOVE THE TOP LAYERS OF DEAD SKIN CELLS, LEAVING DRY SKIN MORE DEWY AND GLOWING.

Alpha hydroxy acids (derived from food), which are used as a skin exfoliant, are most commonly found in face peels but are also found in a multitude of cosmetics products, from cleansers to moisturizers, and are used as a lower concentrate and more gentle ingredient (as opposed to retinoids). They come in the guise of glycolic acid, lactic acid, citric acid, and other fruit acids. It is best to follow use of these acids with a moisturizing sunscreen since the top layers of the skin are exfoliated and, like retinoids, skin is more photosensitive after using these natural chemicals. Also worth noting, some redness and flaking may occur, but don't be alarmed! This is part of the process. (Warning: Read labels carefully before trying at-home acid peels.)

Here are several **Best Bets** I recommend:
- Dr. Dennis Gross Alpha Beta Daily Face Peel
- Jurlique Fruit Enzyme Exfoliator
- Peter Thomas Roth Un-Wrinkle Peel Pads

SALICYLIC ACID

FACT: SALICYLIC ACID TREATS ACNE BY REDUCING SWELLING AND IRRITATION AND UNBLOCKING SKIN PORES.

Salicylic acid (derived from tree bark) is part of the beta hydroxy family. Both alpha and beta hydroxy acids work by sloughing off dead or damaged skin on the surface of your face, encouraging new, fresh skin to appear. The main difference between the two is that beta hydroxy is oil soluble and can penetrate deeper into the clogged pores to actually break up sebum. Salicylic acid is most effective when dispensed in prescription strength by a dermatologist. It has been proven very effective in treating acne, which many of us still struggle with at menopause. There are several over-the-counter strengths of this substance, but it can often irritate the skin, so it must be used judiciously and only as directed.

If you have menopausal skin eruptions, you might try one of these **Best Bets:**

- Olay Total Effects Blemish Control Salicylic Acid Acne Cleanser
- Neutrogena Healthy Skin Anti-Wrinkle Anti-Blemish Scrub
- Vichy Normaderm Triple Action Anti-Acne Hydrating Lotion

SKIN WHITENERS/ AGE SPOT REDUCERS

FACT: SOME PRODUCTS EXIST THAT CAN REDUCE AGE SPOTS AND EVEN OUT THE SKIN'S APPEARANCE, BUT BEWARE OF PRODUCTS CONTAINING HYDRAQUINONE.

Never ever use a skin cream containing this nasty ingredient, which is banned in many countries. Not only can it irritate and damage the surface of the skin, but evidence suggests it can also cause damage at the DNA level. Yes, it does produce results, but at a potentially great cost to your health. There are other products on the market that do not contain hydraquinone and are considered safe. These products require continued use to see a visible difference.

Here are two **Best Bets** worth mentioning:
- Clinique Even Better Dark Spot Corrector
- Garnier Skin Renew Clinical Dark Spot Overnight Peel

MOISTURIZERS

FACT: MOISTURIZERS THAT DO NOT INCLUDE THE PREVIOUSLY MENTIONED INGREDIENTS GIVE A TEMPORARY EFFECT OF PLUMPING UP, LUBRICATING, AND SOFTENING THE SKIN AND RESTORING ITS SUPPLENESS.

The operative word here is "temporary." To retain this effect, a moisturizer must be used at least twice a day, every day. There is nothing appealing about dry, lifeless skin no matter what our age, so it's a good idea to use one. Hyaluronic acid is a popular ingredient in moisturizers because it draws moisture from the air and holds up to 1,000 times its weight in water. This ingredient does NOT eliminate wrinkles when used topically, and it does NOT penetrate the outer layers of the skin. Hyaluronic acid provides only temporary dry skin relief, but, for the sake of comfort and the look and feel of more supple skin, should be used. Some other moisturizing ingredients that are effective emollients are high-quality oils like camellia, macadamia, rosehip, and argan.

Here are some **Best Bets,** effective classics, and newer oils:

Classics

- CeraVe Facial Moisturizing Lotion (my dermatologist's favorite)
- Olay Regenerist Deep Hydration Regenerating Cream
- Crème de La Mer
- L'Oreal Age Perfect Day Cream for Mature Skin SPF 15

Oils

- Rodin Olio Lusso
- Trilogy Rosehip Oil
- Josie Maran Argan Oil

CLEANSERS

FACT: IT'S IMPORTANT TO WASH YOUR FACE BEFORE BED EVERY NIGHT.

Never, ever hit the pillow without clearing your face of the day's makeup, grit, and grime. What we want at this stage of the game is a no-frills, gentle cleanser that does not dry out the face.

Three very simple, good **Best Bets** are:
- Cetaphil Gentle Skin Cleanser
- Dove Beauty Bar
- CeraVe Foaming Facial Cleanser

THE MAIN POINT: Forget night creams, forget toners, forget eye creams, forget neck creams, forget collagen, forget firming creams, forget lifting creams, forget décolleté creams, and forget super expensive creams. Use a moisturizer instead, and stick with the list above. These are the ingredients or products that will move the needle on your skin. Accept the reality that there are no magic bullets, no instant face lifts.

Just ask your dermatologist (if he or she is not contracted as a spokesperson for a cosmetic company).

Read on and be happy to know that help is on the way, that a few simple skincare products, some strategic cosmetic staples and tips combined with a sensible lifestyle, can do more to enhance the appearance of your face than any "miracle" cream, lotion, or potion.

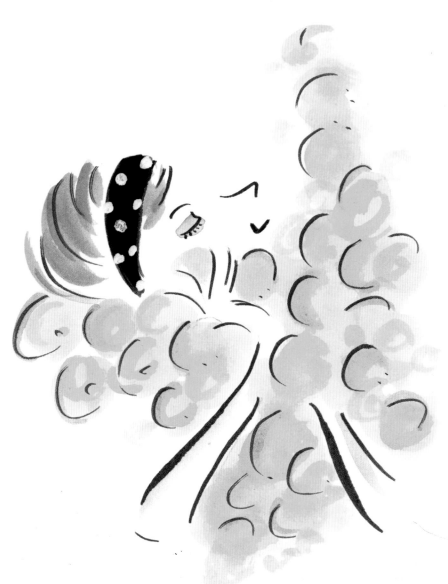

THE PROS AND CONS OF HRT

Menopause, like adolescence, is a fact of life, but it doesn't mean we have to embrace the less glamorous side of aging. I should know; menopause hit me hard and fast in my early forties. As my estrogen levels dipped, so did the collagen in my skin. As my testosterone (the male hormone) increased, so did the hair on my face. And my once-prized dewiness? Done. I was not going down without a fight. My weapon? Hormone Replacement Therapy (HRT). While it is currently the most common way to temper the toll that aging takes on our youthful selves, it does have a dark side—not unlike a menopausal mood swing.

I asked Dr. Michelle Warren, director for Columbia University's Center for Menopause, Hormonal Disorders, and Women's Health, to weigh in on the risks and benefits.

"There are many good things about HRT," she said, adding that while the positive impact on the appearance and elasticity of our skin is very individual, "it generally improves." It also helps combat the suite of symptoms that plague us—from hot flashes and moodiness to painful intercourse and insomnia—and may help offset bone loss and heart disease. Additionally, a recent study she conducted showed that women on HRT were generally happier and more satisfied professionally. But, she cautioned, there are well-documented risks, including blood clots, stroke, and breast cancer (striking 1 in 1,000 women per year).

The takeaway here?

"[The choice] is very individual," she said. Like any health-related decision, it's important to consult very closely with your doctor, since all women's needs and bodies are different.

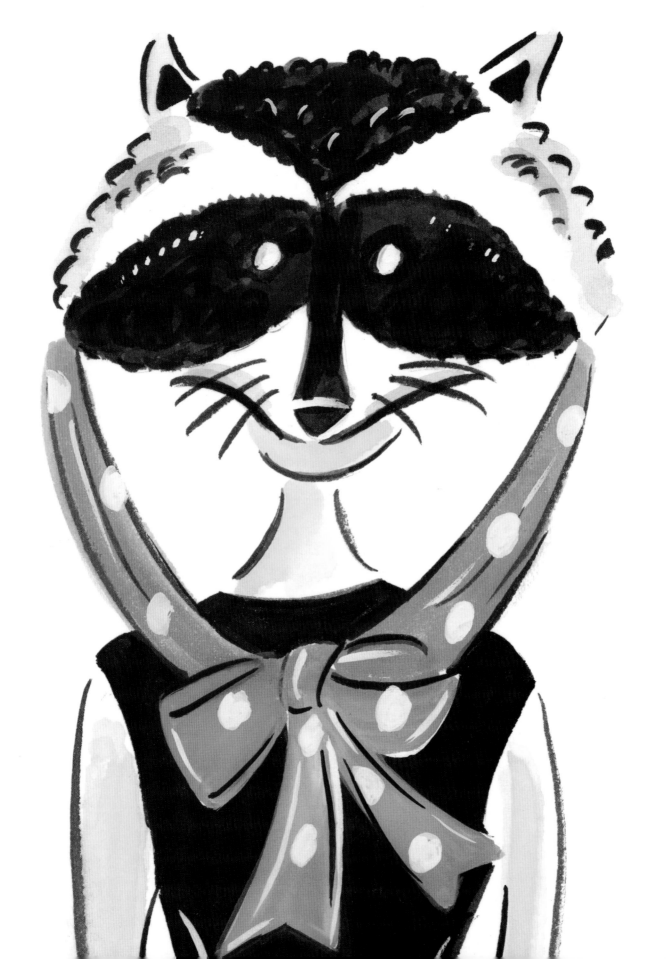

CHAPTER FOUR

Eliminate & Illuminate

concealer, primer, highlighter

REMEMBER WHEN YOU THOUGHT EVERY ACTRESS AND MODEL YOU SAW ON THE PAGES OF GLOSSY MAGAZINES HAD FLAWLESS SKIN? WE'RE A LOT SMARTER NOW THAT WE KNOW ABOUT AIRBRUSHING AND PHOTOSHOP.

And it certainly doesn't hurt that beauty bloggers, gossip columns, news outlets, celebrities, and outspoken models themselves are patrolling beauty companies for truth in advertising—and then calling them out on their practices. Remember when Jezebel.com exposed Faith Hill's unretouched (and still beautiful) photo that appeared on the cover of Redbook? Or when TheCut.com showed a before-and-after shot of an Ann Taylor catalog, and the fashion and beauty industry stopped dead in its tracks?

We no longer have to feel stressed about not looking anything like those celebrities and models who, "au naturel," don't look anything like themselves. We've already established that we *do* want to look like our-

> We're older and wiser, so instead of wishing to be who we were, we're going to embrace the adventure of who we can become.

selves, only better, and by now we should know this book isn't about reclaiming your youth or looking like a model. If you've learned one thing from me so far, I hope it's that aging is *not* a flaw. We're older and wiser, so instead of wishing to be who we *were,* we're going to embrace the adventure of who we can *become.* How? By investing in some minimal cosmetic wizardry via a few simple products, which you will thank me for telling you about later.

But before I reveal this surprisingly simple beauty alchemy, let me share a true story from my magazine days that will give you a laugh *and* a deep appreciation for the handful of cosmetics effective at camouflaging imperfections when necessary:

We were shooting a very big star for the cover of a magazine, and my editor-in-chief insisted the actress look fresh, clean, and entirely natural. This was after the celebrity's very messy and very public divorce, and after she had thrown herself into her work, shooting back-to-back movies. By the time this woman got to us, she looked like she needed a spa week instead of a photo shoot. We had hired a makeup artist whose skills I had admired but I had not yet worked with. The star and the makeup artist met, and within minutes I could cut the tension with a machete. The big dispute: The makeup artist refused to use a concealer to cover the actress's undereye circles, which were darker than the espresso she was drinking. The star abruptly excused herself and disappeared into the ladies room. When she did not return to the set after twenty minutes, I went to the ladies room to see what was wrong—frankly, I was worried she'd blown off the shoot and fled to her car and driver waiting downstairs. But there I found her, in front of the mirror holding a powdered doughnut from the catering table. She wasn't sneaking junk food, she was, believe it or not, delicately dabbing the powdered sugar from the doughnut under her eyes to cover her dark circles! I saved her any additional angst and immediately dismissed the arrogant makeup "divo," dispatched my assistant to pick up the star's favorite concealer, and applied it myself. She stepped in front of the camera and a beautiful magazine cover was created. She looked fabulous, and very natural, but I learned a great lesson from her panicked moment: Always have a concealer on hand.

For women of a certain age—*our* certain age—there is an almighty trio that's going to keep you looking better than ever:

CONCEALER
Think of this as your magic wand. It makes all bad things disappear.

PRIMER
Think of this as Spanx for your face.

HIGHLIGHTER
Your lightening rod, attracting light to key places on your face.

This chapter will teach you how to use all of the above to master the fine art of "concealing," coupled with the even more refined art of revealing, and how to cosmetically cope with lines, wrinkles, circles, and spots so that you get that fresh, youthful look.

get that fresh, youthful look . . .

concealer

Let me repeat a fundamental lesson from a previous chapter. Modern makeup means concealing more by using less. This is especially true for women our age. What exactly do I mean by this? Here's an example: We've all seen people who've used a heavy spackle-type concealer in a shade much lighter than their foundation to hide their dark circles. That never works. Unfortunately, they end up looking like a raccoon. Not a good look, unless it's Halloween. Which brings me to an important . . .

Did you record that? It's so important. Read on for facts and tips that will help you master the blend and conceal.

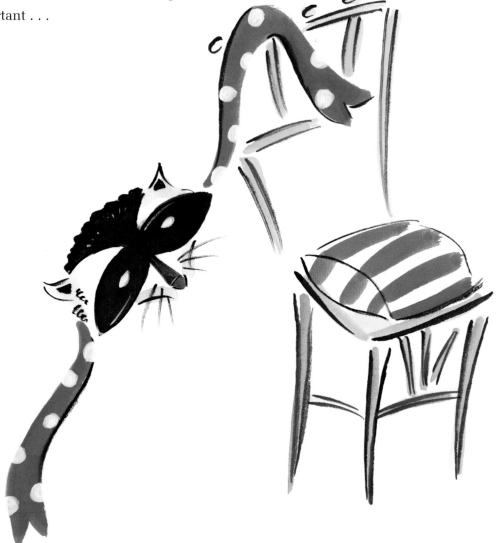

FOR YOUR EYES ONLY

If you have dark circles under your eyes, the worst thing you can do is apply a thick, dry, and pasty concealer in a lighter shade than your foundation! It will only make you look worse because it will emphasize wrinkles and bags. Here's the right way to handle dark circles, in three simple steps:

1 Start by applying foundation to your entire face.

2 Next, layer a heavier dose of foundation over your dark circles. Use a small, stiff, flat brush and build up carefully to an adequate coverage. If this doesn't do the trick, move to a concealer. I repeat, of the same color.

3 Apply your concealer with a light hand, layering it thinly over your foundation and "patting" it in place with the same small, stiff, flat brush (or use your ring finger or a high-quality silk sponge, "patting" with gentle pressure). Concealer for this area of the face should be moist and malleable (liquid or creamy texture).

NOTE: Make sure the concealer blends with your foundation *all the way down to your cheekbones*, and, if necessary, apply a bit more of your foundation on top. Pat, pat, pat away until both are seamless.

Here are a few **Best Bets** for undereye concealers that really work:

- Clé de Peau Corrector Concealer (expensive but worth it)

- Lancôme Effacernes

- Maybelline New York Cover Stick

- Almay Line Smoothing Under-Eye Concealer

REIGNING IN ROGUE SKIN

Our skin suffers countless assaults, from acne, blemishes, birthmarks, and spider veins around the nose, to undereye dark circles and brown spots. You and I probably have at least one of the above. I am always waging war on my brown spots (a.k.a., age spots) and blemishes, and this is when a different consistency of concealer is required. However, I underscore once again how critical it is that your concealer matches your foundation (I know you don't want to look like the Halloween raccoon with freckles, as this concealer requires a spot application). With this type of concealer, I prefer to apply my foundation first (but see below—concealer first is fine, too).

When covering these difficult areas, the best tools for applying concealer are a clean Q-tip, a clean synthetic washable brush, or a clean synthetic washable sponge. I emphasize *clean*; it's best not to use your germ-spreading fingertips, especially when dealing with acne or blemishes. The consistency of your foundation-matching concealer for these special needs should be more opaque, not very malleable, and less creamy, since you want it to stay without moving on the spot you are covering. A more solid, dryish texture works best and is usually found in a pot. Follow the three-step method for flawless coverage:

1 Target with precision and apply the concealer, then wait until it dries.

2 If the blemish is still visible, apply again; wait for the concealer to settle.

3 Reapply a thin layer of foundation to the touched-up areas.

target with precision . . .

You might wonder which comes first, the chicken or the egg? Foundation or concealer? The truth is, either is fine in this case. My preference is foundation first. When applying foundation first, apply the foundation, then dot concealer on the spots where you need extra coverage. But I encourage you to experiment; try applying concealer first. You might discover you don't need foundation, or need only a little to even out your skin tone. Try both ways and see which works best for you.

CONCEALER SPOTS THAT YOU SHOULD KNOW ABOUT BUT PROBABLY DON'T:

- Inner dark corners of the eyes for brightness (especially good for Mediterranean and Latina origins)

- Outer corner of the eyes for an upward illusion

- Either side of the mouth for an upward illusion

By now, you've learned that you probably need two different kinds of concealers for best results: a creamy, moisturizing one for dark undereye circles, and a drier textured one for dark spots, acne/pimples, and redness.

This is my list of concealer **Best Bets** for those "special needs" areas:

- Dermablend Smooth Concealer

- Cinema Secrets Ultimate Foundation (use as concealer)

- Laura Mercier Secret Camouflage

And a couple of **Best Bet** zit-fighting concealers with salicylic acid:

- Neutrogena Healthy Skin Clearing Blemish Concealer

- Murad Acne Treatment Concealer

primer

Now let's talk about Spanx—for the face, that is. You know Spanx's "power panties"? I couldn't exist without them; the über camouflage they provide for my protruding belly and fulsome hips. Well, girls, turn your attention to a power primer. After the diet program for your makeup bag I spoke about in Chapter 2, this would be the first few ounces I would

Take it from me, a good primer makes your foundation or tinted moisturizer roll on more smoothly, filling in wrinkles, lines, and pores. It also covers most dark circles, and makes your foundation last longer.

"put on." Yes, it's another step (swap the powder for this). No, I didn't wear it when I was younger, but, after my skin started to change, primer and I formed a codependent relationship. The key is to test-drive several different types. You need to find the one that's going to work well with your foundation. Primers can be very drying, so look for a hydrating texture (unless you are going to use it on your

oily T-zone), and forego the colored ones (green, orange, and lavender) and the gels. Take it from me, a good primer makes your foundation or tinted moisturizer roll on more smoothly, filling in wrinkles, lines, and pores. It also covers most dark circles, and makes your foundation last longer. Apply primer after you've moisturized and sun-protected your skin. It's like waterproofing your skin; it holds in the moisture and prepares your skin for the next layer—tinted moisturizer or foundation. Primers come with SPFs built in and some can be worn alone without makeup.

My **Best Bets** for a range of skin types:

- Clarins Instant Smooth Perfecting Touch

- Laura Mercier Foundation Primer—Hydrating

- Sunday Riley Effortless Breathable Tinted Primer (can be worn alone)

- MAC Prep + Prime Face Protect SPF 50

- NYC New York Color Smooth Skin Perfecting Primer

- Benefit Cosmetics The POREfessional

- Dior Skinflash Primer Radiance Boosting Makeup Primer

highlighter

Welcome to the land of Tinker Bell, fairy dust, and happy thoughts. I don't know about you, but I could use all three. Highlighters, used subtly, can transport us to Never Never Land. In my book, that's the land of less wrinkles, less gray pallor, less thin lips, and less droopy eyes. We "never never" want to have those issues. Highlighters can diminish features like receding chins and wide noses, and accentuate features like high cheekbones. The secret of highlighters is this: They use light to draw attention to features we want to accentuate and deflect attention from spots we want to diminish— like receding chins, droopy eyes, or a wide nose. Don't underestimate the magic lurking in petite swipes of this versatile product when used in just the right places.

There are many different types of highlighters: sticks, creams, cake powders, loose powders, and liquids. And there are just as many colors and levels of shimmer and glitter. I stick to creams because I find them subtle and easy to control. The color I prefer is a golden or a natural skin tone, with a very low level of shimmer. Highlighters were made to highlight the areas the sun naturally spotlights, so be sure to keep it natural.

> Don't underestimate the magic lurking in petite swipes of this versatile product when used in just the right places.

Avoid at all cost the pearly-white consistencies because they look fake, noticeable, and vaguely stripperish. The rule here is that your highlighter should not be visible. The look we are going for is a good healthy shine and glow where we need it.

a good healthy shine and glow . . .

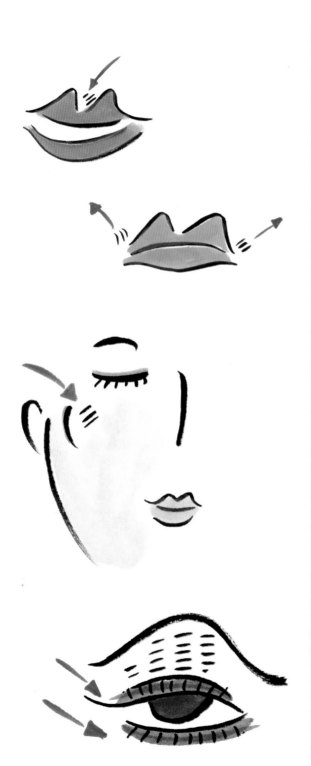

Here are my tried and true tips for how to use highlighter to accentuate or downplay elements of your face:

- Your highlighter has to be lighter than your foundation by at least two shades.

- Apply all highlighter with your finger and blend with patting motion.

- Use for the illusion of a fuller mouth (our lips can start to thin out and lose volume) by applying highlighter to the Cupid's bow (the area between the peaks of the upper lip).

- To avoid a downturned unhappy look to the mouth, dab and blend a small swipe of highlighter at the outer edges of the upper lip at the side of the mouth (concealer can also do this trick).

- After you've applied blush (to the apple of the cheek), dab and pat highlighter across the top of the cheekbone for a luminous, youthful look.

- To emphasize eyes, dab and blend under the arch of the brow. I often work it down on to the lid. There is no need for shadow afterward, just some smudgy dark eyeliner along the upper and lower lash lines. (This tip also helps if your brows make you look angry, disapproving, or tired.)

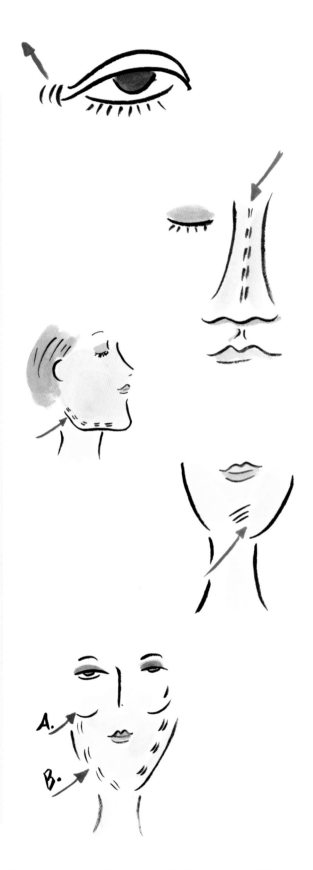

- To avoid drooping eyes, dab and pat a tiny amount of highlighter on the outer edges of the eyes at the side of the upper lids (same idea as the outer edges of the mouth for a slight lift illusion).

- For a wide nose, dab and blend down the center of the nose, starting at the bridge and stopping where nostrils begin to widen.

- For a slackening jaw or jowls, dab and blend along the jawbone, starting where the jowls begin and working your way back.

- For a receding chin, dab and blend a swipe on the middle of the chin.

- For a narrow face, before applying foundation, dab and blend highlighter from (A) the top of the cheekbone (the part closest to the ear) down to (B) the top side of the jawbone. If highlighter disappears, dab and blend on top of the foundation. For a wide face, use a darker shade of foundation or concealer rather than a highlighter.

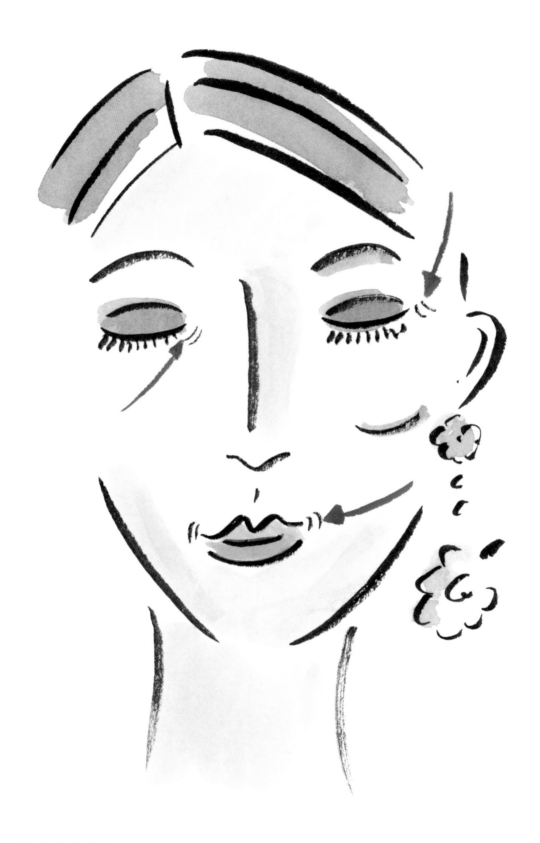

I repeat, a good highlighter will not and should not "read" shimmer in any kind of light. Its purpose is to attract light and to highlight the areas that show you off to your best advantage. Highlighter can be one of the most effective purchases you will ever make, but be very cautious. It's just like overdone plastic surgery: Used inappropriately, this can make you look weird. If you don't know what I mean, think Joan Rivers.

Here are some highlighters worth highlighting:

- Clinique Up-Lighting Liquid Illuminator

- Benefit Cosmetics Moon Beam

- e.l.f. Shimmering Facial Whip

- Yves Saint Laurent Touche Eclat

- L'Oreal Studio Secrets Professional Magic Lumi Highlighter

- Smashbox Halo Highlighting Wand

Concealer, primer, and highlighter, affordable antiaging products with real benefits, are the tools that give us the vision to reimagine ourselves. I am seduced by the magic of their effects and the transformation that comes with the mastery of their use. Here's the lowdown: For the absolute best results, tackle one feature at a time.

The trick to conceal more is to use less product. No circles, spots, or acne? Dump the concealer. No splotchy skin? Ditch the primer. You get the gist. Use the trial and error system to discover what and how much works uniquely for you. And believe in change. That's why you're reading this book. The best news? Unlike more drastic and lasting measures, Kleenex, Q-tips, and cleanser wipe it all off, enabling you to experiment, redraw, and reinvent again without stress.

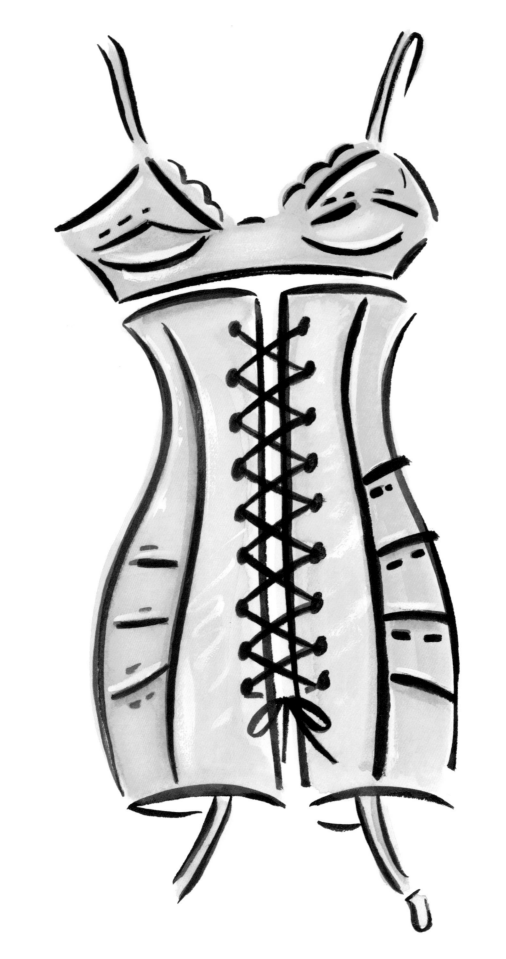

CHAPTER FIVE

Foundation

the (nearly) naked truth

I HATE THE F-WORD—FOUNDATION, THAT IS. IT EVOKES THE CONSTRICTING GIRDLES I USED TO SEE IN MY MOTHER'S UNDERWEAR DRAWER. AND THE WORD *BASE* . . . WELL, IT SOUNDS JUST BASE. CANVAS ISN'T MUCH BETTER.

Is your makeup routine really in the same league as those reusable bags you bring to Whole Foods? Do you really want your face to look like a blank slate: boring, lifeless, and perfect? And anyway, who needs perfect at a time in our lives when we don't want to hold back? We want to be engaging, seductive, vibrant, alive, sexy, and free—anything but blank and perfect. Yes, this chapter is about . . . okay . . . foundation, but there's nothing base about it. Here's the truth. As much as I'm a proponent of all things natural, I don't think foundation is optional. In fact, foundation is almost mandatory; it's the single most important weapon in your cosmetic arsenal. Think of it this way, you know how you're

Well, think of foundation as the perfect white T-shirt of makeup— it's the crucial anchor piece around which you can build the rest of your look.

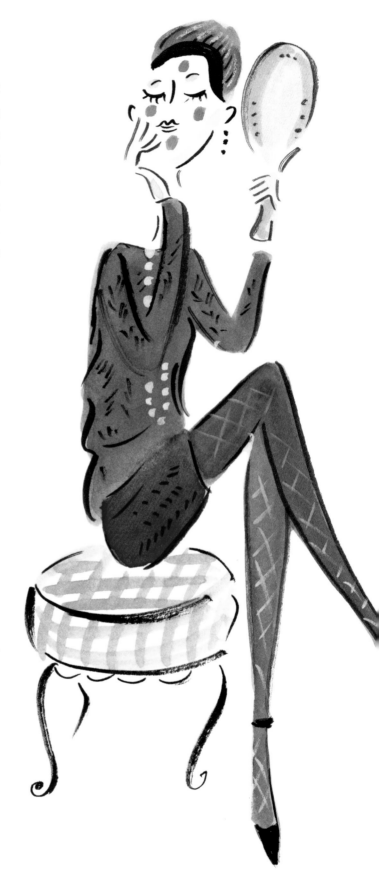

always on the hunt for that perfect white tee? The one that's clean, smooth, lightweight, doesn't pill, and looks as good under your favorite jacket as it does with a pair of jeans? Well, think of foundation as the perfect white T-shirt of makeup—it's the crucial anchor piece around which you can build the rest of your look. I'm going to tell you how to find the foundation equivalent of your dream tee, but the key to success here is to shed your fear of showing your actual skin. Yes, this sounds counterintuitive, but it will make perfect sense, trust me. Read on and see.

less is more

Here's a beauty truth with real face value; commit this to memory: Revealing the right parts of your skin makes you look fresh and beautiful. Attempting to hide the "wrong" parts of your skin makes you look old. And when I say "old," I mean crypt-keeper old. Thick, pasty foundation will make you look dead. And you know the matte look that magazines insist is so chic? That stuff is great—if you're a sixteen-year-old Ukrainian model. Oh wait; you're a real woman? Then toss out those bottles of cement, pronto.

Here's how my less-is-more makeup mantra took root. When I was a beauty editor, I was periodically summoned for tea to the office of the iconic Mrs. Estée Lauder, where she'd introduce the company's new color palette for that particular season. The tea always started out the same way. "Why doesn't a pretty girl like you wear makeup?" (I never told her I was wearing a full face of artfully applied neutral shades). "Here," she would say, "let me show you how to do something with your looks." Out came that season's palette. And there I was, no exit possible—you didn't say no to Mrs. Lauder.

While tea with the legendary Mrs. Lauder was always entertaining, she never really sold me on her "more, more, more" approach to makeup; by the time she finished my "makeover," I wouldn't have been able to pick myself out of a police lineup. Even so, I would thank her profusely, promise to consider the colors for upcoming stories in the magazine, and head straight for the nearest ladies room, where I'd scrub and scrub until I recognized myself again, then surreptitiously make my way to the elevator, hoping she wouldn't catch me on the way out.

For me, those visits were an early lesson in what I *didn't* think worked for modern women: thick, skin-smothering foundation layered under a palette of brights. What *does* work is finding the right foundation, using it where needed, and warming it up with a little color.

Let's get started.

finding cover

Your mission is to discover a foundation that makes every day a good skin day. The key is finding a formula and shade that blends with your complexion perfectly. In other words, your "skin soul mate."

Finding the right foundation takes time. But don't worry, you can strike foundation gold at almost any point on the price spectrum. This isn't about trading up or trading down on the cost spectrum, it's about Cinderella trying on the glass slipper and finding just the right fit. This perfect fit may require a splurge, but think of it this way: There is no cosmetic investment that is more important than your face. Of course, there's expensive and then there's stratospheric. For instance, as I write this, you can nab one of Laura Mercier's much-beloved tinted moisturizers for under $50, or splurge on a liquid foundation from Sisley for a cool $115. Often, the foundations created by beauty

And sorry to be a big buzzkill, but you need to hear this (again): You can't rely on women's magazines for unbiased advice either.

companies with a primary focus on skin care, such as Sisley, La Prairie, or La Mer, are extremely expensive. The rationale is that they're packed with many of the same pricey ingredients used in their serums, creams, and antiaging products, which in my opinion is utter marketing babble (more on this later).

If, after scouring the market, you've fallen head over heels for a foundation that clocks in at north of $100, there's an easy way to reduce your cost per wear: Use it sparingly, with a sponge, and only where you really need it. Remember, less is more.

Now let's head out of the high-end department store beauty counter and make our way over to the drugstore. But first, read this:

I mentioned in an earlier chapter that the mega-cosmetics companies behind your favorite department store makeup brands might also manufacture far less pricey lines for drugstores and other mass-market outlets. Remember, this is a win-win for the beauty companies—when a product "hits" with the customer, they're able to apply the same technology to all of their brands, saving themselves a bundle in research and development costs. But for you, it often just means that you're paying more for a department store product, like foundation, than you actually need to. In my view, you can find a "just as good" foundation in a drugstore.

But cheaper doesn't always mean honest. You know those ad campaigns plastered all over the cosmetic aisles of your local Rite-Aid or Walmart? The ones with your favorite TV star? As an industry insider, I can tell you that the celebrities hawking these affordable foundations aren't necessarily even wearing the makeup they're selling! Celebrities provide star power, period. There is no guarantee whatsoever that they actually wear the foundation they're shilling, so, if you're using the actress from *Modern Family* as a gauge for purchase, you might want to rethink your strategy.

And sorry to be a big buzzkill, but you need to hear this (again): You can't rely on women's magazines for unbiased advice either. Beauty advertising basically supports the magazine business, which is why you'll see countless editorial mentions of a large beauty company's products and very few mentioning the small, independent brands; those niche brands don't advertise—they can't afford to—and therefore aren't helping to fund the magazine's bottom line. And often those cool little "indie" brands get snatched up by the big corporations anyway, because it's cheaper and easier to buy innovation, personality, and street cred than create it themselves. For example, MAC and Smashbox, Kiehl's and The Body Shop, once small stand-alone "indie" brands themselves, all have been "acquired" by the big corporations (Estée Lauder and L'Oreal).

All that information may be a bit of a downer, but the upside to all this makeup madness is that there are a few good products for this stage of our lives at the drugstore *and* the department store. Our first course of action is to determine your ideal shade and the best formula and texture for your skin.

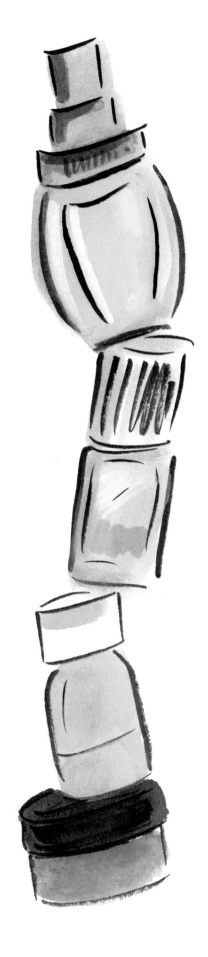

how to shop for the right shade

In your twenties and thirties, the Holy Grail of Hotness is using a foundation that so closely matches your own complexion it all but disappears. But now that we're older, our skin has changed, which means so will the shades that work best for our skin tone. Remember how we touched on menopause in an earlier chapter? Discussing how it changes the elasticity and texture of our skin? Well, it can also change the *color* of

My easy fix to the problem of a fading complexion is to "go for the gold."

our complexion, often making it paler. Since the face is the site of numerous estrogen receptors, any hormonal upset (menopause obviously being the mother of all hormonal upsets) can result in shifts in our complexion, so, after fifty, we typically start to lose the robust color we were once used to seeing. The last thing we want to do is pick a shade that's matchy-matchy with our menopausally challenged skin. (Remember the

pale crypt-keeper? Exactly.) My easy fix to the problem of a fading complexion is to "go for the gold." Simply by shifting into gold and away from those pink-based foundation shades you've been hoarding, you can banish that gray pallor. Foundations with golden (yellow) undertones work magic on your skin. They neutralize any redness and leave your skin looking instantly healthier. Shop for foundation that is a shade darker (two shades, max) than your natural complexion, but decidedly more gold. In other words, run screaming from any rosy tints the salesperson may try to foist on you. They may match your skin color, and they may have looked great on you when you were in your thirties, but that was then and this is now. If you want to look livelier, friskier, and like you're ready to take on the world, gold is the ticket.

Now that you know you need to go gold, you'll still need to find *your* perfect shade for *your* skin tone. It can be a daunting task, for sure. But it's definitely doable.

Apart from made-to-order custom blending (and your options are very limited on this front), how can you get your ideal shade? With all the advances in beauty, you'd think finding the right match would be a snap. It isn't, and one of the reasons involves some inside scoop on the sample situation.

While many of the big cosmetic companies offer a wide range of foundations, they only supply retailers with samples for the three or four best-selling shades. What if the best-selling shades weren't right for your complexion? You wouldn't have the opportunity to take the color home and try it out, so you very well might end up buying a best-selling shade that isn't right for you. It's basically the industry norm to scrimp on samples. But the news isn't all bad. Most department stores (and even a few drugstore chains) have liberal return policies. So if you don't hit a home run the first few times around, don't be shy about making an exchange or asking for a refund. A store that wants your business will be happy to comply. But the goal, of course, is to avoid mistake purchases in the first place. So here are a few quick tips to help you do that:

1 DO AS MUCH ADVANCE-RECON AS POSSIBLE

Before heading to a department store or beauty boutique, pop by a few drugstores (or even one of the "big box" behemoths like Target) and see if you can scrounge up swatch cards or sample-size freebies of shades you think might be right. After testing them at home, you can either head back to the drugstore and buy a full size, or take them with you to use as a shade reference when you're trading up to a pricier brand at a department store like Macy's or at an independent retailer like Sephora. Also, flip through that stack of fashion magazines on your coffee table. These days, some of the mass-market makeup brands advertise by offering a foundation sample that's the equivalent of a perfume scent strip.

2 SHOP WITH A CLEAN FACE

Yes, I know it's scary to expose yourself to the world barefaced, but how else will you be able to sample foundations on the spot? You can mitigate a little bit of that self-consciousness by dressing well, which is not only a great confidence booster, but it's also a sure-fire way to get salespeople to snap to attention.

3 BRING ALONG AN HONEST FRIEND

If you're the type who asks strangers in dressing rooms whether the jeans you've tried on flatter you or not, because, well, you're just not sure and you really need a second opinion, then consider bringing along a trusted friend when you shop for foundation. Be sure it's someone you know will be straight with you, and whose style you admire. Where you see a match they may see a miss.

4 TEST A FEW STRONG SHADE CONTENDERS ON YOUR JAW LINE

Not the back of your hand. Better yet, have the salesperson (if there is one) do it for you. And don't worry, it disappears with one swipe of a makeup-remover towelette. Consider bringing your own wipes, especially if you have sensitive skin, to avoid wearing war paint as you leave the cosmetics counter and head for the shoes.

5 USE THE MAGNIFYING HAND MIRROR TUCKED IN YOUR PURSE

You'll need this when you head outside to play shade detective. The golden shade that looks good in the retailer's fluorescent lighting might look like a topping for hot dogs in daylight. Natural light is the litmus test; make sure any foundation you're considering passes it.

6 BRING A FAVORITE SHADE FROM YOUR BEAUTY STASH

If you're considering trying a new foundation, be sure to bring the one you've been using up until now—as long as the *shade* has been working for you. For example, if your current foundation seems to look dry on your skin and you want to try a product with added moisture and an SPF, having your correct shade on hand will save you a lot of time.

7 DO SOME RESEARCH BEFORE YOU SHOP

Many popular brands have online tools to help you find the right color (L'Oreal Paris even has a new app for that). Or if you know the product and shade, some sites can match it to the equivalent shade in their line.

Natural light is the litmus test: Make sure any foundation you're considering passes it.

One last thought: When you've decided on your shade, you may also want to buy a shade that's one or two shades deeper to accommodate the change of seasons and the months between winter and summer. As the weather begins to change, you can blend the two shades, customizing your palette as you gradually move into the darker shade for the warmer summer weather.

Now that you've got an excellent grasp on the shade you want, the real fun starts: picking a formula that feels great, provides the right degree of coverage, and makes you feel like a million bucks—make that a billion. But to do that, you need to know how to separate the foundation hype from the foundation help. Here's my guideline built on many years of experience:

LABEL LAW 1
AVOID FOUNDATIONS WITH THE FOLLOWING DESCRIPTORS

Anti-Acne
Want an easy way to get dry, cakey, old-looking skin? Apply an anti-acne foundation all over your face. Even if you're experiencing breakouts, I recommend spot-applying an oil-free formula on the problem area only. Beware the "crypt-keeper" look.

Balancing
Aimed at combination skin (i.e., oily in some spots, dry in others), "balancing" foundations seek to level the playing field. But even if parts of your face feel oily at times, your underlying problem is most likely dryness. And for that, you need moisture. Save "balancing" for meditation.

Clarifying
This is just a more ladylike way of saying anti-acne. Most clarifying foundations contain heavy doses of salicylic acid, way too harsh and drying for your "post-M" face.

Long-Wearing
If your goal is a fresh-looking face, this makeup is not for you. Developed primarily for oily types whose foundation tends to slide or melt off quickly, this isn't something you should be looking for. Better to reapply or touch up with the *right* foundation for your skin when and if you need to.

Matte/Mattifying

This could be great if you're twenty-five, but "matte" is makeup code for drying. Trust me, a matte finish is the polar opposite of what you want in a foundation. You're going for glow and radiance.

Oil-Free

Unless you have bonafide adult acne, or a T-zone that's seriously prone to shininess, an oil-free foundation won't do you any favors. Because of hormonal shifts, your skin is likely dry at this stage of the game. Moisture and shine are your friends, so don't fight them.

Powder

A powder foundation looks cakey on dry skin and can be extremely drying (beware of foundations billed as the trendy "mineral powders"). Many powders make claims of hydration, but when you think about it, "hydrating powder" is an oxymoron. At the risk of sounding like a broken record, at our age, we need a *moisturizing* formula.

Self-Adjusting

The theory here is that these wonder brews somehow magically figure out your skin tone and adapt to match it exactly. Don't buy it, literally.

Smart

The kissing cousin of "self-adjusting," smart foundations that go on clear and then miraculously morph into your exact shade are a myth. Until your foundation can tutor your kid for the SATs, don't fall for this ploy.

LABEL LAW 2
BEWARE OF WISHY-WASHY WORDING

I mentioned this before, but it's especially important to remember these slippery words and phrases when purchasing a foundation or tinted moisturizer. They are usually found in the category of "antiaging" foundations, which I don't put a lot of faith in (see the following page). The race is on among beauty companies to lengthen foundation labels with the latest buzz words or ingredients to sound more beneficial than they really are. As with skin care, these phrases are designed to be a block against lawsuits by stating only what a product "might" or "may help" or "appear" to achieve. Avoid these waffle phrases invented to take your money and prey on your insecurities. Companies have made billions on these meaningless claims and ingredients, while covering their corporate asses at the same time. The truth is, the industry uses them to obfuscate the fact that the claim they're making in this antiaging category probably won't do a damn thing for you. Write down this list, carry it with you, and rule out any foundations with the following language:

- "age-defying"
- "appears to diminish"
- "helps to minimize"
- "helps to prevent"
- "improves the look of"
- "may combat"
- "more than smoothing"
- "reduces the look of"
- any phrase that compares the product to cosmetic procedures, such as "lifting," "firming," "antiwrinkle," and "antislackening"

LABEL LAW 3
A CHEAT SHEET OF FIFTY+ BEAUTY-SPEAK

Brightening
Incandescence is the goal of a brightening foundation, and that jibes nicely with the total effect we're after. Just be aware, it can also mean that it contains age-spot diminishers. Read the label carefully—the fewer potentially irritating "treatment" benefits the better.

Dewy
Ah, yes! For all of us, a truly dewy finish is the Holy Grail of foundation textures. Why? Because it means your skin will appear fresh, healthy, and moist. It doesn't get any better than that.

Luminizing
Akin to brightening minus the pigment-diminishing component, luminizing foundations make your skin look like it was lit from within.

Moisturizing
Dry skin craves hydration. End of story.

Radiance
Yet another take on the brightening/luminizing theme. Ergo, a great bet.

Sheer
As long as your complexion is up to the challenge, sheer—the polar opposite of thick, cakey, and masklike—is ideal.

Now that your armed with discerning knowledge about what beauty-speak to avoid and what to look for in product labeling, it's time to introduce you to the refreshingly broad array of foundation products that work for over-50 skin.

YOU, ONLY BETTER
COMPLEXION-FRIENDLY COVERAGE FOR FIFTY+ SKIN

Tinted Moisturizer

Hands down, tinted moisturizer is my favorite formula for women of our age. For starters, it helps with menopause-generated dryness, and, just as crucial, it's much sheerer than traditional foundation. Tinted moisturizer is really the only type of foundation product that can be used all over the face without worry of amplifying the aging effect. For day use, try one that has a built-in SPF of at least 15.

My short list of **Best Bets** for a range of skin types:
- Clarins Hydra Care Tinted Moisturizer
- Dr. Hauschka Toned Day Cream
- Laura Mercier Tinted Moisturizer SPF 20
- NARS Pure Radiant Tinted Moisturizer SPF 30
- Neutrogena Healthy Skin Enhancer Tinted Moisturizer SPF 20
- Philosophy Hope in a Tinted Moisturize
- Sonia Kashuk Radiant Tinted Moisturizer SPF 15

Alphabet Soup: "BBs," "CCs," "DDs," . . .

Beauty Balms, or BBs, are a hybrid of tinted moisturizer and skin care. The BB cream is most often tinted (one to four shades), with light coverage, and, depending on the brand, may offer sun protection, priming, moisturizing, color correcting, and pore minimizing in a single product. CC stands for "color correct," and this form contains more pigment and more skincare ingredients than its predecessor, the BB. That means more coverage (like a foundation) and more antiaging claims, such as clarity and reduction of age spots. DD stands for "daily defense" (or "dynamic do-all" cream). It's reason for being is to include more environmental protection agents, such as sunscreens and antioxidants. Word has it there's already a GG in the works . . . Where's it all going? Who knows? My advice is to stick with the group below.

Consider these **Best Bets:**
- Dior's Hydra Life BB Crème
- Estée Lauder Daywear BB
- Garnier Skin Renew Miracle Skin Perfector BB Cream
- Chanel CC Cream Complete Correction SPF 30
- Olay CC Cream Total Effects Tone Correcting Moisturizer SPF 15
- Clinique Moisture Surge CC Cream

NOTE: All but the Dior products are produced by the same two corporations (L'Oreal and Estée Lauder), so many of the products share much of the same technology.

Liquid Foundation

I'm happy to report that liquid foundations have come a long way since the spackle days of yore. Several glide on seamlessly, delivering sheer coverage that feels virtually weightless. Still, there's no reason to coat your face from stem to stern. Rather, opt for a very light hand on the face, with a slightly heavier application around the nose, cheeks, and chin to cancel out redness.

Check out these **Best Bets:**

- Boots N07 Lifting & Firming Foundation
- Giorgio Armani Beauty Luminous Silk Foundation
- Maybelline Instant Age Rewind Radiant Firming Makeup
- Shiseido The Makeup Liquid Foundation

Cream Foundations

I love cream foundations because they give great coverage, you need very little to see a visible difference on your skin (great "cost per wear" benefit), they blend easily, have adjustable coverage, and, best of all, you can mix it with your tinted moisturizer (which I do).

My short list of **Best Bets:**

- Chantecaille Future Skin Foundation, Cream
- Laura Mercier Crème Smooth Foundation
- Maybelline Dream Smooth Mousse Ultra Hydrating Cream

Whipped Foundation

These foundations look and feel great. They offer super aerated, lightweight, smooth coverage that has the look and feel of whipped cream and the ease of application of a liquid foundation.

A couple worth considering:

- Elizabeth Arden Flawless Finish Sponge-On Cream Makeup
- Sunday Riley Crème Radiance Breathable Ageless Foundation

Stick Foundation

I like foundation sticks for several reasons: They usually have a creamy texture, they're ideal for spot coverage, and they're handy and portable— you can pop one in your makeup bag without fear that you'll later find a puddle of liquid foundation coating your lipstick and mascara.

A few **Best Bets:**

- Bobbi Brown Foundation Stick
- MAC Foundation Studio Stick SPF 15
- Make Up For Ever Pan Stick Foundation
- Shiseido The Makeup Stick

Cream-to-Powder Foundation

A great cream-to-powder formula offers the best of both worlds: a glide-on start, and a nonshiny finish for those of us still experiencing oily skin. Apply with a sponge only where necessary or when going more golden. If you're covering the entire face, apply sparingly, but go heavier on the T-zone area (i.e., to even out redness on the cheeks or chin or to mitigate shine). Because they're housed in a compact, they're also portable and mess-free. One caveat: This formula is not for dry skin. Women with a drier complexion will want a more luminous finish and will be happier with one of the other formulas mentioned above, particularly a tinted moisturizer, liquid, or cream foundation.

Consider these **Best Bets:**

- Benefit Some Kind-A-Gorgeous The Foundation Faker
- Clé de Peau Beauté Cream Compact Foundation

- CoverGirl AquaSmooth Compact Foundation
- L'Oreal Paris True Match Super-Blendable Compact Makeup
- Max Studio Fix Powder Plus

Brightening Foundation

These offer a radiance boost to the skin. Radiance, which is defined as fresh, luminous, glowing skin that looks youthful, is especially problematic for women over fifty, as the turnover rate of our skin cells has slowed and our skin has lost luminosity. However, be careful that the boost of radiance does not look fake or too shiny on your skin.

On my short list of **Best Bets:**

- CoverGirl + Olay Tone Rehab 2-in-1 Foundation
- Lancôme Teint Miracle Foundation
- Yves Saint Laurent Touche Eclat, the Illuminating Magic Light

Now that you've selected the type of foundation that meets your skincare needs, remember that less is definitely more when it comes to how much you use—especially after fifty. Let the fun begin!

mission accomplished . . . almost

To maximize the benefit of just having found the perfect cover for your skin, you should take advantage of a few easy steps to get more bang for your buck. Knowing how to ready your skin, how to choose an application tool or method, and how to assess your needs and make adjustments for even more perfect coverage can go the extra distance to the state of foundation bliss. Consider the following tips to add to your cosmetic skill set:

1 BE SURE TO EXFOLIATE

You are probably thinking, *What does exfoliating have to do with foundation?* A lot. By sloughing off dead skin cells once or twice a week, you are creating a smooth surface for your foundation to sit on. Makeup will go on evenly, and skin will look fresh, smooth, and glowing. But a word to the wise: Don't go heavy on the scrubs; stick with very mild exfoliants which don't irritate the skin like rice powders and InstantPeel (my favorite—and it comes in single-use packets). Or try the Clarisonic (www.clarisonic.com), a sonic cleansing brush that smoothes dead cells away. I use mine without soap or cleanser—just warm water. Heavy scrubs with abrasive ingredients can cause irritation and redness on the skin; anyone with dry skin should beware of those.

2 SELECT YOUR TOOL OF CHOICE

Fingers, sponge, or brush? It all depends on what type of foundation you're using and how much coverage you want. Be sure to consider the following before you choose which tool to use.

Fingertips:
Test used when applying liquid and cream foundations, because the heat from your fingertips warms up the pigment, making it easy to blend.

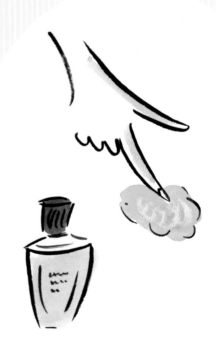

Sponge:

Best to achieve a sheer look, because it absorbs a lot of foundation. Lightly press it into the skin in a blotting/patting motion; don't sweep it across your face unless you want to create streaks. For a dewier look, dampen the sponge with water before dipping it into the foundation.

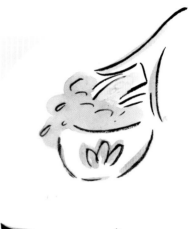

Brush:

Deposits the foundation most evenly and if you choose a tapered brush it allows you to expertly get around your nose and mouth area. "Paint" in light strokes on areas you need more coverage and then in sweeping motions, blend foundation into the skin until it's invisible.

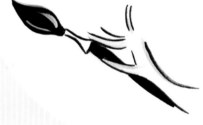

3 ASSESS AND TWEAK

Applying your foundation can be as simple as dabbing a dark spot here and there, or going full-frontal coverage to mask a bad skin day. Before applying your foundation, you need to assess what kind of coverage you think you need. There are bound to be days when you need more or less foundation coverage than usual.

Unless you live in a biosphere, or go around swathed from head to toe like a beekeeper, your complexion doesn't stay the same color year-round. So why should your foundation? It only makes sense that your makeup should shift in tone along with the seasons. When you're paler in the cool weather, you tone it down a shade. When the mercury rises, and your weekend hike has left you with a sun-kissed glow, you ratchet up the über flattering gold factor I discussed earlier.

You can also use a slight shade-tweak to help you fake it till you make it. For example, if you're chained to your desk all summer while all your friends are languishing at the beach, you can "cheat" by using a foundation a few shades darker than your everyday look. (This is why it's always important to buy one or two shades deeper than your standard color.) Nobody needs to know your beauty secrets but you.

Sometimes, your foundation needs will change overnight, literally: Perhaps a Sunday spent outdoors, sailing or skiing has left you a little windblown and ruddy, or maybe you had one too many cocktails at dinner last night and you need that extra face boost. Whether it's seasonal changes

> Nobody needs to know your beauty secrets but you.

or day-to-day shifts in skin tone, don't be afraid to play "mixologist." You can blend a few drops of medium-coverage liquid foundation into your usual light-coverage tinted moisturizer, or even layer a bit of liquid over your crème-to-powder formula.

After applying your primer and concealer to cleansed and moisturized skin (as outlined in Chapter 4), start with a few dabs of foundation and build from there. Just make sure that when you first begin to experiment with mixing and applying your

foundation, you do it in very bright natural light (a window or a skylight, for example). That way, when you step outside or anywhere else, you'll feel confident that your foundation is just the shade you want it to be. Before long, playing DIY makeup artist—and scaling up or down as necessary—will be second nature.

I **HAVE TO** admit, foundation is called foundation for a good reason—it is the baseline for all of your other beauty efforts, and it is *by far* the most important piece of the fifty+ beauty puzzle. Once you nail the right shades and formula, it's transformative in a way that no other product can touch—like a blissful vacation or the morning after. By showing the world the aspects of your face that you really love, and keeping all that other stuff lightly under wraps, you are taking a huge, vibrant, confident leap forward for your face.

Now that you've found the perfect white T-shirt of your beauty routine, read on for beauty tips for eyes, lips, and cheeks. After all, a perfect white T-shirt is great on its own, but paired with a J Crew jacket, it's unstoppable.

YOU SHOULD KNOW

A WORD ON ANTIAGING TREATMENT FOUNDATION

"Treatment" foundations are the darling du jour of the cosmetics companies. A mash-up of skin care and makeup, treatment foundations are often laced with the same high-tech ingredients found in pricey antiaging elixirs. On paper, they sound fabulous—what time-starved woman doesn't want to try to kill two beauty birds with one stone? But while this all sounds great, antiaging treatment foundations don't usually deliver. Simply put, no foundation can lift, firm, or eliminate your lines and wrinkles—period.

A word of caution: Once you start layering treatment foundations on top of the skin care you're already using, you could be setting yourself up for irritation. (Case in point: Retinol, which is frequently included in treatment foundations, should really only be used at night because it renders the skin photosensitive.)

Having said all that, I'm not completely down on treatment foundations. In fact, there are two skincare ingredients that I absolutely swear by in makeup: SPF and hyaluronic acid. Of course you know why you need the former—to short-circuit the formation of additional lines and wrinkles, while hyaluronic acid is a world-class skin plumper and a total moisture magnet. Plump, moist, and sun-protected equals gorgeous fifty+ skin.

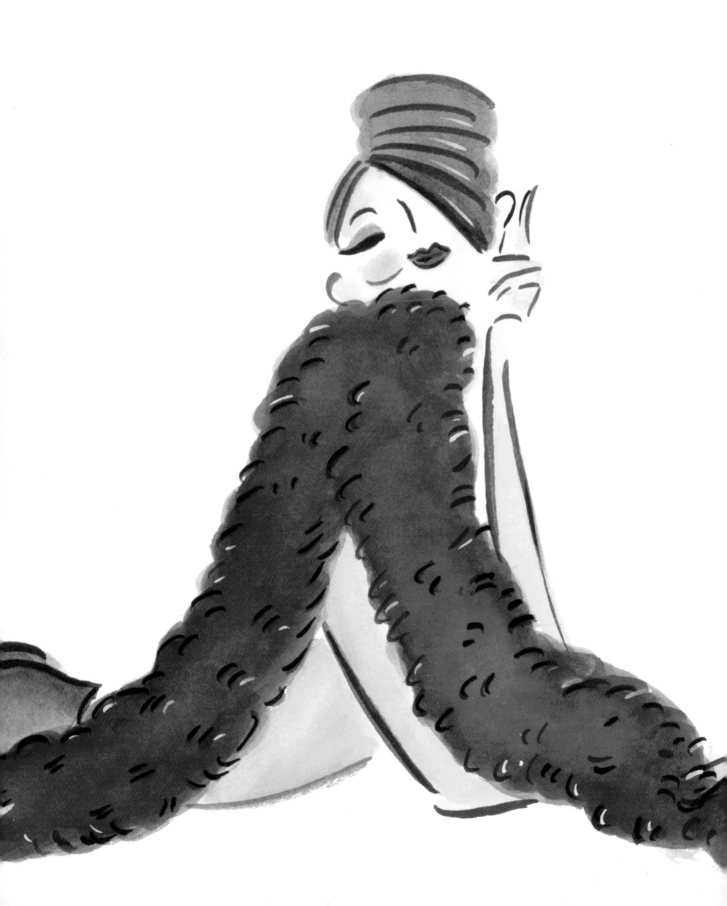

CHAPTER SIX

Blush

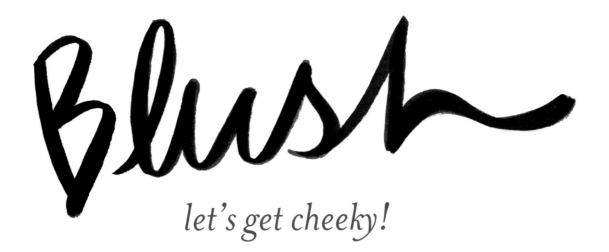

let's get cheeky!

YOUR CHEEKS, UNLIKE YOUR ASS, SHOULD ALWAYS BE PLUMP! PLUMP, FRESH, AND GORGEOUS.

But the cheeks you were born with aren't the same cheeks you see in the mirror once you're over fifty, and, like a host of other body parts, they tend to move south as your birthdays move north.

Like squeezing into a flattering pair of J Brand jeans, knowing how to add the right color and texture where it counts can give the illusion of great "cheeks" and accentuate your assets. Great looking cheeks, both

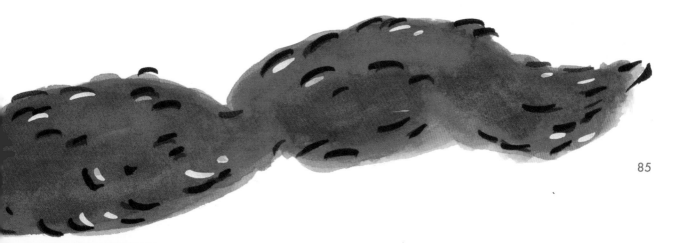

upper and lower, equal good, healthy sex appeal. This chapter will tell you everything you need to know about how to find the right cheek color, how to layer color and use texture, how to highlight, and how to choose the cheek products that will make your face glow because that's exactly what you want now—believable glow, radiance, and luminosity—that "just ran a couple of miles" look.

So, cheeky is a good thing—it really is. Bringing out your cheeks is an easy and essential step for looking your absolute best at fifty+. If you've never worn blush before, you *must* start working it into your daily beauty routine. To me, blush, like taxes, jury duty, and making it to your Pilates class, is *not* optional.

Okay, I'm prejudiced. Blush has always been the cosmetic placeholder of my youth. Perhaps it's my seven-year-old self's memory of my mother with her tiny round cardboard box of what she called "rouge," and her deliberate swirls of the little cotton pad on her face, transforming her beauty. Perhaps it's Julie Christie's cheeks in *Dr. Zhivago*. Perhaps it's because I remember my first kiss on my cheek from Michael Egan when I was twelve.

But even if all my makeup memories didn't somehow circle back to blush, I'd still think it was of primary importance in the grand hierarchy of cosmetics. Because from my experience, there is no other single piece of makeup that is more useful in creating the illusion of youth than blush, when well applied. It is the take-your-breath-away beauty element in your makeup regimen. It is your face's softness, innocence, vulnerability, and natural beauty. For these reasons, using blush and choosing the right color is the face-defining factor—really you, only better. Blush is entirely underrated but incredibly important, so make a mantra of the following . . .

BEAUTY TRUTH:

Getting cheeky is essential to capturing the youth quotient.

For most of us, that is . . . but here's one for the books that gives new meaning to "getting cheeky." This is a true story that happened to a friend (and executive) in the cosmetics industry.

She once had to supervise a campaign shoot for cheek color—a new launch that the company she was working for was sinking a lot of money into with the belief that a certain celebrity spokesperson (who shall remain nameless) with a huge contract (hundreds of thousands, for ten days of work) would do a good job of selling to the public (us). But when it came time to shoot the commercial, the starlet refused to say the name of the product! She even threatened to walk off the set, despite the fact that her dressing room had been stocked with Cristal champagne and Petrossian Caviar at her request. When she finally was convinced to come on set after a heated exchange between the company's legal counsel and her agent, she wanted to keep all the clothes—even the one-of-a-kind original samples we had borrowed from designers. And when the stylist sent her a bill for the shoes and clothing, she promptly handed it over to us and threatened to skip out on the remaining days of her contract if we didn't pay for her shopping spree! She was not the sweet "blushing" girl we all had read about in *People* magazine. No, I will not reveal the identity of this self-absorbed diva, but let's face it—there is cheeky and then there is CHEEKY!

Unlike getting this starlet to cooperate, blush, by contrast, requires very little fuss to get it to deliver. It's an easy-breezy do, and the quickest to apply of all the cosmetic products—just dab, blend, and possibly highlight. Forget trying to contour or sculpt;

it will never look good. Avoid being that woman with the two streaks of color on her face. Run away from this look fast and leave it to celebrity makeup artists. You are not posing for a magazine; you are a real woman living your life!

What *is* critical is choosing your texture and color. Since those buoyant, plump, round cheeks of yore are starting to move downward, we are going to rely on our cosmetic wits to master and restore this lovable part of the face.

the art of blushing

Want to look really old? Use powder blush. Your skin is likely not as smooth as it once was, and perhaps has a few lines and rough patches as well. Powder blush will sit in those lines, and your cheeks will end up looking splotchy and uneven. Never use powder blush again. Go into your makeup closet right this minute and toss that powder blush. Replace it with creams, sticks, and tints—that's all you need. They are mistake-proof, and starting with a little controllable dab, you can easily build to a visible natural color.

Read on for the highlights of how to select and apply blush for best effect.

1 IDENTIFY YOUR COLOR PALETTE

Here are a few color tips that will help you hone in on the right hue for your skin tone:

If you have FAIR skin:

- DO start by trying out dusty pink shades or woody rose tones.
- DON'T choose shades that are ruby or purple in hue, as these shades only create a bruised appearance on the skin.

If you have MEDIUM skin:

- DO go for tawnier tones similar to the yellow undertones in your skin, like apricot, clay, and burnt coral colors.
- DON'T use dark shades, pastels, and very light pinks, which offset the warmth in your skin color.

If you have DARK skin:

- DO try more deep and intense shades, like bronze and golden shades; deep plums, burgundies, and ruby reds work well, too.
- DON'T use pastels and bright pinks, as these shades may create a washed out or chalky appearance on your skin.

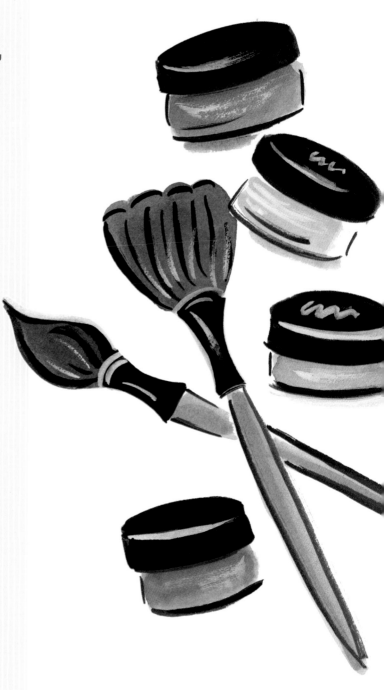

I admit I am a sucker for a neutral palette even on the darkest skin, so make sure the intense colors also have a neutral cast to them. Often, women with darker skin tones feel compelled to use bright colors. Rethink this. There is nothing prettier than a dot of healthy neutral color (in deeper intensities) on the cheeks of very dark skin. Try a burgundy to the brown side; you may be very surprised—the more neutral, the more natural.

Another good tip for choosing a cheek color: If you have a favorite tried-and-true lip color, pick a blush in the same family. This creates more harmony on the face. Also, try to pick up colors that will look good with your hair. For example, redheads should stick with the colors of highlights in their hair (rosy and/or peachy).

Now that you have an idea of your correct color palette, it's time to determine what type of blush consistency will best suit your skin type.

2 SELECT A TEXTURE

Assuming you've all tossed out your powder blushes like I recommended above (Not yet? I'll wait. Done? Okay), it's time to choose a consistency and type of blush that works best for your skin and lifestyle. As I mentioned, both creams and sticks work much the same way, so it's really just finding what type of application form you prefer. Some find sticks easier to use and quicker to apply, while others enjoy the flexibility of creams, since they're easier to mix with foundation or moisturizer. It's up to you.

Cream Blushes:

These products come in a variety of consistencies, from very shiny to more matte creams, so it is a question of finding which works best with your skin type. For example, super dry skin should not use the matte textures because this consistency, like powder blush, will sit in your lines and not move over dry patches. Creams also do not last as long as powder, so know that you may have to retouch a few times a day to hold the intensity. And one more thing you should know is that you can't always count on the color in the pot being the color you get on your face, so trying it before you buy it is imperative. If you can't try it before purchasing and feel you've made a mistake, return it or try this: If it is too intense, blend foundation into the color; if too pale, mix it with darker lipstick.

Here are a few **Best Bets** in cream-based blush products:
- Laura Mercier Crème Cheek Colour (my favorite shade is Praline)
- MAC Blushcreme (my favorite shade is Lilicent)
- Maybelline Dream Mousse Blush
- NARS Cream Blush
- Revlon Cream Blush

Stick Blushes:

This form of blush is similar to a cream blush and most often less oily in consistency; like lipstick, it also comes in a container that is portable, and it aids in controlling the "messy" factor during application. It is a bit dryer in texture than cream, and one quick dab on each cheek usually distributes enough color that can be quickly blended with the fingers. Like creams, sticks come in a variety of finishes that require some trial and error to see what works best for your skin. A word of caution: Avoid the sticks that have a high level of shimmer.

On my short list of good stick blushes:
- Clinique Blushwear Cream Stick
- NARS The Multiple
- NYX Stick Blush

3 FIND YOUR SWEET SPOT AND APPLY

Look in the mirror and smile—just trust me. Now put your
finger on the apple, or "sweet spot," of your cheek.
It's located just a hair under your cheekbone (the apple
might have to move a little higher as time passes). Rub
your fingers in a circular motion on that spot until you
see a small blush of color begin to develop and notice
where it is most intense. This is the "sweet spot" where
you'll dab a small amount of your blush and blend it.
With creams and sticks, your best application tool is your
clean finger or a washable flat silk sponge, and the objective is
to blend your cheek color seamlessly into your moisturized face
(or into your foundation or tinted moisturizer), so the blush is natural
looking and has soft edges. (Note that creamy formulas can warm to a more intense hue with
the heat of our body, so apply sparingly and build the color gradually and carefully.) Dab the
cream blush on with your middle finger and then blend with your pointer, middle, and ring
fingers. Use a circular motion, building color, and feathering the edges for softness. This is the
key to beautiful, natural-looking cheeks. Easy, right? Read on for further tips and tricks to maximize your cheekiness.

Experiment with glow by taking a small swipe of your natural, low-shimmer highlighter (or
another very shiny cream blush) and move it in a circular motion across the cheekbone for an
extra shot of youthfulness. This attracts light the way young luminous skin does. (I use Laura
Mercier Crème Cheek Colour and then use another more shiny cheek color, MAC Blushcreme,
as my highlighter). If you want a healthy, sun-kissed look, apply your blush, and then swipe
bronzer lightly on top of your cheek color. You can also try the reverse—bronzer first with cream
blush on top. Which way looks best? It depends on you and your blush. Another trick, one I
favor, is to catch your foundation or tinted moisturizer before it has completely dried and mix the
blush right into it, forming a completely natural look. In other words, it is the immediate next step
after applying your foundation.

THE TINIEST CHANGE can often make a huge difference, and this is the way I feel about blush. Just moving from powder to cream moves your look forward and into the more natural sphere. You'll also find that it takes less time, and I am a great believer in our hand getting in touch with the planes of our face. That's how we get to know it and love it.

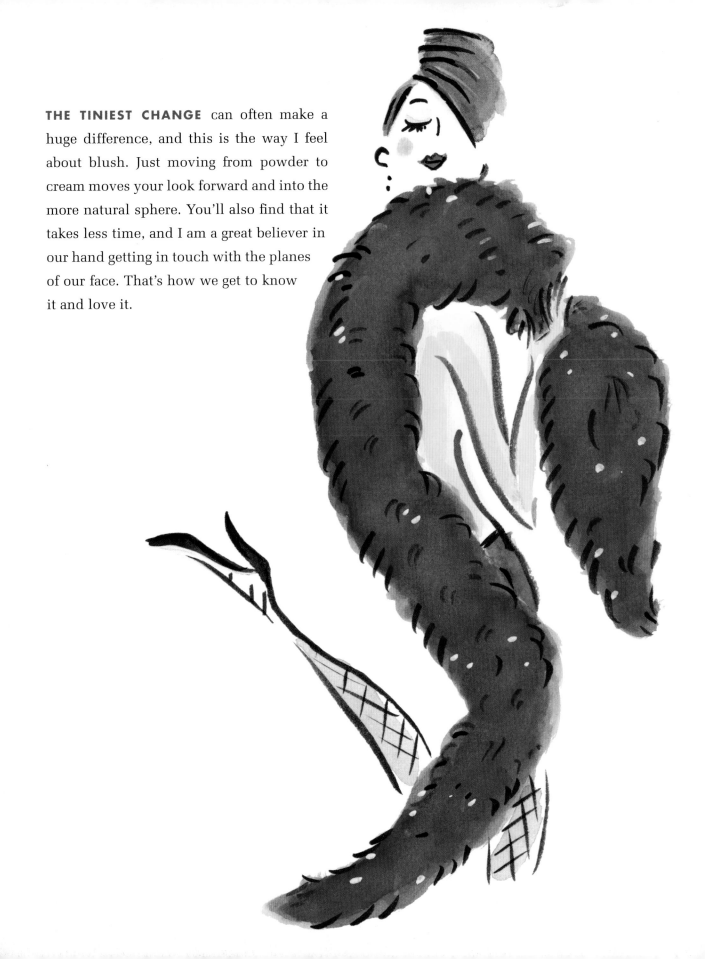

When it comes to shopping for blush products, here's a beauty truth worth knowing about: Cosmetic companies annually (sometimes twice a year) do "category reviews" on best-selling shades among their competitors and then incorporate those bestsellers into their product lineup. The catch? These luxury brands now view drugstore brands as competitors since consumers increasingly shop for cosmetics at both high-end department stores like Saks as well as drugstores like CVS, so you are likely to find the same bestselling cheek shades from brands like Maybelline and L'Oreal as you might from a higher-end manufacturer, like Lancôme.

Additionally, did you know that many companies don't produce or create their own powder cheek colors? They go to a handful of vendors (mostly Italian) with expertise in finely milled powders to source them. The end product you see—whether it's $10 or $75, whether it's headed to CVS or Saks—likely came from the same supplier/factory with many of the same formulas and colors.

Talk about being cheeky!

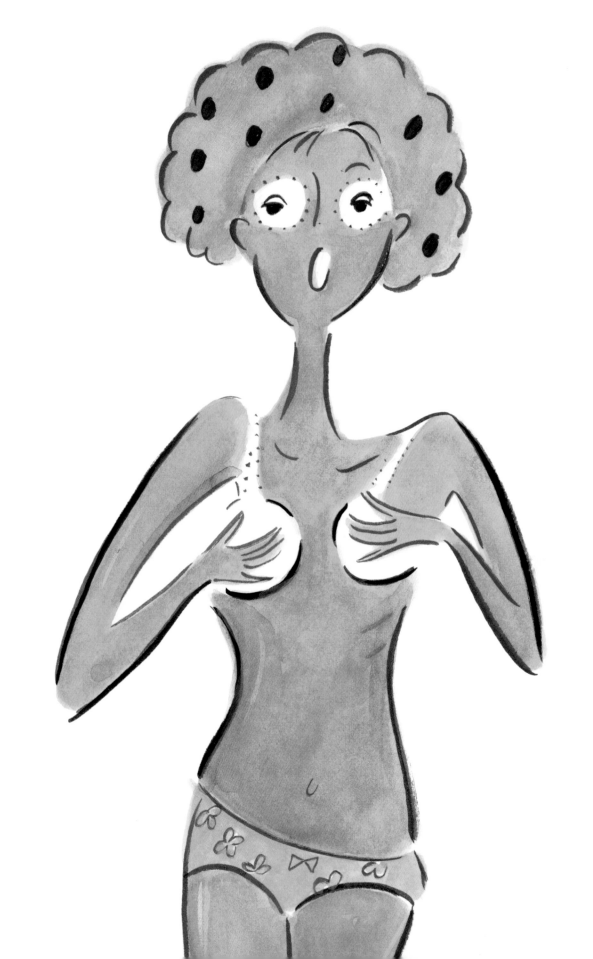

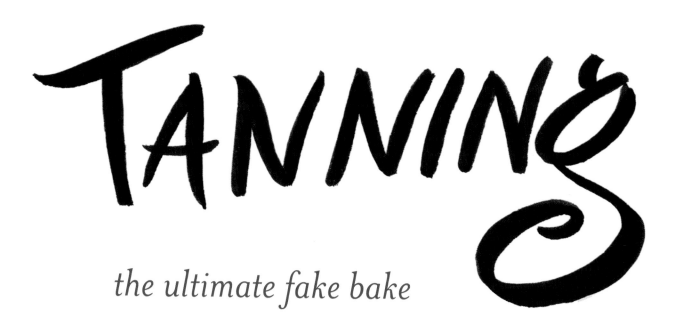

CHAPTER SEVEN

Tanning

the ultimate fake bake

WANT TO KNOW THE MOST GLAMOROUS WAY TO GET SKIN CANCER? LAY OUT ON A YACHT DECK IN SAINT TROPEZ, SLATHERED IN BABY OIL AND IODINE.

Okay, it's a bit dramatic, and frankly, I shouldn't even have to say it—by now you should know: Don't sit in the sun unprotected. Never, never, never!

Tanning is no longer an option unless you want crocodile skin. Though you may find it appealing on a pair of Jimmy Choo boots, you definitely don't want to see scaley skin on your face, so one more time: No tanning! Not on the beach, not in a tanning bed, not anywhere—not allowed. But you are allowed to still have a gorgeous, sun-kissed glow that adds an exotic aura and sensuality to your skin. It's no secret that a good "tan" can hide a multitude of sins, including yellow teeth, uneven skin tone, red spots, and veins. And with a great healthy glow, you don't need to wear foundation, which is a luxury in itself. (It will also make your eye color look more intense.)

A little bronzer is the quickest and easiest way to give your skin a bit of golden color.

This chapter discusses how to achieve that fabulous fake bake using a variety of products without damaging your skin. Of course, that sunny radiance isn't easy to achieve, so you have to start a relationship with one or perhaps all of the following backups: a good bronzer, a great self-tanner, and a golden-tinted moisturizer.

I will teach you how to layer these products to customize just the right tone for your skin so that you can achieve a year-round golden glow. For instance, did you know that you can layer a self-tanner with an illuminating bronzer for even more glow? And, since it goes without saying that you still need to wear sunscreen every day, I'll give you that list, too. But first, let's start with the obvious: bronzer.

bronzers

A little bronzer is the quickest and easiest way to give your skin a bit of golden color. Remember, golden is the path to radiance and youth, but be careful. Going too orange or too red with your bronzer can make you look like an Oompa Loompa, so avoid this pitfall. The trick is choosing the right golden hue for your skin tone and applying it properly. If you are fair, select a bronzer that has rosy-gold or peach undertones. If you have medium skin, use a bronze or copper shade, and, with dark skin, go for a bronzer that has deep rust and deep copper undertones. Steer clear of sparkle, glitter, and high shimmer—that's for high school.

a great healthy glow . . .

CREAM BRONZERS

These will give you a glow that you won't get from powder, and they are especially great for dry skin, which most of us have after age fifty. This consistency may come in a stick as well as a pot. Apply it on the areas of the face and décolletage where the sun would naturally fall. Blend it on the cheek bones, lightly on the temples, and sweep it across the bridge of your nose—but only if it has a low-level or no shimmer. Most bronzers do have some shimmer pigment, so if you choose one with shimmer, skip the bridge of your nose. I love the look of bronzer mixed with blush—try mixing the two (cream with cream) for a subtle, healthy flush. Best application tools are fingertips and/or a sponge.

Best Bets:

- NARS The Multiple in Lamu, South Beach, and St. Bart's
- Sally Hansen Natural Beauty Sheerest Cream Bronzer

LIQUID BRONZERS

These come as gels, tints, and serums and are usually the sheerest formulas, great for everyday wear. Gels (which also come in stick form) are best suited for oilier skin types, which few of us are at this stage of life. They are packaged in a tube or bottle and often look darker than the color that you want, but they are often more translucent and lighter than they appear, and give your skin the sheerest wash of color. Try mixing your foundation or tinted moisturizer with a liquid bronzer, but again make sure the bronzer has little to no shimmer if you are going to use it all over your face. Start with a small amount and build from there. Here, too, sponge and fingertips work equally well for application.

A few **Best Bets:**

- Dr. Hauschka Skin Care Summer Impressions Bronzing Fluid
- Giorgio Armani Fluid Sheer 10 (good for medium to dark skin tones)
- Givenchy Mister Radiant (good for light skin tones)
- Laura Mercier Bronzing Gel
- MAC Lustre Drops in Sun Rush

POWDER BRONZERS

As you've probably gathered, I am not a fan of powder for cheeks, face, or for bronzing, and, unfortunately, powder bronzer is probably the most common form found in department stores and drugstores. Those big compacts that won't fit in a purse have enough product to last Snooki and JWoww combined for the next decade. Plus, powder on top of dry skin will make you look old and cannot be easily blended. Most often it looks really fake. So if you cannot find a bronzer that's anything but powder, go for a finely milled dewy bronzing powder that will blend seamlessly with your tinted moisturizer or foundation, once they have dried after application, and try lightly dusting it over your blush for just a hint of a healthy glow. Use a big fluffy brush and tap off any excess product before using. Concentrate the color at your temples and along your cheekbones. And without double dipping, lightly brush across your nose and chin. As always, do not choose a powder with detectable shimmer or glitter!

Choose among these **Best Bets:**

- Benefit Hoola Bronzing Powder
- Bobbi Brown Bronzing Powder
- Guerlain Terracotta Bronzing Powder
- NARS Bronzing Powder in Laguna
- Tom Ford Bronzing Powder in Terra

Whatever bronzer you choose to go with, the key to getting that perfect faux glow is not just about having the right product, it's also knowing how to apply it well and use it properly. Here are a few tips to achieving the right amount of radiance:

do not choose a powder with detectable shimmer or glitter . . .

1   A bronzer should be used to look healthier, not tanner.

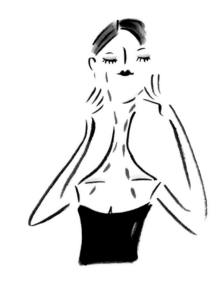

2   Avoid ending up with a different colored face and neck by extending your bronzing strokes lightly down the face to the neck and on to the collarbone.

3   Apply your bronzer lightly, building up your color slowly; it's easier to add color than it is to take it away.

4   Skip bronzer altogether if you have any skin eruptions, large pores, or your skin is misbehaving.

5   If you can't find a shade of bronzer that looks perfectly natural on your skin, try mixing two colors of the same consistency.

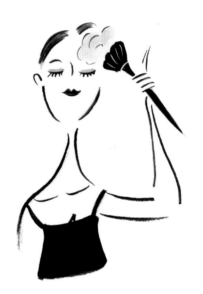

6   For a more subtle glow, mix liquid bronzer with your moisturizer or your primer, and then follow with foundation or tinted moisturizer.

7   For a more intense glow, skip the primer and try mixing liquid bronzer with your foundation or tinted moisturizer.

8   If your hair will be styled in a ponytail, twist, or knot, use bronzer on the ears and the back of the neck.

9   Always apply bronzer in natural light.

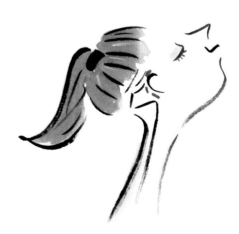

self-tanners

Here's a confession: I had gotten the message early about the damaging effects of sunbathing and tanning beds, so I became a spray-tan addict—along with Lindsay Lohan and every other reality TV star and red carpet disaster. I was hooked—I mean *really* hooked. At least once a week, I would step into a booth, strip down to nothing, extend my arms out like a scarecrow, and hold my breath as the tanning spray misted me from head to toe. Then I'd turn around and do it on the other side. I felt like one of those rotisserie chickens at Whole Foods.

> And much like dessert portions, the method for finding the line where a little becomes too much is the key to success.

But then one day, I discovered something unsettling that made me go cold turkey (or cold chicken, in this case). Sure, I'd been willing to suffer through the embalming solution smell for the first six hours and had put up with it when the tanning solution stained my Egyptian cotton sheets orange, along with my ankles and heels. I was undaunted! Unstoppable! Even after my blond highlights went umber in that mist, ruining Louis Licari's sophisticated handiwork on my hair. What ultimately undid me, after a year of addiction, was being handed a pair of nose clips to wear when I checked in at the salon for my weekly spray down. With this little gesture, my beauty routine was transformed into a HazMat situation. I panicked! What exactly was I breathing in? Were Lindsay and I going to be victims of "orange lung" disease—or worse?

Once I discovered the deleterious side effects of indulging in spray tans (beyond orange heels and ruined sheets, I was inhaling possible cancer-causing chemicals), I quit and moved to at-home DIY self-tanning. Better to have "orange hand" than "orange lung."

Despite all this drama, nothing beats a little healthy glow on the body and face at this stage of life. The operative point here is "a little." And much like dessert portions, the method for finding the line where a little becomes too much is the key to success.

The best way to navigate this category without looking like a pumpkin is by using tanning lotions that provide *gradual* color, and by applying them properly. Here are some take-home tanning tips that will help you avoid the orange menace:

TEST

If this is your first adventure into the world of sunless tanning, test the product on a hidden spot on your body to be sure the color and shade is right for you and that you have no allergic reaction.

EXFOLIATE

This is often overlooked and it is a very important step. By exfoliating in the days before applying a self-tanner, you will ensure your tan looks even and lasts longer. When you rub away dead skin cells, the new layer of skin will absorb the formula more efficiently.

MOISTURIZE

After each exfoliation you need to hydrate the skin to expedite the absorption of the formula and to leave skin looking ultra smooth and glowing.

WASH HANDS

To avoid orange stains or streaks, wash your hands every five minutes when applying the self-tanner, and don't forget the area between the fingers, fingernails, cuticles and knuckles. Or use surgical gloves. Personally, I find it difficult to apply lotion with gloves, but many have mastered this.

BEWARE OF BENDABLE AREAS

Go easy when spreading the self-tanning formula around your knees, armpits, ankles, feet, and elbows, as the thicker the skin, the more it absorbs the color, which then leaves you with dark-orange areas. You can also apply a light layer of lotion to these areas beforehand to help dilute the product.

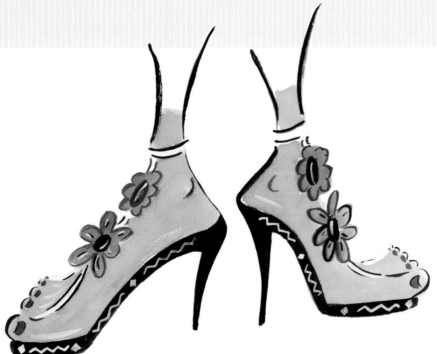

Now that you know the best practices of self-tanning application, you'll need to choose among the dizzying array of products out there and decide whether you want instant gratification or a slow-to-grow glow. All come with manageable pros and cons, and most brands offer a standard skin color range: fair, medium, or dark.

GRADUAL SELF-TANNING LOTIONS

As mentioned earlier, the key to good color, in my opinion, is to build the glow slowly with daily use. Like any beauty venture, there are pros and cons to different methods. With gradual color, the advantage is that you'll see minimal streaking, blotchiness, and buildup on ankles, souls of the feet, and knuckles. The downside? Patience. You're going to have to be patient—it takes a few days to arrive at the color you want, and you must reapply the self-tanner every day. The good news: These products are made to moisturize, so you can cut the moisturizing step out of your daily beauty routine. Also, they often contain a sunscreen, so you can eliminate this step as well. This category is very affordable, almost foolproof, and can be found easily at your local CVS, Duane Reade, or Walgreens.

Consider these **Best Bets:**
- L'Oreal Sublime Bronze Self-Tanning Lotion SPF 15
- Physician Formula Sun Shield Sunless Tanning Lotion SPF 20
- Coppertone Sunless Tanning Gradual Tan Moisturizing Lotion

In my opinion, *gradual* self-tanning is the way to go. BUT, if for some reason you jump immediately to an instant self-tanner, I would exercise extreme moderation until you have found a color and method of application that's right for you. I am not trying to be a killjoy, but these products can get us into trouble. And by trouble, I mean Oompa Loompa orange: dark-orange elbows, orange knuckles, orange knees, orange ankles, and even face, if you apply too liberally. Guard against getting it in your eyebrows, as well, as blond eyebrows will turn orange. Also, instant self-tanners are not so instant; they usually take several hours to activate to full color and will last several days (a week)

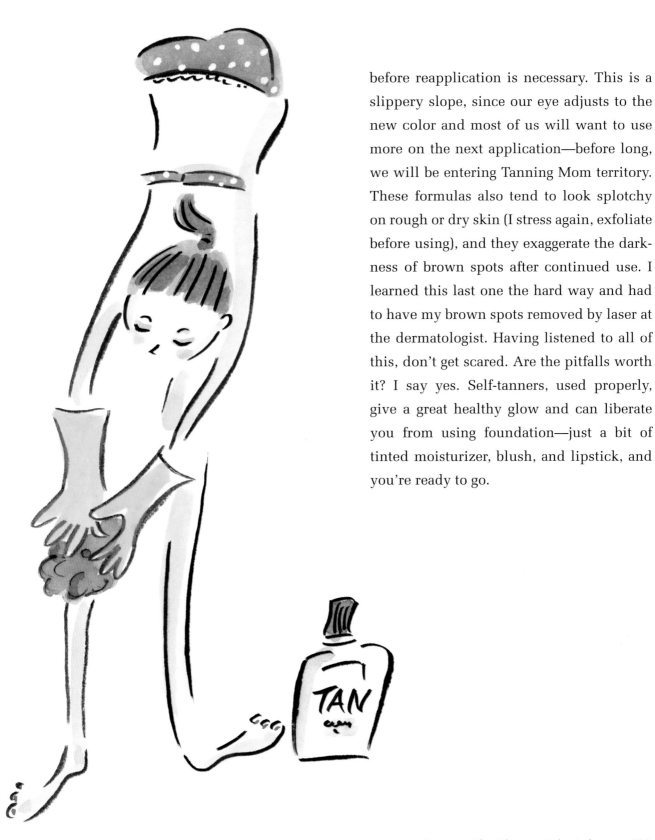

before reapplication is necessary. This is a slippery slope, since our eye adjusts to the new color and most of us will want to use more on the next application—before long, we will be entering Tanning Mom territory. These formulas also tend to look splotchy on rough or dry skin (I stress again, exfoliate before using), and they exaggerate the darkness of brown spots after continued use. I learned this last one the hard way and had to have my brown spots removed by laser at the dermatologist. Having listened to all of this, don't get scared. Are the pitfalls worth it? I say yes. Self-tanners, used properly, give a great healthy glow and can liberate you from using foundation—just a bit of tinted moisturizer, blush, and lipstick, and you're ready to go.

INSTANT SELF-TANNERS

Within the world of instant self-tanners, there is a wide range of choices and forms available—lotions, creams, liquids, gels, mousses (foams), aerosol spray tans, and tan towels. Your selection should be based on the easiest application method for you to handle, your natural skin color, and the hoped-for result, which should be an even, healthy glow. Like the gradual tanning lotions (which by far are my first choice), they most often come with a skin-color code. You never want to go more than a couple of shades darker than your natural skin color—more than that begins to look fake.

Self-Tanning Towelettes

I personally prefer the tan towels, since they can be used easily with surgical gloves (no orange palms), and their solution spreads evenly and dries quickly. They come in packets for different parts of the body (face, arms, or legs), which is a great benefit for travel. When using the towel, be sure to reach into corners of the face and cover the surface of the ears. Use very carefully around the hairline and around the neck and décolletage. The downside of the tan towel is that it is drying, so it's wise to use a liberal dose of moisturizer once the color has reached its full potential.

Best Bets:

- Dr. Dennis Gross Skincare Alpha Beta Glow Pad
- Kate Somerville 360 Degrees Face Self-Tanning Pads

Lotions and Creams

These products are convenient, and, if you have really dry skin, they're better than using self-tanning towelettes because they bring instant moisture to the equation. The downside? The chances of streaking, uneven color, and blotching are greater because, as you rub the product in, it's hard to know what areas you have already covered until it begins to show up. So you'll need to establish a routine for your application, working your way either up your body or down. As you become more adept at your application, this routine will become habit, and you'll find that you miss fewer spots and provide more even coverage over your skin. Be aware—that like spray tanning, these self-tanning products can stain your clothes, towels, and bed sheets, so be sure to let the product dry before getting dressed or going to bed.

Best Bets worth considering:

- Aveeno Continuous Radiance
  Moisturizing Lotion
- Jergens Natural Glow FACE Daily Facial
  Moisturizing with SPF 20
- Jergens Natural Glow Revitalizing
  Daily Moisturizing
- Nivea Sun-Kissed Radiant Skin Gradual
  Tan and Daily Lotion

Gels and Mousses

People with oily or eruption-prone menopausal skin usually prefer a gel or mousse (or tan towel) because they usually contain less oil, making them less likely to clog pores. An added benefit— they spread and dry quickly. These forms offer the same coverage power of lotions or creams without the downside of too many humectants.

Here are a few of my favorites:

- Clarins Delectable Self-Tanning Mousse
  SPF 15
- L'Oreal Sublime Bronze Clear
  Self-Tanning Gel
- Neutrogena Sun Fresh Sunless Foam
- St. Tropez Bronzing Mousse

Aerosols

Personally, spray tans in an aerosol remind me too much of the tanning booth. I don't like breathing in the mist, the notion of ruining the ozone layer, or doing damage to the walls of my bathroom and shower, which will take on a vague orange color like the pollution haze at sunset in Los Angeles. Be forewarned about this. That said, they . . . enough said.

HOW LONG DOES a faux tan last with any one of the above choices? Five to seven days. Reapplying before that (other than touching up missed spots) will start you on that very slippery downhill slope that tripped up Lindsay and me.

So proceed with caution and learn how to master the fine art of tanning without the fears that accompany harmful ultra violet rays of the sun. Of course, it goes without saying that you *must* still wear sunscreen every day. It's like a credit card or a fully charged cell phone—you don't want to leave home without it. Used wisely, self-tanners are a great tool for the warm weather months and a healthy pick-me-up for changing skin tone and color. And yes, if you *really* are daunted by the self-tanning trial and error, simply stick to your tinted moisturizer or foundation in a golden shade. But I didn't dedicate an entire chapter of this book because I wanted to skip my grueling Pilates workout—I did it because I know it's one of the best things you can do to look more vibrant, sexy, vigorous, and youthful. The bottom line? A great self-tan can do wonders for your confidence. But much like cheesecake and chocolate mousse, it's best to indulge in it with moderation.

a great self-tan can do wonders for your confidence . . .

YOU SHOULD KNOW

Odor alert! The chemical agent (DHA) that triggers the tanning action of many self-tanners has a distinct and pungent smell similar to that of hair color chemicals in salons, but in my darkest thoughts I imagine it smells a little like embalming fluid. Then again, I have no idea what that smells like. This smell takes several showers to eliminate, so be prepared to camouflage that odor with your favorite fragrance—or avoid mingling in close quarters with others until it dissipates. Some products, however, boast mild to no smell. If after-scent is an issue to you, be sure to test it with your own nose before purchasing.

Sometimes, self-tanning goes wrong: streaks, blotchiness, and dark-orange smudges on the ankles, heels, and between the fingers, to name a few. Don't hide behind gloves, socks, or a muumuu if this happens to you! There *are* remedies. While the newest self-tanning formulas are easier to apply and somewhat foolproof, mistakes do happen. Should this happen to you, here are a few tips for dialing down the damage:

- Rub lemon juice, rubbing alcohol, or an alpha hydroxy acid cream over the area to minimize the smudging and/or streaking.

- Exfoliate and try to get the pigments out by sloughing off skin cells. Whether you use a loofah, body scrub, or plain old baking soda on a washcloth, this action will allow newer (untanned) skin cells to surface more rapidly.

- Use a self-tan remover. Several companies offer tan remover pads or creams to help lift the pigment away from the skin. Try St. Tropez Tan Optimiser Remover for your palms or Uh Oh Self Tan Remover.

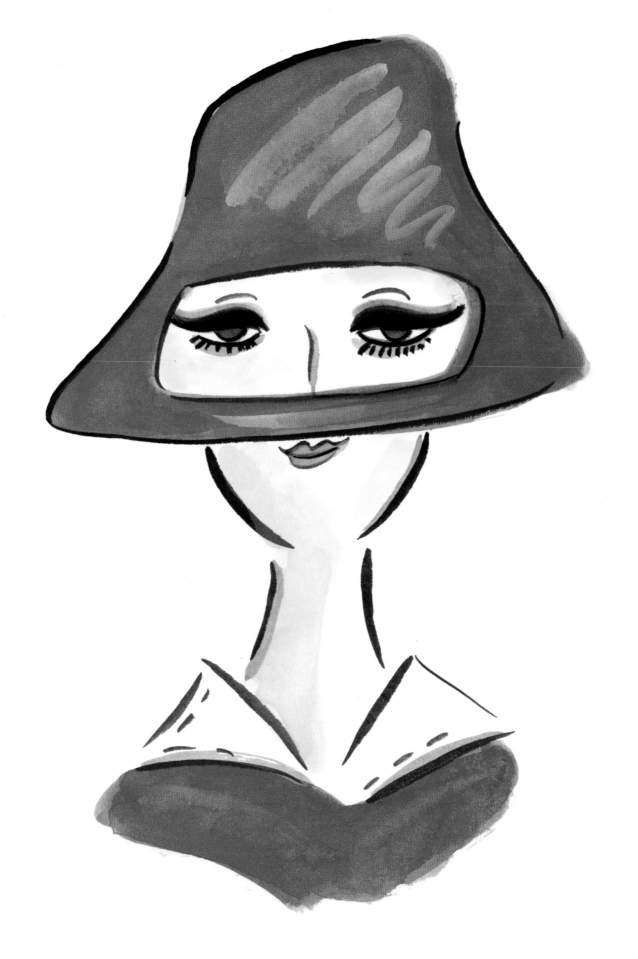

CHAPTER EIGHT

The Eyes Have It

eyeliner, eye shadow, mascara

A FEW YEARS AGO, I OBSERVED A "WOMAN OF A CERTAIN AGE" SURROUNDED BY THE MOST ATTRACTIVE MEN IN THE ROOM, ALL OF WHOM SEEMED OBVIOUSLY CHARMED BY HER.

It was at a cocktail party given by my boss and his wife, whom I was staying with for the weekend. There were plenty of "pretty young things" at the party (emphasis on the "young"), so I wondered what made her so alluring. I later found out from the hostess that she'd already had five husbands! (I wish I could tell you who this very social Mrs. X was, but revealing her name would put me in the witness protection program.) Having recently come out of a divorce myself, from a husband of many years, you can imagine my curiosity. As it turned out, she was staying the weekend as well, and, being fresh on the dating scene, I took the occasion to ask her for some advice. Here's what she told me: "It's all about the eyes. When I see someone attractive across the room, I stare

"I may not always have the right shoes, but I always have the right mascara."

until they notice me. When they do, I smile, and most often they follow." And wow oh wow did she work those eyes! She said, "I may not always have the right shoes, but I always have the right mascara."

For many of us, when we look in the mirror, our eyes do the opposite of wooing—they trigger a litany of complaints instead: bags, crow's feet, crêpe-y lids, and wimpy lashes. Here's where you want to take a deep breath, inhale, exhale, and listen: Eyes should be celebrated, not disparaged, so let's embrace this thought and learn how to love the eyes that we have.

In this chapter, I'll teach you simple, eye-opening makeup tips to help you accentuate the most expressive part of your face. It will include the products, the tools, and the application instruction you need to turn your eyes from tired to glamorous. If eyes can provoke battles, inspire songs, seduce lovers, and be the windows to the soul, don't you think it's worth the effort? Mrs. X got this concept in spades.

That said, Mrs. X wasn't *completely* candid with me on the mascara thing, as I found out later when I asked to borrow a hairdryer from the closet in her bathroom. She made the mistake of leaving her cosmetics bag out on the counter, and of course I locked the bathroom door and determined very quickly she wasn't just wearing mascara. Most of the products in her cosmetics case were indeed eye makeup, but she did such a great job using it that all you noticed were her gorgeous eyes and not her makeup. This is what I discovered in Mrs. X's makeup bag:

it's all about the eyes . . .

- A duo eye-shadow palette in a neutral pair of light and medium tones (flesh and medium brown)

- A single shadow in a deep brown

- Three brushes: a shadow brush, a very thin liner brush, and an angled brush

- Lid primer

- Concealer

- Mascara

- Brow gel

- Eyelash curler

- Eyelash comb

Quite a lineup for our natural-looking, mascara-wearing Mrs. X, wasn't it? As the weekend progressed, I felt comfortable enough to ask her what she did with her eyes, besides flirting. She offered to share her tricks (about eye makeup, that is) and here's what I learned: She stated at the outset that the overarching goal was to use eye makeup in an upward and outward motion so the eyes looked bright, youthful, and open. I registered this as a very important clue since I had already noticed that it wasn't in my best interest to follow the downward direction of my upper eyelids. Here's Mrs. X's routine in more detail:

1 She reached for the primer first and applied it lightly to the lid all the way up to the brow to smooth and camouflage the fine lines. She gently patted it in with her ring finger.

2 This was followed by mixing the duo colors together with the shadow brush and applying the blended shades to the upper lid, up to the crease. This gave a very soft and pretty definition to the eye.

3 She then took the angled brush, dipped it into the dark single shadow, and applied a thin line along the upper lash line.

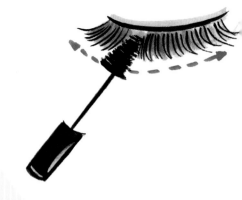

4 When she reached the outer corner of the eye, she blended in a bit more of the dark shadow and "winged" it out in a barely visible stroke. The goal of this, she mentioned, is to give the illusion of "lifting" the eye up, but not true cat eyes effect. (Leave that to your daughter along with liquid eyeliner.)

5 She then dipped the thin brush into the dark single eye shadow and lightly lined the lower lashes from the outer edges to three-quarters of the way to the inner corner of the eye, making the soft line thinner as it moved toward the inner corner.

6 Before using mascara, she curled her lashes. Her mascara routine was unlike any I had seen before—she applied the wand close to the lash line and moved it back and forth several times before pulling it through the lashes and followed up by holding the wand vertically and moving it back and forth like a windshield wiper (she claimed this rid the lashes of excess mascara and ensured that the tips were coated).

7 Next, Mrs. X applied a dot of concealer on the outer edges of her eyes, just under the uplifted shadow to emphasize the upward direction of her eyes.

8 She then added a dot of concealer on the inner corner next to the nose and blended it well to remove any darkness there (she emphasized that this step makes the eyes stand out).

9 Mrs. X finished her routine with a tiny bit of brow gel, which she used to gently sculpt her brows in—yes, that's right—an upward and outward direction, just like her shadow routine.

I can't say this routine will get you five more husbands (and really, who wants THAT), but I can say it's the easiest and most foolproof route to beautiful eye makeup. I've passed this lesson on to several grateful friends and colleagues, including makeup artists. Mrs. X was not a makeup artist, not a model, not a magazine editor, nor a beauty company executive. She was a woman of a certain age who had taught herself to master the art of eye makeup. The makeup was brilliant because it made you notice HER: her expression (happy and youthful), her beautiful eye color (green), and her pretty lashes. You didn't notice her crêpe-y eyelids or her crow's feet, which were there but camouflaged with the few strategic steps I've just outlined. But the most important piece of information I can share is that none of the steps had to be precise. The shadows she selected were so subtle (flesh and browns) that they blended seamlessly on to the lids, and a little bit of smudging did not harm the overall effect, which made for the most perfectly imperfect *Wabi-Sabi* eyes.

This is the method I have used every day (well . . . almost every day) since my encounter with Mrs. X, who luckily still remains married to her most recent happy husband.

Here are a few additional tips I picked up along the way as a beauty editor:

TO MAKE SMALL EYES BIGGER:

After primer, use the flesh or light gray part of your duo to cover the upper lid. Use the darker brown or dark gray/black to line the crease of the upper eye lid (A). Next, shade the outer corner of the lid and the crease with the darker brown or dark gray/black and blend well (B). Use the same color to line the lashes on the upper lid only (C). Curl the lashes and finish with two coats of mascara on the upper lashes only, concentrating the mascara in the middle and outer corners of the eye using upward strokes. Use a flesh or white liner to line inside of lower lashes.

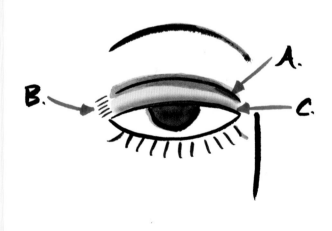

FOR CLOSE-SET EYES:

Like moving furniture around your house or apartment, the goal with close-set eyes is to give the illusion of more space (between the eyes). Use a lighter shade to the inner third of the lid from the lashes to the brow bone (A). Next, apply the dark shade to the outer two thirds of the eye from the lash line to the brow bone (B). Concentrate color on the far corners of your eyes, extending slightly past your natural line (C). Blend. Apply liner to only the outer third of the upper lash line (D). Apply mascara.

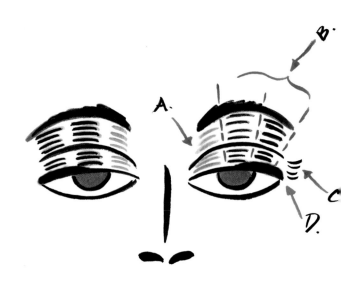

FOR WIDE-SET EYES:

The goal is to give the illusion of less space between the eyes. Just know that wide-set eyes are currently in vogue. Check out the current crop of models used by *Vogue* and other fashion magazines. But our goal is to make you look and feel great, so the hell with what they are dictating. This tutorial aims to make the space between them narrower. Begin by applying the lighter shade to the outer two thirds of the lid (A). Start at the lashes and blend upward, stopping at the brow bone. Next use the dark shade on the inside third of the eye, from the lash line to the brow bone and blend upward (B). Apply eyeliner from the inner to outer corner of the upper lid (C). Apply mascara.

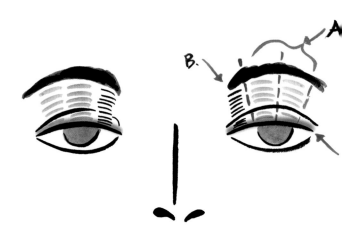

Now that we've had a few lessons in how to apply this trio of eye products, let's open our eyes to the simple truth about eye shadow, eyeliner, and mascara: Despite the ridiculous number of products and colors and blends out there vying for your attention and your wallet, if you keep it simple, you can't go wrong.

eye shadow

The truth is, all powders are pretty much equal. Powder products are tricky products to produce; it requires the right amount of milling and pressing to create a finely milled, soft, and blendable product. The equipment to do this is expensive, and there are key "outside" vendors that are able to do this with great expertise, thus, many of the big companies use these same few vendors to produce their shadows and then simply label it as their own. So it is hard to say one product is better than the other. Additionally, the same ingredients are generally used to create the base of the shadow, which generally contains talc, mica, ethylhexyl palmitate, zince stearate, methylparaben, propylparaben, and silica, plus added minerals and colorants to create the shade. One big difference, however, is that some of these powder eye shadows claim to be made with minerals that are said to be less irritating and safer for the eye—but be forewarned, some people find these mineral products to be more irritating.

A word to the wise: Many "drugstore" brands use these same outside vendors for their eye shadow as higher-end brands, so see if they have your favorite shade in a finely milled and pressed powder before you drop a bundle for a shadow in places like Sephora, Nordstrom, or other higher-end retailers.

> A word to the wise: Many "drugstore" brands use these same outside vendors for their eye shadow as higher-end brands.

When it comes to color, what I've discovered since my eye-opening weekend with Mrs. X is that the best shadow duos are the beige to brown for dark eyes, or the gray to black family for light eyes. One or both of these shadow families will look good and appropriate on everyone. Unless you want to look like a peacock, forget the plums and pinks, greens and blues. Neutral tones are more natural, letting your eyes do the magic. Leave the garish look for Halloween. And much like my rule for lipstick colors, your eye shadow should not contain high levels of metallics, shimmer, and glitter. Dark shades combined with lighter neutrals are the most forgiving and youthful choices for the lids.

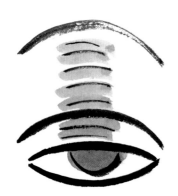

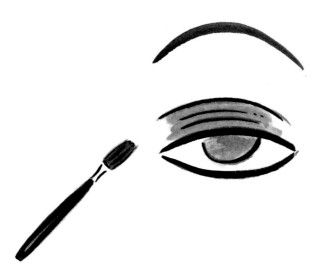

HERE ARE A FEW BEST BETS:

Singles:

- CoverGirl Eye Enhancers 1 Kit Shadow in Brown Smolder or Swiss Chocolate
- L'Oreal Paris Studio Secrets Professional Eye Shadow Singles in Lush Raven (smoky black)
- Lancôme Color Design Singles: in Mochaccino or Ciel du Soir
- Nars Single Eye Shadow: Fez and Coconut Grove
- Rimmel London Glam'Eyes Eyeshadow in Jet Black or Night Jewel
- Trish McEvoy Eye Shadow in Soft Grey or Glamorous

Duos:

- Chanel Ombres Contraste Duo in 47 Nuit-Clair
- Clinique Colour Surge Eye Shadow Duo in Like Mink or Double Date
- CoverGirl Smoky Studio Blast in Onyx Smoke
- Maybelline Expert Wear Duo Eye Shadow in Browntones
- Sonia Kashuk Eye Shadow Duos in Heaven and Earth

eyeliner

Eyeliner does for the eyes what a good accessory does for clothes: It enhances and completes the look. What would Chanel suits be without gold chains and pearls? Good, but much more FABULOUS with them. Some women depend on eyeliner to change the shape of their eyes, while others value the way it seems to open the eyes and draw attention to make them appear bigger. In either case, used properly, eyeliner is a great asset.

That said, there are only a few occasions when I will say NEVER in this book, and this is one: Never ever use a liquid liner—it looks hard and emphasizes the delicate (often crêpe-y) and fine skin surrounding your eyes. Soft pencil liners (that can be smudged) are my preferred form because of their manageability. Powder liner will work as well, but they tend to flake and leave a mess under the eyes, requiring additional cleanup. Here, too, neutrals work best. The bright blues, purples, and greens are best to put on hold . . . forever.

MY PICK OF BEST BETS:

- CoverGirl Perfect Blend Eyeliner
- Elizabeth Arden Smoky Eyes Powder Pencil
- L'Oreal Paris Le Kohl
- MAC Kohl Liner

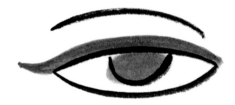

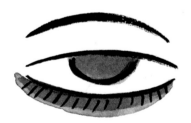

mascara

When it comes to makeup, mascara is always a subject of great interest to women: Who among us wouldn't love to have long, thick, voluminous, beautiful lashes? As we get older, however, our lashes become sparse, making it more difficult to create the look that we once had. But don't get caught up in the mascara hype. Claims like "400 percent more volumized," or "100 times thicker," or "extreme-length" have to be taken with a grain of salt. Instead, experiment with a formula and brush that covers the "grays" and combs through *your* lashes, making them look the most natural, well-defined, and clumpless. Trying to create more lashes with unreasonable expectations from your mascara will most likely create more of a problem than a solution. There are a few go-to mascaras that work extremely well for the average set of lashes, so it might be helpful to start with the following **Best Bets**:

- CoverGirl Lash Blast
- CoverGirl Lash Blast Clump Crusher
- L'Oreal Voluminous
- Lancôme Definicils

Most everyday formulas wear well throughout the day without smudging and are easily removable with soap and water or simple eye makeup remover. These are your best bets. Avoid regular use of waterproof formulas. Save those for special occasions, like tears at your daughter's wedding. They are too tough to remove for everyday use—you'll have to rub hard to loosen the color, and in doing so you risk breaking your fragile lashes.

makeup tools

Never underestimate the power of a good tool to get the job done. Thankfully, we don't need anything complicated or hard to operate—just a few brushes and other simple applicators. While some products, like eye shadows and powder liners, often come with their own application brush, they're generally poorly made, not the right size, and difficult to hold. It's worth investing a few dollars in high-quality makeup tools to, yes, get the job done—and well.

PRIMER SPONGE

In lieu of your finger, a well-shaped sponge works wonders at reaching the tight spots around the eyes and nose.

A few **Best Bets:**
- Beauty Blender (these are allergen and latex-free, with no harsh chemicals)
- Sonia Kashuk Blending Sponge

BRUSHES

You might be surprised to know that the material of your brush plays a role in the quality of your makeup application. The makeup formulas you use will help you determine whether to choose natural (real) or synthetic (fake) hair. Natural brushes are better for dry products like blush and eye shadow, and synthetic brushes are best suited for cream or liquid because they soak up less formula than natural hair.

To keep them clean and to avoid bacteria build-up, wash with soap and water (or baby shampoo) one or more times a week and air dry on a clean towel. Since buying a good set of brushes will set you back a hefty sum, be careful not to let water touch the shank of the brush where the hairs are held together, otherwise the metal will rust and the brush will start to disintegrate.

Shadow Brush

Use a flat, round-tip, natural-hair brush that is firm enough to pick up the shadow yet soft enough to spread it gently without being harsh to our delicate lids. Pony and goat hair brushes don't shed and give a precise application.

Best Bets:
- CoverGirl Make-Up Masters Eye Shadow Brush.
- Sephora Pro Shadow Brush
- Trish McEvoy Brush 45

Angled Eyeliner Brush

Use a slim, tapered, synthetic, firm-bristled brush. The hairs should be tightly packed and have a sharp-angled straight edge so they can, with some precision, distribute the dark color along the lash line, and into an up-and-out direction.

Best Bets:
- Benefit Hard Angled Definer Brush
- EcoTools Bamboo Angled Eyeliner Brush
- Trish McEvoy Brush 50

Thin Eyeliner Smudge Brush

Use a flat, short-haired brush with a rounded tip that is dense and tightly enough packed to pick up the shadow color and distribute it along the lash line with soft, smooth strokes. These brushes do a great job in softening the look of eyeliner.

Best Bets:

- Jane Iredale Smudge Brush
- NARS Smudging Brush
- Trish McEvoy Brush 54

DUAL ENDED Q-TIPS

These old-school bathroom staples do an exceptional job at doing double-duty as makeup applicators. Use the pointed end to pick up highlighter or concealer to place under the outer edge of the shadow and on the inside corner of the eye. Only a dot is needed. Blend with the rounded corner of the Q-tip.

EYELASH CURLER

Last but not least, I want to mention the value of a good eyelash curler. It opens up the eyes, making them look bigger, wider, and brighter, and these are extremely valuable qualities as we cut back on the heavier eye makeup we most likely used in the past. To avoid eyelash breakage, curl the lashes *first*, gently and close to the root, and then apply mascara. Be sure you use a good curler with a comfortable grip and a high-quality rubber piece.

Best Bets:

- Kevyn Aucoin Eyelash Curler
- Maybelline Expert Tools Eyelash Curler
- Sally Hansen Flirty Eyes Classic Eyelash Curler
- Shu Uemura Eyelash Curler

only a dot is needed . . .

bad hair days

During and after menopause, thinning hair often becomes a concern. Turns out, our declining estrogen levels don't just affect the hair on our heads; our lashes and brows also tend to thin and gray as we age. While all mascaras will cover gray and help mask thinning lashes, there may come a time when mascara alone won't suffice in making so-so lashes look super. The good news is that when lashes thin out or break, or there's simply not enough hair to coat evenly with mascara, there are many weapons you can do battle with, relative to your cosmetic regimen.

FALSE EYELASHES

Having supervised so many editorial and ad campaigns throughout my career, I always appreciated what false eyelashes did to a model or celebrity for the camera, but I never put much stock in wearing them for real life, despite the influence of Liza and Twiggy. Tammy Faye kind of put the kibosh on that one—that is, until my friend Gloria showed me her eyelash technique, which came in handy when she had chemo and lost all her hair! So here are Gloria's foolproof steps for buying and wearing false lashes that look undetectably natural, with or without your own lash hair:

1 Shop at the drugstore and pay no more than $2.99 a pair for real hair lashes. Gloria's favorite brand for the most natural-looking lashes is Andrea #53, and for a little more fullness, Elite #18. Buy a few at a time because stock runs out on these two favorites.

2 Unless you wear brown mascara, look for black lashes.

3 Buy a tube of dark Duo Adhesive and a box of toothpicks.

4 When you get home, take them out of the box gently and lay them along your lash line (this step is essential whether you have lashes or not).

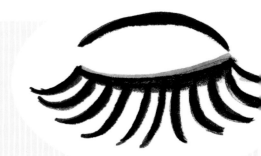

5 Invariably, they will be too wide for your eyelid, and you will have to cut them from the longer lash side to fit your lid.

6 Save the lashes you've trimmed. You'll need them later.

7 Before proceeding, put your eye makeup on. If you have lashes, apply one thin coat of mascara (before using the false lashes) to establish a good base.

8 Squeeze a miniscule dot of Duo adhesive on the top of your hand. Dab the tip of a toothpick into the Duo and apply a very thin layer along the base of the false lash strip. Wait about 30 seconds, then apply to your own lash line. Work from the outer corner in. Gently press with ring finer to set the lashes in place.

9 For fuller day lashes or for evening wear, take the lashes you've just trimmed off and apply them to the outer corner of the eye on top of the already applied lashes, using the same glue technique. If you are lucky enough to have fairly full lashes, use these trimmed pieces for daily use on the outer edges of the eye and use the full strip for evening.

10 Keep the tube of Duo and a toothpick in your cosmetic pouch for a quick touchup, should one of your lashes detach.

Like your first week of yoga classes, the first few times you try to apply false eyelashes can prove daunting, but, with a little practice, you'll become a pro. And don't worry, you will never look like Tammy Faye or Ru Paul with this routine. This is one of those moments when less (your lashes) is really more (with false lashes), in terms of its benefits. A pair of lashes should last at least a week if you remove them gently each night, take off the adhesive with your fingertips, and place them back on the form they came with.

EYELASH EXTENSIONS

A lot of women use eyelash extensions, but be aware that, while they are attractive, the procedure is time-consuming and costly (between $50–$100 for the initial application) and maintenance is required every three weeks. Like hair extensions, there are risks to using them, and, when not applied properly, it puts one's natural lash in danger of falling out or breaking off—even permanent loss of hair. And like hair extensions, the long thick lashes can be addictive. When Gloria's eyelashes were growing back after chemo, she was advised by the extension technician to continue using false eyelashes, since her own lashes were too weak for extensions at that stage of growth. Now, even though she's a candidate for extensions, she's happy to stick with her false eyelashes. She's perfected the method, taking only a minute per eye to apply them, avoiding the expense and time involved in getting extensions.

Having said all of this, here are a few vital pieces of information to know if you decide to pursue extensions:

- Do your research. Go to a reputable salon (preferably one recommended and tried by friends). Consider having a free consultation first, and, while there, check to be certain the lash artist is a licensed aesthetician or cosmetologist.

- Be sure the technician is not applying "cluster lash" extensions. It should be one single lash applied to each one of your own lashes.

- Avoid getting the extensions wet for 24 to 48 hours after application. The adhesive will reactivate and may cause the lashes to stick together and look like caked-on mascara.

- Don't touch! No pulling, tugging, or twisting. You can damage your lashes or even your lids. Don't try to remove them yourself; always have them professionally removed.

- Stay away from oil-based and moisture-rich hair products and face creams—they will loosen the bond. When washing hair, tilt head back.

EYELASH TINTING

This procedure, which is more affordable than extensions (from $15–$50 dollars), works best if you have lots of lashes, very light lashes (blond, red, or gray), and/or light tips on your natural lashes. You can achieve spectacular eye definition with lash tinting, allowing you to skip wearing mascara all together, but don't expect longer or thicker lashes—only darker and more defined lashes. To maintain your tint, you should have your lashes retouched every four to six weeks, but it only takes thirty minutes in a salon. I am a convert and regular user for many years, and here's what I've learned:

- Never use DIY, at-home products; you risk eye infections and irritation. It's always great to save money, but your eyes are important and delicate—treat them as a precious investment.

- Before tinting, research the salon's reputation, and the skill and experience of the aesthetician.

- Be sure to do an allergy and sensitivity patch test *before* making a commitment.

- Have some saline or lubricating solution to apply after the treatment (my aesthetician supplies a generous dose of this at the end of the treatment).

- Black is by far the most effective tint color, as it really makes lashes stand out.

ALERT: Eyelash tinting may be illegal in your state because there is a history of irritation caused by the misuse of coal-tar dyes on the lashes. Never allow your eyelashes to be tinted with anything other than vegetable-based dyes.

EYELASH GROWTH TREATMENTS

If you have thinning or short lashes, and you want longer, fuller lashes that don't require upkeep, you should know about Latisse, which is an FDA-approved, prescription-only drug (originally used for treatment of glaucoma and ocular pressure). It is not a perfect solution because, while it effectively enhances lash thickness and length of lashes, Latisse does have proven downsides: In some patients, the drug company reported a permanent brown pigmentation of the iris and eyelid skin darkening, as well as redness, itchiness, and dry eye. So be forewarned, and take my advice: Consider safer, over-the-counter products that condition the lashes and provide moisture and shine.

Best Bets:
- RapidLash Eyelash Enhancing Serum
- Prevage Clinical Lash and Brow Enhancing Serum

eyebrows

Have you ever noticed how downturned eyes are often accompanied by downturned brows? This "pairing" can often age a face, but a well-groomed brow can be a subtle and effective way to enhance the eyes and give your face a more youthful expression. Like a picture frame enhances a painting, the brow draws attention to your eyes. Fuller, more natural, brows give a youthful look, and well-shaped brows open up your face, bringing out bone structure and giving eyes the illusion of being bigger than they actually are. Groomed brows add definition to eyes, and it should be considered a key step in your makeup regimen.

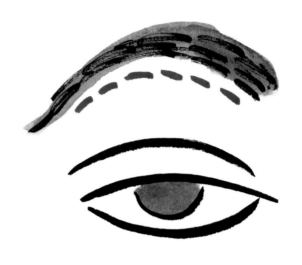

EYEBROW SHAPING

While many of us are adept at plucking our own brows, I highly recommend leaving this important grooming technique to a professional. Even if you ultimately want to be in control of your own brows, it is helpful to get started with a good professional. Once the shape is determined and set, you can easily maintain them, leaving less of a margin for haphazard plucking errors.

Droopy eyes can be changed by slightly arching the brows and extending them outward toward the temples (rather than having the tail curve down around the eye). The arch is an important part of the brow and should be a gradual and very gentle lift in line with the outer third of the eye.

The three standard techniques for shaping are tweezing, waxing, or threading (a salon method of hair removal with a thread). I say choose the method that hurts you the least! I prefer the speedy, at-home maintenance of tweezing, but the key takeaway here is that groomed, well-shaped brows are as crucial as eye makeup for a youthful appearance. Yes, taking care of your brows is that important.

BROW COLOR

Brows should never be lighter than your hair color. This dulls the face and gives a pale pallor to your complexion. The brows can be up to two shades darker than your hair, but, if you are using a pencil to fill in some missing brow hair, choose a shade lighter than your eyebrow hair color, otherwise it will look fake. Use short light strokes to fill in the gaps, and extend the outer ends just beyond the eyes. For a natural look, try dual-ended pencils that give you the choice of blending two colors together.

If you have patchy spots, another option is to use a brow powder. Just make sure the outer edges of the brows don't disappear. The tail of the brow is important, as it creates the youthful outward direction for the brow and gives some emphasis to the arch, but it should never be a hard, dark line. What about gray brows? Never ever pluck. Not even one stray. Hide gray strays either by dyeing at your local hair colorist, spa, or brow bar, or by using a brow marker. The felt-tip point lets you paint hairs precisely. You can also use a mascara-type "brow tint" to help camouflage all the grays (see below).

Best Bets:
- Benefit Brow Zing (eyebrow powder)
- Lancôme's Le Crayon Poudre Powder Pencil
- Milani Brow Tint Pen
- Paul and Joe's Eyebrow Pencil
- Paula Dorf Brow Tint
- TouchBack Brow Marker

the tail of the brow is important . . .

WHILE I MAY never reveal the identity of the fabulous Mrs. X, I am thrilled to spill the details of her eye makeup regimen. Learning it was a game changer for me, and not just because she taught me a quick and foolproof cosmetic routine for my eyes. More important, she taught me the power of the eyes, not only to seduce and flirt, but also to see and to learn, to embrace and to enhance, what we've been given. She was undaunted by crow's feet, unalarmed by wrinkles, undiscouraged by dark circles, and unflinching when it came to taking hold of her talents—in this case her eyes—and using them to the max. And now that you know her secret, why shouldn't you take advantage of it, too?

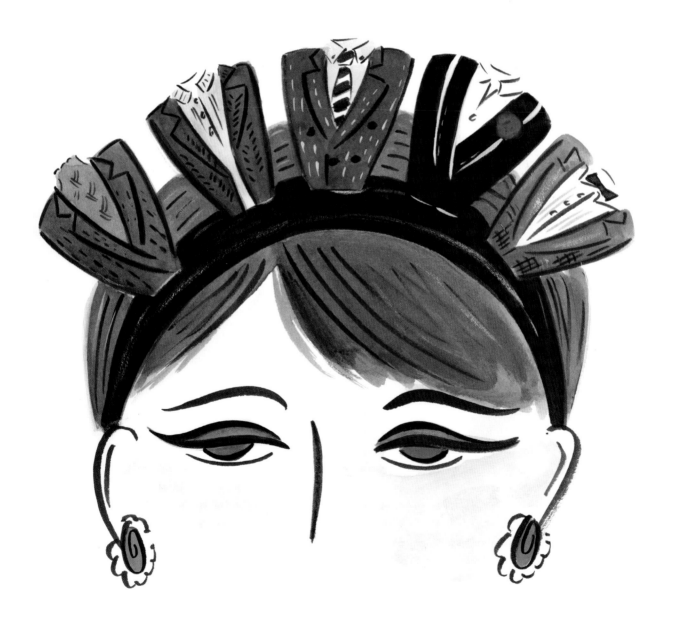

In a hurry but don't want naked lids? Skip the eye shadow routine and just use a natural shade primer on your lids, followed by a soft line of dark shadow along the upper and lower lashes. Or use a soft eye pencil in a dark shade, smudging it along the lash line in the same upward and outward direction.

If you are in a *real* hurry, mix primer and concealer to diffuse lines and wrinkles on your eyelids, then finish with mascara.

If you're like me and have very heavy brows with rogue hairs, here's a great trick to keeping them looking neat and groomed, which I learned from Kevyn Aucoin. Brush all your brow hairs up using a spoolie brush, then use brow scissors to cut the tips of the hairs that extend above the top of the brow. Tweezerman Brow Shaping Scissors are one of the best tools to use for this purpose. Their slanted, stainless-steel tip firmly grips hair at the base so that you can ease them out without pinching. They are light and easy to handle and come in bright colors, making them easy to find in your makeup bag. Another added bonus: Your Tweezerman comes with a lifetime guarantee and free sharpening.

MASCARA WARS

A little inside "dirt" is always fun to know. L'Oreal Paris and CoverGirl are long-time rivals in many cosmetics areas, but none so competitively as mascara. L'Oreal has been the all-time leader in the category for well over twenty years, and here is how they did it. They had a particular gentleman in their product development department who invented all their mascara brushes and developed winner after winner that was immediately patented so that competitors could not copy or imitate these designs (or "masterpieces," in the world of cosmetics). This mascara master would come to meetings that I attended with a briefcase full of his latest designs and pull out a mirror and demonstrate on his *own* lashes the benefit of each new brush he had invented. Many cosmetics companies tried to invent competitive products, but L'Oreal held the leading edge—and the patents—on the designs, thereby blocking the competition. That is, until CoverGirl invented the big, orange, molded plastic brush which became an overnight winner with CoverGirl LashBlast, breaking the L'Oreal winning streak and starting the legendary "Mascara Wars." And they are still duking it out today, with every new mascara launch.

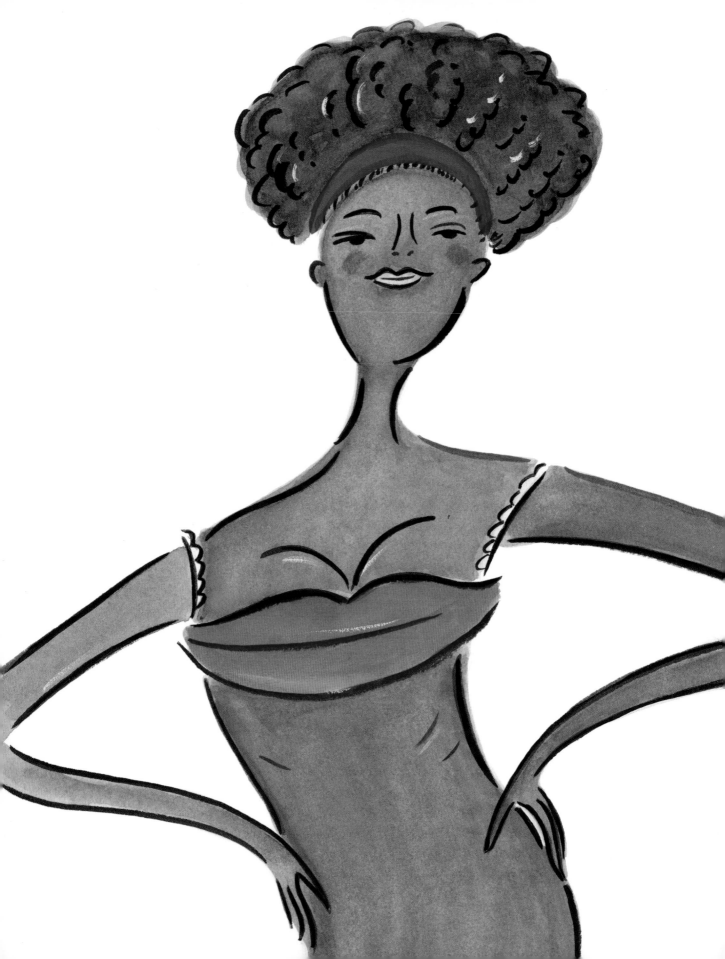

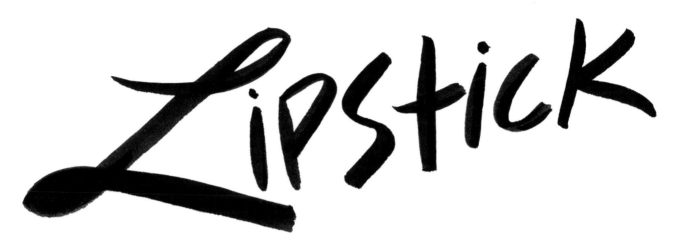

CHAPTER NINE

Lipstick

the magic bullet

IT'S TIME TO GET RID OF THOSE STICKY, TACKY, HIGH-SHINE, LACQUERED TUBES. SIMPLY PUT: TOSS THE GLOSS.

If foundation is the perfect white T-shirt of your cosmetic bag, then lipstick is the push-up bra, giving you added sex appeal, and radiating sophistication and confidence. But let me be clear: I'm talking lipstick, not lip gloss.

If you're one of the millions of women who've hit fifty and think gloss is the answer to fabulous lips, boy am I glad that we've found each other. If you have those nasty little vertical demon lines above your upper lip, you can't use it anymore. Sorry. The same thing goes for all dark lipsticks. See also: red lipstick. Unless you have rich dark skin or plump lineless lips, toss those deep shades. They may seem sexy and sophisticated in the tube, but dark shades creep into those lines around your mouth and nothing ages you more than "bleeding" lipstick. I know this seems counterintuitive. You're embracing your sexuality, your confidence, and your inner goddess, and you have to renounce

It's time to take those sticky, tacky, lacquered tubes of high gloss and shine and toss them out!

the very makeup item that symbolizes all of that. I feel your pain. I remember how great that little black dress looked on my thirtieth birthday, wearing nothing else but my red lips. I remember "Cherries in the Snow" and "Fire and Ice" and that rush of sexual confidence that came from swiping a bit of red on my lips before a date with Mr. Guess Who.

But if you want to look good now, wearing red lipstick will kill your game. It looks like you're trying too hard—there are other ways to exude sex appeal. BUT—that doesn't mean we have to forget about our mouths and call it a day. Au contraire . . .

Neutral is the new name of the game. The right shade of neutral can compensate and draw attention away from our less-attractive features, while red lipstick or very dark shades can emphasize dark circles under the eyes and make your lips look thin. Whether it's a silky taupe, creamy caramel, nude pink, dusty fawn, or light chocolate, it's time to embrace neutral lipstick and learn how to work our most feminine feature in a different way.

It all goes back to my twelve-year-old memory of Tangee. Remember that lipstick? It was orange in the stick, but, as you put it on, your mouth was magically transformed into the most perfect shade of "lip"—not orange at all, but a rosy, natural shade that somehow gave my adolescent lips a luscious, smooth, naturally-tinted fullness that transported me into the world of

i was hooked . . .

sophisticated women. I was hooked, and so was every boy on my street—I kissed them all that summer. This was the beginning of my love affair with subtle naked lip shades.

Many of us will remember when it was nearly impossible to find a good neutral shade. That's why, as I mentioned in the opening of the book, I created The Nakeds and The Naughty Nakeds when I was president of Ultima II. Since I am the quintessential au naturel "babe" at heart, I wanted to create a group of neutral lip colors that were good for women of all ethnicities, a group of colors that spoke up for our deepest beauty instincts, a group of colors that shouted, "This is who we are!" Now more than ever, with the confidence and wisdom of experience and the arsenal of beauty info I'll supply, we are going to enjoy looking like ourselves, only better. To loosely paraphrase Gloria Steinem, "This is what 50, 60, 70, 80, 90 looks like, and it's pretty damn good."

This chapter is about the seduction of that magic shade range, and how your lips can be just as powerful, compelling, and sexy with neutrals as they were with bright reds and pinks. Getting the lips right can give the entire face a more youthful appearance. After all, at a time of life when you have a lot to say, why not call some extra attention to your mouth.

drawing the line with lip shaping

Let's start with an indispensible tool—lip liner—and learn how to build a fabulous mouth. Personally, I am an ardent and faithful devotee of lip pencils. I would even choose one over straight-up lipstick, because with a good lip pencil I can create (draw) the mouth I want, and then add lip balm to make them look moist and plump. Be sure to select a neutral matte pencil (wood-clenched is best, where the color is imbedded in the wood, just like in a lead pencil), and choose a shade that's close to your natural lip color.

Sharpen the pencil (the line must be very thin and fine). Use the pencil to draw a line just above the outside edge of your natural lip line. If you can't see your lip line any more (as we age, many of us lose our lips or our lips become very thin), get out some old pictures of yourself that you like, and, with the help of a magnifying mirror, try to imitate the natural line of the mouth you once had. This requires practice, so don't get frustrated if your lips aren't perfect right away.

If your lip line has faded, follow this simple ten-step process to redefine your lips. Practice makes perfect!

1 Place your index finger vertically under one of your nostrils (right nostril with right hand, left with left hand), with your fingertip resting just beneath the nostril opening.

2 With the lip liner pencil, place one dot on the upper lip area aligning the dot on the inside edge of your finger next to the first joint of your finger.

3 Repeat with the other hand and nostril. Draw a short vertical line in the middle of the two dots on the upper lip (it should be a bit shorter than the height of the two dots).

4 Next, starting on one side of your mouth, draw a line from the outside corner of your mouth, up to the dot on your upper lip area.

5 Repeat on the other side.

6 Draw a diagonal line down from each dot to the top of a short vertical line in the middle of the dots. This forms the peaks of the upper lip.

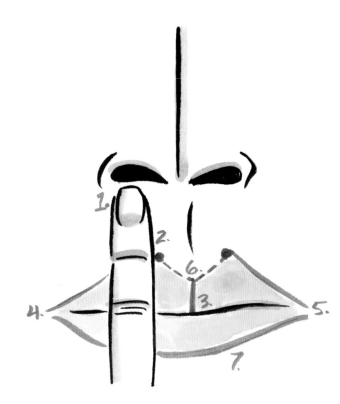

7 Line the outside of the lower lips, since it is most often the upper lip that disappears.

8 Once you like what you see, fill in the lips with the lip liner and take a picture with your phone. (When I am unsure about a piece of makeup I've used—or even a new hairstyle—I always take a picture. It's better than looking in the mirror where one can lose perspective.)

9 Last, apply your lipstick. Start in the middle of your lips to avoid color clumping at the corners of the mouth. I usually just swipe it on hurriedly from the tube, but, when I really want to look good, I go the extra distance and use a lip brush. (See sidebar for information on lip brushes.)

And that's it! Just make sure that the lip line you created is lightly covered with lip color, as is the rest of your mouth. You want to avoid the look of a heavy lip liner at all costs.

HERE ARE A FEW OF MY FAVORITE LINERS:
- Chanel Precision Lip Definer in Nude (a creamy, mauvey, midtone brown liner that comes with its own sharpener)
- L'Oreal Colour Riche Lip Liner in Au Naturale and Forever Rose (neutral enough to work with many shades in the neutral palette)
- MAC Cosmetics Lip Pencil in Spice or Stripdown (looks great on everybody and blends well with virtually any shade of neutral)

inside the lines

Now that you've mastered the art of lining your lips, it's time to focus on the finishing touch: lipstick. Depending on your lip shape and condition, sometimes lipstick is all you need. But now that traditional darks most likely no longer do it, how do we determine the best color for our skin tone and coloring? And what about texture and wear? Like most cosmetics, the "choice effect" with lipsticks can leave us paralyzed when it comes to choosing the appropriate products. There are just too many to select from. Often, we default to our tried-and-true colors and brands, but, as our skin color changes through the years, these colors and styles may no longer suit our needs. Additionally, it's important to know the inside scoop on the labels and formulas before investing in lip products. Remember how I mentioned before that makeup and skincare formulas for the large cosmetic corporations are most often developed in a central research and development laboratory that services all divisions or brands in the corporation? The same applies here. So be aware of the following: A few years ago, a lipstick breakthrough formula would have first been applied to the most upscale brand of all the divisions. The theory behind this was that a brand like Lancôme (sold at department stores) was the most prestigious and fashion-forward brand, so Lancôme might get the technology first, and then, for example, L'Oreal Paris (sold in drugstores) might utilize the same technology some period of time after that. The cosmetic industry called this the "trickle down" effect. In other words, the customers who shopped for high-end brands were thought to be the most fashion-forward, and they bought their products in department stores. By selling these "high-end" brands at department stores, companies ensured their prestige status. Later in the shopping cycle, the wisdom went, that style preference would "trickle down" to the less fashionable drugstore shoppers. But consumer behaviors changed, as did the market, and cosmetics corporations soon discovered that time-starved women (often raising a family and holding down a job at the same time) began cross-shopping in drugstores and anywhere else she could meet her beauty and shopping needs, thereby diluting the high-end market. Today, corporations are more likely to give new lipstick formulas to their lower-end brands first! And by the way, the lower-end brands have stepped up their fashion quotient dramatically over the last decade. The lesson: Don't be fooled by fancy packaging and shade names—you may very well find the same formula in less expensive brands. So check at CVS first!

LIPSTICK SHADE

Finding the right lip color can be tricky, so use the following guide to help you select the neutral color family that will look most flattering:

Fair or Pale Skin Tones

Look for neutrals with soft pinks, pale peaches, and apricot undertones and avoid beige lipstick that can wash you out.

Here are your **Best Bets:**
- Jemma Kidd's Peggy
- NARS Dolce Vita, Barbarella
- Revlon Super Lustrous Lipstick in Demure
- Rimmel London Moisture Renew Lip Colour in Dreamy

Golden Skin Tones

Go for creamy, caramel, and clay-toned nudes and warm beiges. If your skin is deeper, look for midtone beige, like mocha and rich latte. Avoid anything cool in undertone, like mauve.

Consider these **Best Bets:**
- Chanel Rouge Coco Shine in Canotier
- Dior Rouge Dior Lip Color in Angelique Beige
- L'Oreal Paris Colour Riche Lip Color in Gilded Pink
- Maybelline Color Sensational Lip Color in Warm Me Up

Olive Skin Tones

If your skin is deeper than golden, but not dark, look for midtone beiges like mocha and rich latte. Avoid anything cool in undertone, like mauve. The Tom Ford recommendation below hits the right amount of beige without going too dark.

Best Bets:
- Maybelline's Color Sensational Lipcolor in Totally Toffee
- Nuance Salma Hayek Color Vibrance Lipstick in Nude
- Sonia Kashuk Satin Luxe Lipcolor with SPF 16 in Barely Nude
- Tom Ford Lip Color in Sable Smoke

Dark Skin Tones

Opt for chocolate tones, such as rich golden-browns like coffee, and avoid anything remotely orange as it makes skin look drab.

Best Bets:

- CoverGirl LipPerfection Lipcolor in Delish (a nice deep beige)
- CoverGirl Queen Collection Lipcolor in Coffee Break
- Laura Mercier Crème Lip Colour in Espresso and Brown Plum
- Wet 'N Wild Mega Shield Lip Color SPF 15 in Bare-ly Legal

LIPSTICK TEXTURE

Now let's discuss texture, since the right texture choice is the make-or-break factor on your mouth. The three most common choices are matte, frost or shimmers, and creamy/shine. Here's the lowdown on the pros and cons of each:

Matte

Want to look really old? No? Then run away from this pasty, drying look as fast as you can.

Frost

Want to look really cheap? No? Then if you move to shimmer, make it very subtle, or prepare to resemble Blanche from *The Golden Girls*.

Creamy/Shine

Ding, ding, ding! You've found the winner! Rich, moist-looking lips that make your mouth look full and soft, satiny and youthful. Forget about high gloss, metallics, and glitter—save those for costume parties only.

Best Bets worth considering:

- CoverGirl LipPerfect Lipcolor in Darling, Delish, and Sultry
- Dolce and Gabbana Classic Cream Lipstick in Petal, Mandorla, and Cashmere
- Maybelline New York Color Sensational Lip Color in Born With It, Nearly There, and Totally Toffee
- N.Y.C. Ultra Moist Lipwear in Petal, Café, and Mocha

Now that you've narrowed your choices down to shade and texture, here are a few insider tips to help your lip color look even better:

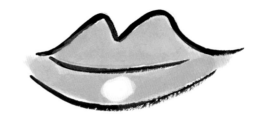

- For a fuller mouth, dab the slightest bit of Vaseline or shiny moisturizing lip balm (don't buy lip gloss) on the middle of the lower lip.

- For a fuller upper-lip look, dot highlighter between the peaks of the lips (the Cupid's bow).

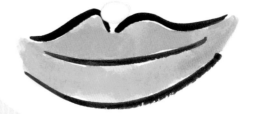

- When choosing between two colors, opt for the lighter one. Pale colors make lips look fuller.

- For a longer-lasting color, avoid using matte lipsticks and use instead a lip stain before applying lipstick.

- For a longer-lasting color, apply lipstick straight from the tube, blot with a tissue and apply the lipstick again. The second swipe will also add shine and coverage

- Before using your lip liner, cover your lips with foundation, concealer, or primer—this will also help the color last.

- To avoid hard edges, roll the tip of your lip liner around on the palm of your hand before using.

- If you've made a mistake and your lips are too dark, gently blend in some foundation or concealer to lighten them.

- Test lip color in the store on your fingertip—not the side of your hand!—as that is closest to your natural lip shade.

ALL DAY LIPSTICKS

No one knows more about the birth of this category than I do since it was invented by my team at Revlon's Ultima II when I was president. The first product entry in the market was called LipSexxxy. This category caused a minor sensation in the marketplace, especially with working women, who wanted to have lipstick that they didn't have to apply during the day, that didn't come off on drinking glasses, and that didn't come off on fabric. The lipsticks flew off the store shelves and our competitors rushed to copy us. The tradeoff compared to regular lipsticks on the market was that they were rather dry on the lips. Since then, several companies, including Revlon, have come up with liquid lipsticks that are available in intense pigments with long-lasting polymers and moisturizing ingredients like vitamin E and argan oil to keep lips hydrated.

Consider these **Best Bets:**

- e.l.f. Essential Luscious Liquid Lipstick in Bark
- Hourglass Opaque Rouge Liquid Lipstick in Canvas
- Revlon ColorStay Ultimate Liquid Lipstick in Perfect Peony
- Yves Saint Laurent Rouge Pur Couture Vernis à Lèvres Glossy Stain in Beige Aquarelle

And while we're on the subject of hydration, one of the best sources for great-looking, super-hydrated lips without having to resort to lip gloss is tinted lip balm. Not only do they come in lip-enhancing natural shades that soothe and condition, but some also come with a sun protection factor.

Try these **Best Bets:**

- Burt's Bees Tinted Lip Balm in Caramel Daisy
- Clinique Chubby Sticks Moisturizing Lip Color Balm in Curvy Candy
- Maybelline New York Baby Lips Moisturizing Lip Balm in Peach Kiss

lip rehab

Our lips aren't always fit for color. In fact, sometimes they need serious intervention before color even comes in to the picture. Weather, neglect, age, even illness can wreak havoc on our soft-skinned kissers.

If your lips look anything like mine have looked on occasion—cracked, wrinkled, chapped—they need a good stint of therapy. Sometimes, they require a little help to spring back to the sexy little place they once held on your face. Here's what to do:

EXFOLIATE

Yes, you can—and should—exfoliate your lips. They, too, get dead-skin buildup. Getting rid of all the dead cells will make your lips look smoother and plumper and help foster new cell turnover. If they're chapped, a quick, soothing, and effective at-home remedy for ridding your lips of the flaky bits of skin you're so tempted to chew off is to hold a warm, wet washcloth (with texture) against them for a couple of minutes, then rub the washcloth (or a soft toothbrush) in a circular motion to gently slough off the moistened dead skin. Follow up by coating them with a good lip balm with SPF. I suggest avoiding commercial lip plumpers, as they irritate the skin for none to minimal results. Instead, just keep lips hydrated. And NEVER lick your lips to moisten them, especially in windy conditions! Though it may alleviate dryness in the moment, it's like drinking saltwater when you're thirsty: It

just dries them out further. There are a number of good lip balms and exfoliants on the market. Some **Best Bets:**

- Aquaphor Lip Repair and Protect SPF 30
- Bliss Fabulips Sugar Lip Scrub
- Fresh Sugar Lip Polish
- Neutrogena Instant Lip Remedy

It's also worth noting that good old-fashioned Carmex does the trick, as does Vaseline—both excellent agents for dry lips. We often get so used to using a lip balm when our lips are chapped that when we stop using it we have the sensation that our lips have dried out. After several days of using lip balm, it's better to ease off and get back to our regular moisturizing lipstick.

Now, let's "chew the fat" about more permanent solutions for problems like disappearing lips and those nasty vertical lines that plague our upper lips.

LIP INJECTIONS

Lips gone entirely? In this case, if your budget can afford it, I would opt for help from a good dermatologist. The operative words here are "good" (someone with proven skills on this part of the face) and "budget" (it's expensive). You certainly don't want to end up with "trout pouts" like Lisa Rinna (she just had hers corrected, at great expense) or Goldie Hawn in *The First Wives Club*. You need a reputable expert who will build up your mouth gradually, using Restylane or Juvaderm (both hyluronic acids). This is a very precarious undertaking, one that can easily go awry in the hands of a doctor who lacks experience or a good eye. You can end up with much-too-much (the Angelina Jolie look on steroids) or not enough (a big waste of your money). Dr. Gervaise Gerstner, a well-known board-certified New York dermatologist and expert in the world of fillers, has saved many faces by injecting lips that have all but disappeared.

When is it worth considering this procedure? When the upper lip has rolled inward and is disproportionate to the lower lip. Dr. Gerstner's guideline for the "ideal size ratio of lips should be 1/3 top lip versus 2/3 bottom lip." She adds that patients should know that "lip filler doesn't last as long as filler lasts in other areas of the face,

as we use the lips so much." What does she use to battle the tiny little lines above the lip that cosmetics have a difficult time camouflaging? She favors a filler called Belotero.

Warning: Lip injections in the wrong hands are very obvious. An over-inflated mouth, and the little curl or roll back on the edge of the lips, is the dead giveaway. It has ruined the face of many a starlet, celebrity, and average Joe, so buyer beware. If your lips are merely thin, I would simply employ the less-permanent cosmetic remedies outlined above. As with any cosmetic surgery, there are downsides to lip injections:

- It hurts (while it's being injected)

- It's temporary (lasts three to six months)

- It will cost $500–$975 (the latter when two tubes of filler are used)

- You could end up with bruises that take days to go away

WRINKLE REMOVERS

Lip wrinkles are real demons. Once you notice these little vertical lines begin to appear along your upper lip line, they seem to turn into grooves and craters overnight! That said, I truly believe that they come from a life well-lived—a lot of smiling, talking with emotion, eating good food, drinking good wine, and generally lots of fun. But we are not going to let them have their way with us, are we? Here's what can be done.

Start by using moisturizers around the lips. Extra moisture can temporarily plump the skin and make the lines much less noticeable. Retin A and Renova work quite effectively in areas prone to wrinkles, like the eye and mouth area, but they are prescription-only and take several weeks to months to notice a softening of the lines.

Deeper lines can best be addressed by fractional lasers, dermabrasion, chemical peels, and fillers (Restylane and Juvaderm), Botox (the latter should be used with great care as there are many downsides, including drooping mouth and impaired speech), and Dr. Gerstner's favorite for this part of the face, too—Belotero. My advice? Avoid Botox on this area of the face, and go with one of the other technological advances I've mentioned instead—but bring your wallet. Like fillers for the lips, it is an expensive proposition ($500–$800). I have a friend who ended up in the hands of the wrong dermatologist when she was searching for a solution to her deepening lines above her mouth. She looked like she had an enlarged monkey mouth by the time he got through with her. He injected too much filler, and it took her six months to start looking halfway "normal" again. Lasers and microdermabrasion (for less severe lines) can be very effective, but be prepared for downtime and discomfort. I have another friend who opted for a very strong laser solution, and she was out of commission for over two weeks—a severe burn, painkillers, face bandages, peeling skin, and a Michael Jackson–type mask covering nose to chin. But the outcome, in her words, was "spectacular," and she would do it again if necessary. The result was that good. But it, too, is costly ($2,500).

Ultimately, your doctor will determine which laser procedure, chemical solution, or filler is appropriate—as will your budget and your tolerance for discomfort. I can't stress enough how important it is to make sure you go with a skilled doctor who has lots of experience and a good eye. Make no mistake, just as makeup is an art that requires trial and error to get it right, so are fillers and lasers. So choosing a doctor, in this case, becomes more than looking for a good medical technician, it is looking for an artistic eye and hand.

How do you identify a good dermatologist? Here are a few clues:

- Make sure the dermatologist is board-certified (check the American Academy of Dermatology: www.aad.org). This is a must and should be identified by the online presence of the doctor.

- Look for a dermatologist that practices primarily in the area of cosmetology; he or she will have much more experience than a general dermatologist. (The doctor's website should give you this information.)

- Arrange a consultation with the doctor and ask to see before-and-after photos of the procedure you are interested in pursuing.

- Get recommendations from friends who've had natural-looking procedures done.

I STARTED THIS chapter by saying that lipstick is the pushup bra of your makeup bag. There is nothing better to give your face a sexy boost than a great-looking lipstick that's been wisely chosen and well applied. Just like the Victoria's Secret catalogue says, there's "one for every moment and mood." But buyer beware in your quest for sexy smackers. Just as breast implants in the wrong hands can make your chest look like you are wearing water balloons, lip fillers can make you resemble a duck more than a duchess. Instead, read my lips: Your magic bullet is a creamy natural lipstick, outlined with an evenhanded lip liner, and carried with the confidence of a beautiful woman. (That would be you.)

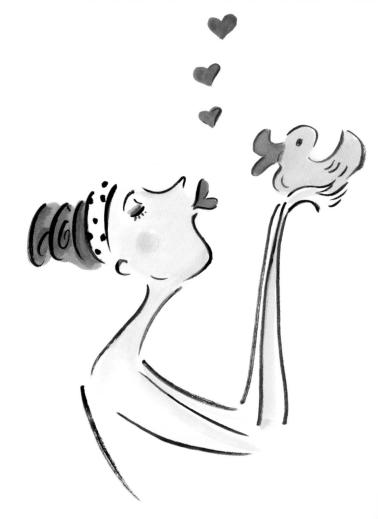

Some might consider lip brushes superfluous. Not so—just ask any good makeup artist. They have staying power worthy of investment. A mouthful of moist lipstick applied with a lip brush trumps the tube anytime for last and beauty—just try it. I love the Tom Ford Lip Brush #21 because it's taut enough to pick up a good amount of lip color from the tube but gentle on the lips and flexible enough to spread the color easily. That said, Tom Ford is a luxury beauty splurge, and you may want to try something less pricey. For that I suggest the following:

- Kevyn Aucoin Retractable Lip Brush—great for the purse and foolproof precision

- MAC #306 Lip Brush has lots of color pickup and is great for blending

- Scott Barnes Retractable Lip Brush—great for not having a mess in your cosmetic pouch

Here's a surprising ally in the quest for younger-looking lips: A good cosmetic dentist specializing in veneers.

Veneers can be contoured or built out to widen the lip's arch and increase lip support, resulting in a permanently plumped-up looking mouth. But like most cosmetic procedures, it is a pricey remedy: Veneers can cost up to $1,500 per tooth!

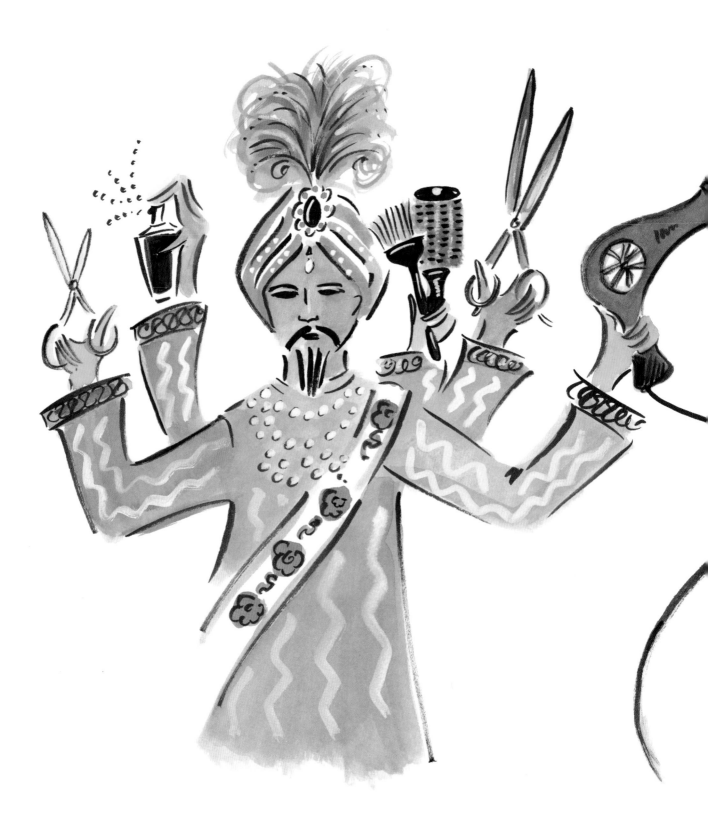

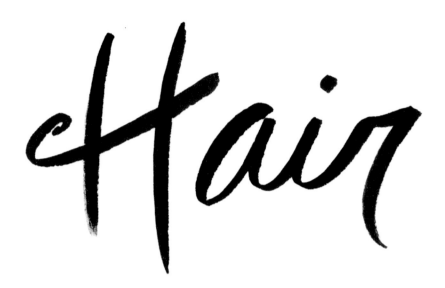

CHAPTER TEN

Hair

hair dos and hair don'ts

FIRST THINGS FIRST: ALL HAIR, YOURS AND MINE INCLUDED, SHOULD LOOK EFFORTLESS. YOU DON'T WANT YOUR HAIR TO BE SO OVER THE TOP THAT IT LOOKS LIKE IT'S HEADED TO A RED-CARPET RENDEZVOUS WITHOUT YOU.

At our age, casual, natural elegance is what we're going for—not helmet heads, shoe-polish mops, frosted frizzies, teased tresses, or highlight ODs. If you recognize your own hair in this paragraph, you may need a good hair guru to come between you and your current coiffure.

The truth is, unlike lipstick or eyeliner, hair is the only cosmetic you can't simply wipe off, so isn't it worth getting

147

it right? Because getting it wrong can be a major beauty disaster. You can throw out an impulse purchase, or wipe off a frosted lipstick, but you can't just shampoo a cure into a bad coif—a few wrong moves with the scissors and you've got shear disaster. A cut too layered, too short, or too long can exaggerate the lines in your face and make your whole body seem out of proportion. And the wrong color can give you the Morticia Addams look, aging you instantly.

The truth is, unlike lipstick or eyeliner, hair is the only cosmetic you can't simply wipe off, so isn't it worth getting it right?

When it comes to women of a certain age, there are so many bad hair dos, and even more hair don'ts, that it's easy to get confused. For instance, you probably recognize some of these "rules" about hairstyles after fifty:

- "You shouldn't wear long hair."

- "You shouldn't wear bangs."

- "Get rid of the dark hair."

- "Add blond highlights to cover the gray strands."

But I don't believe in those rules, and neither do the famous hair masters I consulted. Take, for example, hairdresser Gad Cohen, who knows everything about haircuts and makeup (see www.gadcohen.com). He's styled great beauties from Jaclyn Smith to Jane Seymour. Or Louis Licari, Manhattan's go-to color genius and *Today Show* regular. (I've seen Ellen Barkin and Susan Sarandon in his Fifth Avenue habitat.)

Louis says, "The most common faux pas I see is when a woman says, 'I am this number of years old, so now I have to have lighter hair.'" And Gad says: "When you have good quality hair and the silhouette is right, you can have any kind of hair—including long hair. The right haircut is better than the scalpel."

Louis adds, "Hair is the best kind of makeup for the face." The right shade can enhance skin tone, complement a well-composed cosmetic palate, and, yes, even make you look more youthful.

This chapter will focus on how to determine the right cut and color that works best for you, and how to work with your hairdresser and colorist to help them make you look like yourself, only better.

I will also shed some guiding light on how to determine the right length for your hair, how to achieve the most realistic color, and when you can get away with doing color at home. And while I'm at it, I'll also explain why you should never cross your legs at the beauty salon, along with why lace is good for thinning hair. First, let's start with an important . . .

Don't look back! Don't attempt to freeze-frame the cut or color of your past. After years of time and sun exposure, your skin color has changed. That means your hair must change, too, in order to complement your face. As our faces morph, so must our hair.

But where do you look for inspiration? Certainly, models and celebrities have been setting hairstyle trends for decades. Remember Julie Christie's bob, Mia Farrow's pixie cut, Diana Ross's afro, and Farrah Faucet's feathered layers—not to mention Jennifer Aniston's "Rachel,"

which remains the most requested cut in history? But be forewarned: What you see isn't always what you get. Often, the pumped-up tresses you see on models and actresses in fashion magazines are not altogether real. I speak from experience when I tell you that many of those women are wearing wigs, hairpieces, hair extensions, or some combination of the above.

Case in point: I once had a photo shoot with a major pop music diva. Her iconic beauty look had a lot to do with her very large and thick head of hair, so of course we had brought along one of the best and most celebrated hairdressers in the world to work with her. But she declined his services, explaining that she worked exclusively with one hair artist who arrived glued to her hip, along with a huge suitcase of unknown contents.

"Hair is the best kind of makeup for the face."

Our hairdresser could not have been more gracious. He expressed his regrets about having missed the opportunity to work with the celebrity, and she seemed genuinely remorseful. But those of us who watched her getting ready for the camera learned that under that thick crown of hair and in that hairdresser's suitcase, a big dark secret lurked: She was almost bald! Her signature tresses, the ones that inspired a huge amount of hair envy and imitation and defined her physical presence, were in fact a series of wigs and hairpieces! When I saw her without the fakes, it took my breath away. That, of course, was why the chanteuse wanted no one except her own hairdresser—more accurately, her own wig master—within blow-dry distance.

Get a color that complements your skin tone, a cut that complements your body type, and don't get obsessed with what you can't have.

The lesson here? Don't be influenced by trumped-up celebrity styles. Find your own style that works with the hair you have, not the seemingly voluminous hair you see on celebrities of a certain age, because we now know that much of the time their hair isn't real. Get a color that complements your skin tone, a cut that complements your body type, and don't get obsessed with what you can't have—especially since a quick glimpse in the mirror should prove you've likely got plenty to work with. Let's start with the essentials.

it's all about the cut

Here's the truth: A good haircut cannot—and should not—be underestimated. Back in the day (let's say the '50s and '60s) when hair salons were called "beauty parlors," you got a "hairdo." Your "beautician" set your hair in pincurls or rollers, put you under a dryer, and then "teased your hair" and "combed you out." An asphyxiating application of ozone-destroying hairspray was usually involved. Young women spent a lot of time worrying how they'd manage to look good after they got married. No, they weren't worried about "letting themselves go," they were trying to figure out how they'd manage their hair if they couldn't climb into bed each night with a helmet of pink rollers.

Enter the swinging '60s, when Vidal Sassoon changed the world with a pair of scissors. Though there aren't many people still

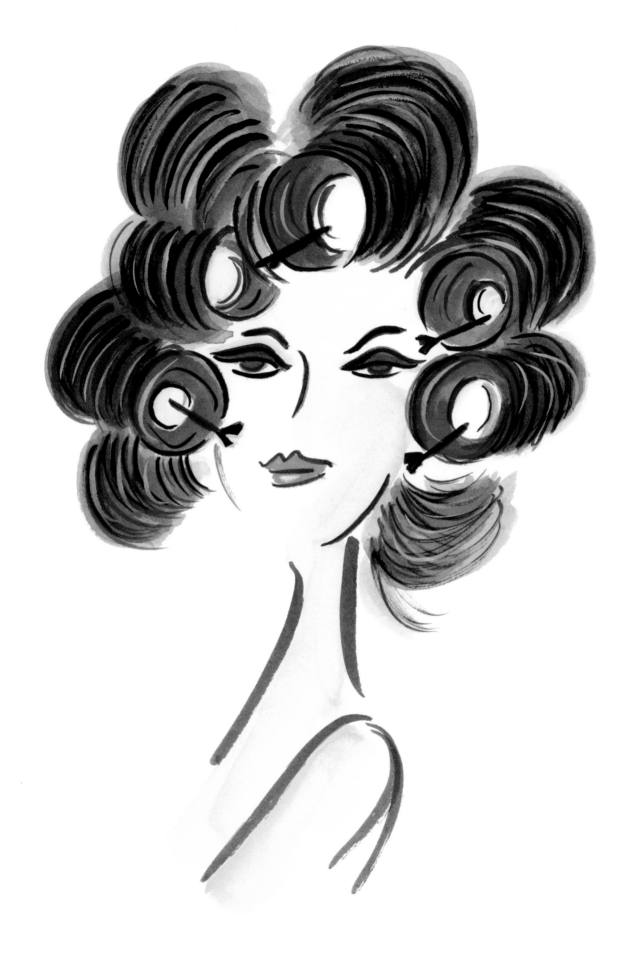

sporting the geometric cut he made famous, we're all benefitting from his revolutionary notion of ready-to-wear hair that required no rollers, hairdryers, or hairspray—but this assumes a lot of skill from the person doing the cutting.

"Length and volume should be dictated by your height and your weight—your shape."

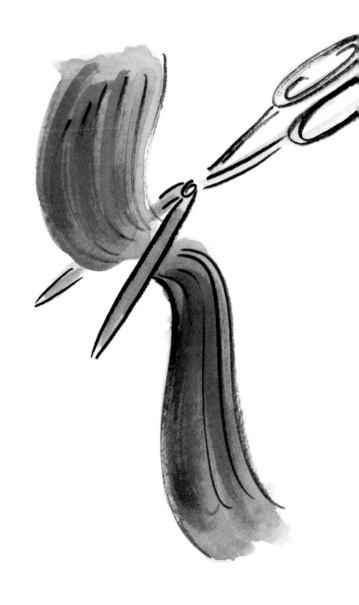

Here's the trick to getting a good haircut: proportion and balance. Hair should relate to the silhouette of your body. Gad says, "Length and volume should be dictated by your height and your weight—your shape."

His general rule of thumb: The larger and taller the body, the bigger the hair can be. If you're lean, your hair most likely will benefit from being the same: sleek and close to the head. If you're curvy, as a general rule, you need longer, fuller hair so your head doesn't look too small in contrast to your body. If you're shorter, you'll want a cut that gives height at the crown. The whole image must be taken into account, including your natural neckline and jewelry choices. For example, if you have a short neck, wear minimal jewelry. Keep earrings and necklaces simple and small and avoid big collars on blouses, sweaters and coats. Hair should be layered gently around your face.

Most women over fifty look best if they choose a length somewhere between the chin and just grazing the shoulder, with a cut that adds volume. And Gad says, "Use bangs instead of Botox." He suggests hair looks best at this stage of life with soft, imperceptible layers that are cut on the bias—that is, not in choppy layers, which are too artificial looking, unflattering, and dated.

Black women have a unique elasticity to their hair, which can be styled and worn close and cropped tightly to the head or stretched out for a longer look. Gad uses the shape of the head to determine the shape of the cut. Michelle Obama and Oprah Winfrey both wear longer hair that's been chemically relaxed, to great effect. As an alternative to that look and length, pull the hair back with a band and allow the hair behind it—on the crown and sides—to go unrelaxed and free. "That's a modern, totally empowering look," that Gad says is "wearing your essence." And if it works with the overall silhouette, shorter hair can look great on black women because they often have beautifully shaped heads and wrinkle-free skin.

the basics of color

"The main purpose of hair color is to complement and give contrast to your skin color so your facial features will come alive and you look fresh, younger, and vital," Louis Licari says. "If you have to wear more makeup to make a new hair color look right, you picked the wrong color."

So how do you get the right color if you're doing it at home? Louis says that all the big-brand, at-home DIY products are pretty good. What really matters is the shade you pick. And he warns, be careful. "Hair color is a bit like drugs. It's easy to become addicted, and a little goes a long way."

One great side benefit of using color on your hair is that it looks thicker. Individual hairs are covered with microscopic scales, like fish scales, and when you dye or bleach the hair, the scales open and never lay flat as they did before the chemicals were applied. Opened hair cuticles can become three times their usual size, but you will sacrifice shine and smoothness.

When it comes to making your color choice, the hardest person to get a good, objective opinion from is the one with the most at stake: you. Most of us view ourselves through a mental scrim that does for us what Vaseline or gauze on the camera lens did for movie stars back in the day—everything looks a bit blurry and not quite in focus: better, kinder, but not very precise and true. That's where smartphones come in. The pictures you can take on a cell phone are not always flattering (they don't call them kindphones), but you can really see what's right or wrong. So be brave! Click and delete later.

Asking a trusted friend for advice is also helpful, but only if you know she's going to be completely frank with you. (This is a much bigger decision than what color to paint the living room walls. Not everyone gets to see your living room.) Better yet, leave it to a professional whose aesthetic you trust. In the world of beauty salons, word of mouth can't be beat. Ask friends, acquaintances, or coworkers whose hair you admire for the name of the person who colors her hair. Admittedly, sometimes it's a bit tricky to ask someone you're not close to for this information, so resort to stealth compliments, and perhaps they'll fess up.

For salons in your vicinity, you can also refer to Yelp.com for business reviews from real customers. Often, stylists within these salons will be lauded (or criticized) for their area of expertise. You'll discover quickly whether there's a color connoisseur in your neighborhood or a shade charlatan leaving a trail of brassy tresses in his wake. As with any big change you embark upon—whether it's finding a painter for your living room or a colorist for your hair—always get a consultation and estimate before making a color commitment. Most experienced stylists will certainly accommodate your request to get an initial (free) consultation before you schedule an appointment with them. If not, take this as a bad sign! Short of that consultation, here are some color tips from Louis, based on skin tone, worth heeding:

VERY FAIR SKIN

Just about any color looks good unless you go to extremes. It's best to avoid deep browns and black (remember Morticia?). You want to avoid that witchy look. Also, pale skin is prone to ruddiness, and dark hair will only draw attention to redness in your undertones. Instead, choose blond, strawberry blond, and light brunette.

RUDDY SKIN

Avoid bright, red hair color; however, auburn would be a good choice, along with medium brown and golden brown.

CREAMY SKIN

Choose medium red tones, along with light browns and golden blonds. Avoid the harshness of dark browns and blacks.

MEDIUM TO OLIVE SKIN

Deep shades like mahogany will warm up your skin tone, but it's best to avoid red or copper tones, which can make your skin look sallow or orange—and avoid becoming blond. Make your hair too light and it can look like gray hair and drain color from your skin. Make it too dark and it can become monochromatic and shout, "I'm a wig."

DARK OR BLACK SKIN

At one time, African-American women thought their only color option was a semipermanent color to cover the gray, adding a tinge of red or going darker. "I think once hairpieces, extensions, and weaves became popular, Black women found a lot of other possibilities and became very creative with their hair, and they certainly started thinking in terms of different colors," Louis says.

And like fair skin, it works with a large range of colors. If you have golden undertones in your skin, try weaving caramel or cinnamon highlights around your face and through the ends, where the sun would hit. If you are more adventurous, you can even go blond (check out Rihanna in one of her hair color transformations, or Beyonce's blondish hues). Take care when mixing color with other chemical products like relaxants, and be aware that Black hair absorbs color much more quickly than Caucasian hair.

No matter what color your skin is, if you'd like to avoid the saturated, monochrome shoe-polish look that a bad dye job can bring, select a translucent color—not like an opaque paint, but rather more like a varnish, where each hair takes on a different tone. Louis says, "Tell your colorist, 'I'm a brunette. I'm happy as a brunette. But I don't want to look harsh. I want to see nuances in my hair. I would like to have most of my gray hair covered, but, if a strand or two shows through, that's all right.'" He explains, "This approach helps ensure your hair won't be too dark—and if it's too light, the colorist can always add color."

If you want a variegated look, you can put in highlights. But if there is too much contrast between the dark hair and the highlights, you'll look like an old-fashioned "frosty," which will make you look older and tacky. "Highlights shouldn't be too perfect or too bold," Louis says. "Perfect is imperfection." (Remember what I said in Chapter 2, about the concept of *Wabi-Sabi?* If not, reread.) What you're going for is a random collection of color, a thin stroke here, and a thicker stroke there that mimics what nature does.

Next to picking the wrong color, the second biggest hair color error, says Louis, is this: "Hairstylists think they have to work color from the roots to ends every time. But when you get a touch-up," he says, "get color on the roots only." And only work the color through to the ends for the last few minutes before taking it off. He recommends that everyone's hair should go from darker on top to lighter at the bottom.

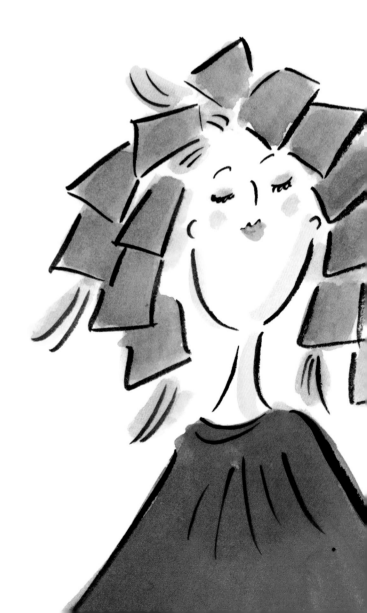

between appointments

In between salon visits, to cover up those gray hairs that sprout near your face and at your part (where they can make you look as if your hair is thinning), ask the salon to give you a formula to do minor touch-ups at home, or to give to the local salon in your winter or summer community. Don't be shy. Louis says he does it all the time to accommodate his customers when they are going away for extended periods of time and can't get in for a touch-up.

Also, friend and colleague formerly from L'Oreal, Joan Lasker, invented a brilliant product for gray roots between salon visits or DIY hair-color sessions called TouchBack. It is temporary hair color in a mistake-proof marker that bonds to the hair and holds its color until shampooed out, and it's available in eight shades.

This product was born out of Joan's personal need to cover the gray roots of her own beautiful hair. Joan had a fabulous career in the beauty industry and reinvented her professional self after fifty by starting her own business out of her house after her son went off to college. **Best Bets:** Women across the country have tried TouchBack (touchbackgray.com) and love it. And the product has been the recipient of Allure's Best of Beauty Award three times. Clairol Nice 'N Easy Root Touch-Up comes in a variety of shades as does Rita Hazan Root Concealer, and both work well for those times between.

DIY color

Thanks to the do-it-yourself trend of at-home products that imitate salon procedures, coloring has hit a high note in popularity. Advertisements make it look so effortless and easy. Who wouldn't want shiny, swishy hair like Andie MacDowell and Eva Longoria? For a fraction of a salon fee, a box of hair color is a steal and can deliver great results—but lest you want to end up with orange highlights or green hair, you MUST know what you are doing. If you're ready to color your hair at home, don't start before reading these simple rules.

1 BE CONSERVATIVE

It's best to go only a couple of shades lighter or darker than your natural color.

2 TRY BEFORE YOU DYE

Do a strand test before committing to the entire box. If the color turns out to be a bust, you only wasted $12. That's a bummer, but it's nothing compared to the hundreds you'd have to fork over to get it color-corrected by a professional! (See OOOPS! section later in the chapter.)

3 CHOOSE THE RIGHT SHADE

The color you see on the pack isn't going to look like the same shade on your head. A color expert once shared with me that if the hair color on the package picks up the pink or gold in your skin, then it's a shade that will suit you.

4 GO A SHADE LIGHTER

Select the ideal shade you are looking for, and then go a shade lighter because it's easier to go darker if you make a mistake than it is to make a dark shade lighter.

5 PREPARE YOUR HAIR

For color-staying power, be sure your hair is clean and well conditioned before you put color on it. It's best to wash your hair the night before you color.

6 ENLIST A FRIEND TO HELP

You don't want miss a spot on the back of your head.

7 CONDITION YOUR HAIR

After you rinse out the color, be sure to condition your hair, then do a deep-conditioning treatment at least once a week to preserve the color and nourish your hair.

Here's how to select the at-home color product that's right for you: It all depends on whether you're simply flirting with color changes, need gray coverage or a color boost, or you want something more permanent. Choose from those that wash out after a couple of shampoos to those that are permanent:

TEMPORARY COLORS
(LASTS 1–3 SHAMPOOS)

- What they will do: Add temporary color highlights and wash out quickly.

- What they won't do: Cover gray, lighten hair, or last very long.

SEMIPERMANENT
(LASTS 4–8 SHAMPOOS)

- What they will do: Can be used regularly to subtly enhance your natural color by adding a red tone to brown hair or a gold hue to blond, for example, or to disguise the first signs of gray. If you don't like the effect, these colors will eventually wash out.

- What they won't do: Lighten hair or give a dramatic, lasting color change or cover a high percentage of gray.

PERMANENT COLOR
(LASTS THROUGH 28 SHAMPOOS)

- What they will do: Give you a permanent color change—which means you'll need to touch up the roots every 4–6 weeks. Most will cover up to 100 percent gray (check the pack for details).

- What they won't do: It can't be washed out, period. If you make a mistake, visit a salon and hope for the best.

Once you have an idea of the level of color permanence you're looking for, you'll have to decide on what level of processing you want. Do you want all-over color or highlights? A quick pick-me-up, or a shine boost? Here are some facts to help guide you:

SINGLE PROCESS

A new color or toner is applied all over to create a new base color. The hair color is lightened and a new color is added in one easy step.

DOUBLE PROCESS

Typically used when lightening hair by more than two shades. First the hair is bleached to remove natural or colored hair pigments, and then pigment is added into the hair to create the desired shade. Since color is adjusted more than two or three shades, it's best to leave this process to the professionals.

HIGHLIGHTS

Adding highlights gives you more visible contrast than a regular single-process dye. Remember, less is more, and a few strands framing your face can offer you just the right amount of light to give skin a healthy glow.

GLAZES AND COLOR-ENHANCING SHAMPOOS

Use glazes, including tint formulas and color-enhancing shampoos, to help intensify a fading shade between salon visits. They revitalize color, smooth the cuticle, and add vibrant shine. To reduce hair damage, look for products that are ammonia-free. John Frieda offers a good selection, including Glaze Luminous Color, Glaze Clear Shine Gloss, Brilliant Brunette, Sheer Blonde, and Radiant Red, so one's bound to work for you.

Don't forget to wear something old when coloring your hair (if it stains your hair, it will certainly stain your silks, cottons, and polyester blends!), and smooth Vaseline along your hairline, on your ears, and on the back of your neck to create a barrier to keep dye from staining your skin.

OOOPS!

When hair color goes bad, I highly recommend you visit your salon for a quick fix rather than concoct another mixture to mess up your hair color even more. Remember, just dyeing over a color that might have gone too dark isn't a quick fix. Color cannot lift color. What does that mean? You can't remove black hair dye with light brown, blond, or any other lighter shade of hair color. You need special products to remove the color from your hair before it can be recolored. Purchasing other colors is a simple waste of time. There are products like Color Corrector by Salon Care Professional, which is a gentle, nonbleach blend of chemicals that oxidize permanent dyes. The kit comes with two, one-fluid-ounce bottles of product, which cannot be mixed until they are ready to be used. You choose your option according to your need. But again, I stress and recommend you visit a professional for best results. If you have any concerns, many at-home brands offer hotline numbers with consultants on call to answer any questions or problems (Clairol 1-800-CLAIROL and L'Oreal, 1-800-361-7358) are two of the most popular ones.

gray's anatomy

As for going totally gray: I think it can be dazzling on the right person, like my beautiful friend and colleague Jade Hobson, who is a former *Vogue* editor. But it only works if you have a complexion that has color and depth. It's best for someone with a slightly olive undertone and a lot of style. But you still have to take care of gray hair with the proper maintenance, including regular cuts, nourishing conditioners, and the occasional hair mask. Gray hair tends to be drier and coarser than hair that has retained pigment. Clairol Lights Shimmer or Artec White Violet Color Shampoo are great at-home treatments that contain bluing tints to prevent that "avoid-at-all-costs" yellowing effect, which comes from overexposure to certain elements like the sun or chlorine. Purchase moisturizing shampoos and alternate these with the above-mentioned products. Get occasional deep conditioning treatments or glazes at your salon; this will add shine while toning the hair to keep the brassiness away. Gray hair left unattended will never measure up to the beautiful statement it can make about entering your middle years, and it really will make you look old. But do it right, and this can qualify as another "wear your essence" moment, and thank you, Gad, for that concept!

hair quality and texture

Here is one of life's little injustices: As we age, the only body part that seems to get thinner is our hair.

After menopause, you have only about three-quarters the amount of hair you had as a younger person. (Though a few of the missing strands may turn up on your chin. But that's another story.) So what's the solution, other than hats? The medical options (at least for now) are limited to Rogaine or hair transplants (both show good results), and I'm not convinced that any of the home remedies or alternative medicines work.

Simpler and less costly approaches are products containing hair fibers and powders. Hair fibers, like Super Million Hair Enhancement Fibres, can be sprinkled on to thinning hair and will help camouflage trouble spots. They are available in a wide array of hair colors and seamlessly blend in with your natural hair. Hair powders not only color the scalp to conceal thinning hair but also help boost fine hair at the root.

hairpieces

Another option is to have a hairpiece made. But don't let the word fool you: it's more hairnet than wig, with large holes for your own hair to be pulled through. Real or synthetic hair that matches yours is tied onto the hair netting in very thin layers so it does not look bulky or wiglike. Once placed strategically on your head (usually on the crown or bangs, where it is often needed most), it secures into place with a flat small clip. It can be made to cover the entire crown, or just partially, and it blends easily with bangs. This is especially effective for hair that is curly, but it also works for straight hair.

While some might scoff at the idea of a "wig," you'd be surprised by how many celebrities with thinning hair use similar products. According to Louis, the high-end solution for celebrities these days is something called a "lace" hairpiece. It's a custom-made and imperceptible bit of lightweight fabric that looks something like a veil. It blends seamlessly with the skin of the scalp and with hair (real or synthetic) that has been matched to the natural hair.

SOME BEST BETS WORTH TRYING:
- Bumble and Bumble Hair Powder
- Nexxus Youth Renewal Rejuvenating Dry Shampoo
- Pssssst Instant Dry Shampoo
- TRESemme FreshStart Dry Shampoo

If your retreating mane could use a little mending, check local listings for wigmakers and have a consultation done. Prices and options vary, depending on the retailer, hair quality, and size.

hair extensions

Another more long-lasting solution to thinning hair can be found in the world of hair extensions. You need longer hair (chin to shoulder length) to camouflage them, and, if your hair is too layered, they show, but done properly, they're very effective. The process is somewhat laborious, as the hair extensions must be glued, woven, braided, or wrapped into your own tresses a few strands at a time. A good extension "job" should last two to three months and can withstand frequent shampoos and blow-drying. But you need strong hair to maximize the life of the extensions, so heed this warning from personal experience: My hair is very fine, and, when I tried extensions, the weight of the hair and glue put too much stress on my strands, and I ended up with a bald spot. If you have fine hair, it's better to avoid this nightmare altogether and instead opt for imperceptible clip-on extensions, especially if you want the extra confidence booster of full glorious hair for a special occasion. Many a red-carpet walker uses this subtle technique, and only her hairdresser knows.

One caution: Whether you're using extensions, hairnets, or lace hairpieces, these remedies are expensive ($300–$5,000, depending on the choice and whether hair is real or synthetic). Be prepared.

a primer on hair products

What if you're not interested in faux tresses, but you could use some help finessing the hair you have? The shelves are full of hair-care products that promise all manner of magic—some that deliver and some that don't. The selection can be overwhelming, but it's helpful to know that all of them are designed to serve just one of five purposes: to add volume, to add shine and smoothness, to enhance natural curls, to strengthen weak hair, and to prolong hair color. You might find that you have several hair issues to address at once. You may want to add volume to smooth hair or want to preserve color and strengthen hair. There are several good products that work like cross-trainers and cover many bases when it comes to hair needs.

FOR VOLUME

This category of products creates the illusion of thickness and is designed for people with fine, limp thin hair. The easiest way to get volume is to invest in a volumizing shampoo because it is the most familiar form of hair product and therefore the simplest to manage. A volumizing shampoo works by leaving out most of the ingredients in regular shampoos and conditioners that weigh hair down and by removing the excess debris from around the root, allowing the hair to flow freely and unencumbered by weighty ingredients, giving the illusion of more volume. Since these products often compromise shine, it can be replaced by rubbing a dot of argan oil between the palms of your hands and fingers and stroking it through your hair. Or choose a modern formula that uses botanical alcohols to add lift, take away dryness, and compensate with ingredients such as wheat proteins that soften and add texture and shine.

Other volumizing products come in mousse, gel, and spray forms. These work by depositing hair thickening agents, such as proteins, keratin, and polymers, which coat the strands, increase the strand diameter, and temporarily make the hair feel and look thicker. Sprays seem to be the newest form, which help lift the hair at the root for volume and texture. A word of caution: Use these products sparingly because they can have the opposite effect when applied too amply.

Try these **Best Bets:**
- Oribe Dry Texturizing Spray (oribe.com)
- Oribe Shampoo and Conditioner for Magnificent Volume (oribe.com)
- Pantene Expert Age Defy Collection (Thickening Treatment, Shampoo, Conditioner, and Masque)
- Phytovolume Actif Volumizing Spray (sephora.com)

FOR SLEEK, FRIZZ-FREE, SHINY HAIR

You need hydrating shampoos and conditioners that contain conditioning oils such as argan oil to even out the hair shaft and create a smooth cuticle surface to promote shine. Finish with a leave-in hair conditioner to make hair less frizzy and more manageable. The newest versions are very effective and lightweight, using natural oils or silicones that allow hair to breathe and prevent a greasy or oily look.

Best Bets:
- Argana Mon Tresor (gadcohen.com)

- Garnier Fructis Sleek and Shine Fortifying Shampoo and Conditioner, Sleek Finish 5-in-1 Serum Spray (at most drugstores)
- Living Proof No Frizz Leave in Conditioner (livingproof.com)
- Matrix Biolage Smooththérapie Deep Smoothing Shampoo, Conditioner, and Leave-In Cream (matrix.com for salons)

FOR SOFT, DEFINED CURLS

In the past, harsh gels were the only tool in the arsenal for hair that is tightly curled, making the curls look hard and crisp. Research into the unique structure of curly hair has shown that it can be very fine, yet needs super conditioning to calm down the frizz. In general, the new prescription for this hair type is gentle shampoos with low or no harsh surfactants, coupled with lightweight creamy conditioners or sprays that coat the hair, defining curls and locking them into place.

Best Bets for Curl "Girls":
- Bumble and Bumble Curl Conscious Smoothing Shampoo and Conditioner (bumbleandbumble.com)
- Devachan DevaCurl Low-Poo Cleanser, One Condition and DevaCurl Set It Free Spray (devachan.com)

- John Freida Frizz-Ease Dream Curls Curl Perfecting Spray (at most drugstores)
- Motions Define My Curls Crème (at most drugstores—a fave for ethnic hair)

FOR STRONG RESILIENT HAIR

One of the biggest signs of aging (giving our neck and hands competition) is our hair. Since our hair is dead protein, it cannot repair and renew itself. It gradually wears out from environmental factors like sun and wind, chemical treatments, heat styling, and plain old brushing and combing. Untended hair at a certain point can look dull, lifeless, and broken. The solution is serious deep moisturizing and conditioning with proteins like keratin or fatty acids, which have ceramides that coat the strands and bind to the cuticle, filling in the cracks to help prevent breakage. Here are a couple of my favorites for the look of strong, beautiful hair:

Best Bets:
- Kerastase Bain Force Architecte (shampoo), Ciment Anti-Usure (conditioner), and Masque Force Architecte (kerastase-usa.com)
- TRESemmé Platinum Strength Strengthening Shampoo, Conditioner, and Heat Spray (at most drugstores)

FOR COLOR-TREATED HAIR

Most of us do color our hair, and, if you are anything like me, I try to stretch out the time between visits to my hair-color guru, Louis Licari. What I've learned is that normal cleansing agents in shampoos can sometimes literally strip away color, so, if extending the life of your hair color is your biggest issue, the best shampoo to use is a sulfate-free formula that employs a different cleansing system that doesn't "chelate," or extract the hair color molecules from the hair shaft.

Two on my **Best Bets** list:

- L'Oreal Paris EverPure Sulfate-Free Color Care System (at most drugstores)
- Pureology Hydrate Shampoo and Conditioner for dry, overprocessed hair (ulta.com)

UV light can also fade hair, especially in the summer months, so try a treatment spray like Redken Color Extend Total Recharge (redken.com)

THERE'S A REASON when we came of age that the biggest thing on Broadway was called *HAIR.* We're the first generation to embrace our "shining, gleaming, streaming, flaxen-waxen" birthright, and the ones who first understood that ready-to-wear hair is chic-er and more modern than anything created with pink, plastic rollers. There's no reason to allow a few gray hairs to make us give up now, especially with so many advances in at-home coloring and styling products. There's also no shame in walking into a salon and telling them exactly what we want—we did it with our male bosses decades ago, so this part should be easy. And taking charge of our own beauty, including our hair, is truly the ultimate 'do.

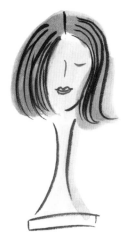
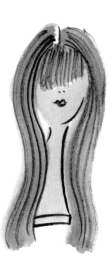
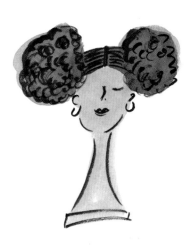

According to famed hairdresser Gad Cohen, never cross your legs when you're getting your hair cut! Crossing your legs makes your spine shift, causing one side to be higher than the other. Instead, sit up straight and keep your shoulders even with one another.

When it comes to at-home hair color, some trusted brands have created new formulas that are healthier for your hair and easier to use. For instance, Clairol's permanent hair colors—like its Perfect 10 line—don't contain the ammonium hydroxide that's in most formulas. It smells a whole lot better and has a lower pH, which means it's gentler on the hair. Other formulations now also come in foam, making application much easier and less messy, thanks to its mousselike texture. Try John Frieda Precision Foam Hair Color for foolproof, drip-proof color. Another new advent in hair color is oil-powered color. Try Garnier's Olia line, which uses a blend of natural flower oils that improve hair health and shine, in addition to color.

Your hair isn't alive, but your scalp is! Treating your scalp like skin (which it is) can affect the look of your hair. Your scalp is aging just like every other part of your skin and probably experiencing excess dryness like you might have on other body parts and your face, due to the fact that cell turnover is slowing down. This can lead to a buildup of excess skin cell debris around the hair shaft and follicle, along with sweat and dirt, impeding the look of a healthy head of hair. If you treat your scalp like your face—with deep cleansing and moisturizing—you'll provide a smoother platform and environment for healthier-looking hair.

BEST BETS:

- Clear Scalp and Hair Beauty Therapy, Damage and Color Repair 7 Day Intensive Treatment

- John Frieda Root Awakening Hydrate + Nourish Shampoo and Conditioner

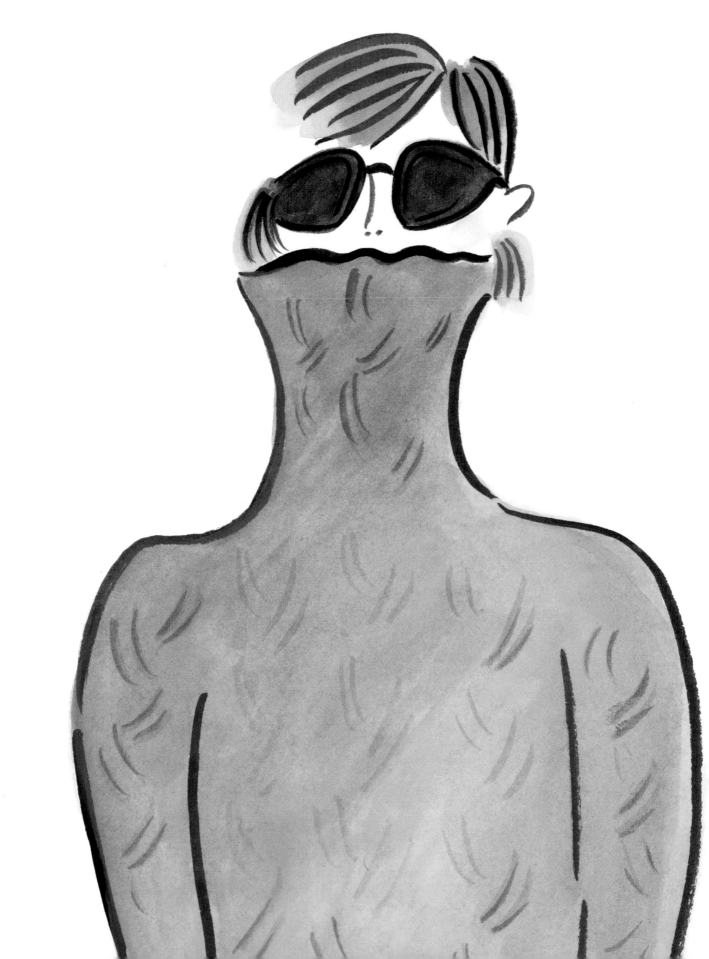

CHAPTER ELEVEN

THE FORGOTTEN ZONES

from the neck down to the hands up

I SPENT MOST OF MY ADULT LIFE WORRYING ABOUT MY BUTT AND BUST, NEVER ANTICIPATING THAT IN MY FIFTIES, MY ATTENTION WOULD BE DIVERTED TO ANOTHER BODY PART.

Alas, the moment arrived when I realized that the Thanksgiving turkey and I began to look like those "separated at birth" photos, and that my long, lean neck had to have been stolen by the body snatchers, who forgot to take my oversized butt at the same time.

The late Nora Ephron got this feeling completely, and that's why her book, *I Feel Bad About My Neck*, soared to the bestseller list. For many of us, this troubled drop zone, the increasingly declining curve between the neck and jaw that used to be a taut right angle, has made us feel, well . . . bad. Whether we wrap it in scarves, or hide it under a turtleneck sweater, many of us have become conscious of an area that only used to get attention during perfume application and jewelry shopping. Only a privileged few are granted an elegant, swan neck like

> Only a privileged few are granted an elegant, swan neck like that of Audrey Hepburn— the rest of us fall into the "hide-the-slide" group.

that of Audrey Hepburn—the rest of us fall into the "hide-the-slide" group. Ephron was one of us, a reluctant participant, no doubt, in the acquisition of more scarves, chokers, and turtlenecks that accumulate steadily after one's fiftieth birthday. She nailed it when she said, "I often do what so many women my age do when stuck in front of a mirror: I gently pull the skin of my neck back and stare wistfully at a younger version of myself."

The neck is very delicate because, next to the eyelids, the skin in this area is some of the thinnest. As you age, it loses elasticity faster than anywhere else on your body, taking on the dreaded crêpe-y look. You should be every bit as diligent and careful about taking care of your neck and décolletage as you are about your face.

The same goes for your hands, which age just as quickly and require as much care and protection as our necks and chest.

The looming question: How do we prevent further "droppage" and bring back the illusion of a tight chin line, and how do we handle our fifty+ hands, now that gloves are no longer a "go-to" accessory? I wrote this chapter to answer these quandaries. You can start by heeding the following . . .

BEAUTY TRUTH:

It's okay to feel bad about your neck— and it's also okay to do something about it!

Let's discuss what you can do to prevent any real disasters from the chin down— without going under the knife.

neck neglect: what to do about it

We spend so much time and money trying to stave off the look of aging on our faces, but we often completely neglect our necks and chest. It's not until later, perhaps in our mid forties, that we begin to notice slight changes in the elasticity of the skin beneath our chins, or discover a growing tapestry of spots and lines on our once smooth and unmarked chests. By then, nature will have played some havoc with this delicate area, but the good news is that it is never too late to start damage control. If you don't already follow the basics of skin care from the neck down, begin NOW. Here's what you should be doing on a regular basis to help preserve—and refurbish—this sexy part of your body.

MOISTURIZE

Make sure you slather lotion or cream on your neck and chest every morning and night, and treat these areas to the same care you give your face. Moisturizers provide protection for the skin by limiting the evaporation of water from the epidermis, lubricating and softening its surface and therefore providing a comfortable and healthy appearance. Why deprive the neck of such nurturing?

EXFOLIATE

By getting rid of the surface cells and encouraging cell turnover, you will lessen sunspots and diminish the crêpe-y texture that suddenly seems to appear on your neck and chest. Specialty treatments like Retin A cream or glycolic peels work best but will only effect skin tightening, not the fatty skin lurking there. You should exfoliate once or twice weekly with gentle, nonirritating solutions and avoid grainy scrubs that can tear skin. Regular exfoliation equates with clean healthy glowing skin.

PROTECT

Slather on sunscreen. Like your face, the ultraviolet rays of the sun will take its toll on the elasticity of the skin on your neck if it's not protected. A sunscreen with an SPF of 15 is best and adequate since this will filter out about 93 percent of the skin-damaging UVB rays of the sun. This Sun Protection Factor will give you theoretically fifteen times the protection of your skin in the sun without any sunscreen. As mentioned in Chapter 3, anything over SPF 30 is a waste of money, since SPF 30 filters out 97 percent of UVB rays. Also consider wearing a brimmed hat when you're outdoors for long stretches—whether it's gardening, hiking, or lounging by the pool. The sun is strongest and most damaging between the hours of noon and 3:00 PM, but you should never leave the house without sunscreen, even if it's overcast. If you're active, be sure to reapply your sunscreen. Sweat will quickly wash the layer of sun protectant away, leaving your skin vulnerable to UVs.

Here are a few **Best Bets** for handling the basics:

- La Roche-Posay 40 Sunscreen Cream
- Lancôme Bienfait Multi-Vital SPF 30 Sunscreen
- Olay Complete All Day UV Moisturizer Cream—Normal

Now that you have the preventative-care routine down, it's time to address the existing problems that have crept up over the last few years. See the common complaints below, and consider the cosmetic fixes before making the leap to lasers, fillers, and peels.

JOWLY CHIN LINE

A jowly chin line, the fatty tissue, or sagging area that begins to rear its droopy head on the lower jaw line, is most often noticed in its early stages in our forties and becomes progressively more noticeable during and after menopause. Jowls come from muscles slackening over time, and weight gain.

The Fix

Try using a color cosmetic to help camouflage jowls. Dark contouring powder or a darker foundation used under the chin creates the illusion of slimness and a tight jaw line. Or apply a self-tanner under the chin carefully along the jaw line and down the neck, continuing to the décolleté area for a longer-lasting effect.

Best Bets:

- Make Up For Ever Sculpting Kit
- Neutrogena Sunless Tan

MOTTLED AND SPOTTY SKIN

Mottled skin is skin that has splotchy discolor-ations and age spots on the neck and chest. These patches and spots could be the result of changes in blood vessels, age spots due to over-exposure to UVB rays, or hyper pigmentation (when the body produces too much melanin).

The Fix

Various methods can help mitigate this situation, including microdermabrasion, chemical peels, or laser therapy. This condition is best addressed by a dermatologist after the cause of the spots has been determined.

WRINKLY SKIN

At this stage of life, we all know what wrinkles are.

The Fix

I repeat, what works on your face should be used on your neck and chest, including sun-screens and those night products containing reti-nol, which over time can subtly help build col-lagen to improve elasticity and tone, reduce age spots, and smooth the skin. The most effective retinols, however, are prescribed by a dermatol-ogist. Lasers have also been helpful by removing the top layer of skin and diminishing the surface wrinkles.

Best Bets:

- L'Oreal Skin Expertise RevitaLift Complete Night Cream
- Neutrogena Rapid Wrinkle Repair
- Your dermatologist

*we all know
what wrinkles are . . .*

For a more advanced turkey neck, the only effective tactic is to get yourself to a good dermatologist who knows how to use lasers, fillers at the jaw line, and Botox at the neckline where the chin meets the neck, to re-create that 90-degree angle. Botox will lift the sagging skin; filler (done in tiny doses along the jaw line) will improve the look of the chin line, and lasers will firm and tighten loose skin. It's not for everyone—and it's certainly not cheap—but if you look in the mirror and see that your chin and neck have formed a bigger merger than JPMorgan Chase, take action. Educated action, that is; make sure your dermatologist comes highly recommended and has thorough experience with injectables. (See Chapter 12 for detailed information about these and other cosmetic procedures and how they can help offset a host of other age-related skin issues.)

Now that we've figured out how to stop pulling our turtlenecks up, let's talk about how to stop pulling those sweater sleeves down and move on to the other telltale area of aging: our hands.

talk to the hand

You may wear sunscreen on your face every day, but does it make it on to your hands? Probably not, and then they suffer from sunspots and lines—and while we may feel at the top of our fifty+ game, our hands are suggesting otherwise. Prior generations turned to gloves to hide this spotty problem, but it's time to bring in the heavy artillery—not the lace and leather.

This section calls attention to your hands as an important part of your cosmetic routine. When hands are photographed in magazines, they look flawless, lineless, and veinless. Do you know why? Because the industry hires special hand models who will never touch a dish without a rubber glove, who will never expose their hands to the sun, who wear gloves most of the day, and who have their hands insured for gazillions of dollars. Right before the model's hands are photographed, the standard protocol is that she hold them above her heart for one minute. This trick reduces the amount of blood flow to the hands, making them appear smooth and perfect. These women are often not young like the fashion models seen in *Vogue* and *Vanity Fair*. They're generally in their thirties and forties, which illustrates how good hand care can keep your hands youthful forever. One hand model I know swears by almond oil (Waleda Almond Soothing Facial Oil), which has high amounts of vitamins E and A. She's tested hundreds of creams and believes this inexpensive emollient penetrates the skin better than any hand cream. That said, many celebrities (as they move into their forties) swear by something else—Photoshop—to erase signs of aging from their hands that appear in magazine profiles, product endorsement ads, and movie posters. Fortunately, you don't need high-tech hijinx, just a few quality products and some common sense. Here are some other tips that make the most of our most-used extremities.

PAMPER YOUR CUTICLES

Keep your cuticle pusher in the shower, and, while your cuticles are warm and wet, push them gently back so they frame the nails. Avoid trimming, which only makes them look ragged if not done correctly. Apply an oil afterward (CND Solar Cuticle Oil is a cult favorite and seems to work on the driest and roughest cuticles—which would accurately describe mine).

CUT AND SHAPE YOUR NAILS CONSERVATIVELY

Use an extra-fine emery board and file to a rounded shape. Forget square or pointy—shapes come and go, but the best nail shape to use is the classic curve. This gives you the most natural look. Added benefit: Rounded nails are less likely to break than square shapes. (And nothing looks worse than overly long, unkempt nails of various lengths. As for nail art, leave that to your daughter—along with lip gloss and texting "LOL" to your boyfriend.)

WEAR GLOVES WHILE WASHING DISHES

Madge was right, protect your hands. Chemicals and hot water can strip away the protective lipid barrier on your skin, making it susceptible to irritation and dryness. And remember to apply a layer of lotion to your hands each time you put on your rubber gloves—not only will it protect them, it'll give you an extra dose of moisture.

KEEP LOTION EVERYWHERE

Place a hand-cream pump at every sink in your house, on your bedside table, and stash travel-size tubes in your desk drawer and purse so you'll never forget to moisturize. Nivea Cream's travel-size tube is around a dollar and it's the perfect size for portability.

MOISTURIZE YOUR HANDS EVERY NIGHT

Always go to bed with a layer of moisture on your hands (Kiehl's Hand Cream and Jurlique Rose Hand Cream offer good dry hand relief), and/or use the excess on your hands after moisturizing your face. Every now and then, slather your hands in moisturizer and add cotton gloves to your night of sleep (yep, just like your grandmother did) for the added benefit of an at-home spa treatment.

KEEP YOUR HANDS AND NAILS MAINTAINED

Another must for youthful hands: Take them to the manicurist once a week. And BYOB—or shall I say, BYOP, for "Polish"—as many salons dilute their nail polish formulas. But who else is going to spend ten minutes giving you an amazing hand massage? The boyfriend? Well, maybe on the first few dates. The husband? I don't think so. And while you're there, pamper your toes and feet. They need some TLC any time of the year—no need to wait until sandal season.

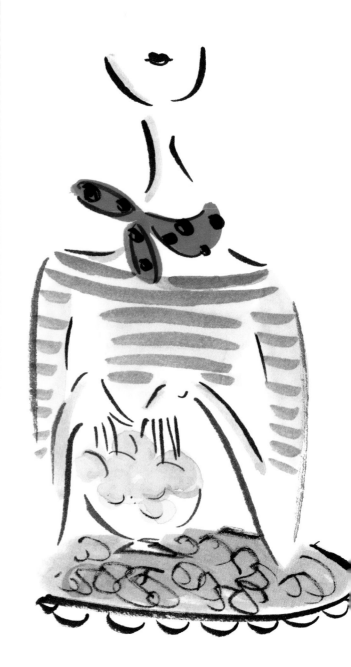

Of course, your nails are just as big a give-away as your skin. It's a rare fifty+ hand that can pull off a bright red, fuchsia, or orange polish. Darker skin allows for broader choices, but, if you fall into the fair-skinned category, bright colors will only emphasize veins and skin discolorations. Leave those fun colors to your toes. That said, it doesn't mean you can't "nail" a good color for your fingers. You just need to consider what works and what doesn't for your skin tone. Read on for the scoop on the nail-polish color spectrum, and what's right for you.

fingernail facts

Let's start with some inside dirt on fingernail polish: Did you know that most American brand name nail color is made in just two labs in the USA? Most large cosmetic companies, with the exception of Revlon, which makes its own, don't create their own nail color formulas. I recall attending a meeting at a nail laboratory, and being amazed at how many big cosmetic companies used this lab to fill their bottles and claim the formula as their own product. The nail polishes themselves are created by the nail lab—it's only the nail brush that each cosmetic company owns. Like with mascara, the brush is all important. Why? The brush

can add to the formula's performance in application, and many companies have patents to protect this asset—L'Oreal Paris and Sally Hansen, for instance, have some of the best brushes in the business. But don't

Like with mascara, the brush is all important.

believe the hype when a label tries to justify outrageous prices with claims about longevity and chipping, especially since your favorite salon brands, like Essie and OPI, are owned by mass cosmetic companies (L'Oreal and Coty, respectively). So the next time you make a nail polish purchase, make it color-driven and price-worthy. No need to splurge on a Chanel polish. Save your money for a Chanel handbag instead, and try Essie nail color, which has a funny way of resembling the Chanel fashion shades we love so much.

But which "P" should you keep in your purse for manicure days? Finding the right nail polish for your skin tone can be as tricky as finding the ideal foundation shade. And choosing the right nude is harder than you think. Here are some tips to keep in mind while selecting color:

FAIR SKIN

This skin tone allows you to wear a bevy of colors, from light to medium. For barely-there shades, choose a clean, nude color, which counters any redness in your skin. Stick with pink or purple undertones for skin tones that are bluish white, and yellow undertones for skin tones that are creamier. Unless your hands are smooth and vein free, avoid anything bright or flashy, which will make your hands look old.

Best Bets:

- Essie Ballet Slippers
- L'Oreal Colour Riche Nail Polish in How Romantic

MEDIUM SKIN

Brighter shades will look better on you because vibrant shades enhance your skin tone and will make it appear tan or darker than it actually is. Brighter shades of pink, as well as orange with a warm neutral base, are your best choices. Avoid undertones that are too silvery or cool; they will clash with your warm skin tone. A good natural midtone nude to look at is Essie Nail Polish in Not Just a Pretty Face. But consider the following

Best Bets:

- CoverGirl Outlast Stay Brilliant Nail Gloss in Peaches and Cream
- OPI Nail Lacquer in Tickle My France-y

DARK SKIN

Very dark skin looks fabulous with dark shades of polish. Deep plums, reds, and browns tend to look great when the hand is smooth and veinless (you can even get away with bright shades on smooth dark skin). The deeper your skin, the darker the nude should be. Avoid shades of white or very pale colors. Essie Nail Polish in Jazz offers good depth of color and is nude in undertone. For a little more neutral sizzle, try these:

Best Bets:

- L'Oreal Colour Riche Nail Polish in Greyt Expectations
- OPI Nail Lacquer in Metro Chic

When I worked at Revlon (where, as I mentioned, they *do* make their own nail polish), I had a male boss who was extremely insistent on my nails always being done (after all, it was Revlon!), and he noticed when they weren't. I'd walk into a big meeting, and, instead of focusing on my marketing plans, he'd say, "Andrea, nail color is one of the hallmarks of this company, and you have bare nails? Not acceptable." I've always worn clear polish, or natural if anything, but, while I had this job, I kept a stash of nail colors in my desk drawer. Before a big meeting, the nail polish fumes gave me away as they followed me down the corridor and into the boardroom. I was never very good at painting my own nails, and my desk looked more like a "Spin Art" station than an executive's workspace, with splattered lacquer and acetone remover stains everywhere. Once, I spilled an entire bottle of "Fire and Ice" on it, just as he was coming into my office—I was literally caught red-handed.

Don't follow my rushed example. Get a manicurist you trust, and visit her often. I always think that a good mani-pedi is better than a visit to the shrink. And though you should certainly pay the few extra bucks for a massage, my version of a "happy ending" is ten perfectly lacquered nails, and polished hands worthy of gesturing and flirting over the next seven days.

YOUR HANDS AND your neck can reveal telltale signs of age faster than a driver's license—but they can also continue to be hallmarks of your natural elegance and beauty. Leave the turkey necks for Thanksgiving dinner. Like Nora Ephron says, it's okay to feel bad about your neck

> Your hands and your neck can reveal telltale signs of age faster than a driver's license—but they can also continue to be hallmarks of your natural elegance and beauty.

and to worry about your hands, the good news is that you can do something about it. Just remember your VIPs (Very Important Parts) are still alluring and sexy, just like the rest of you.

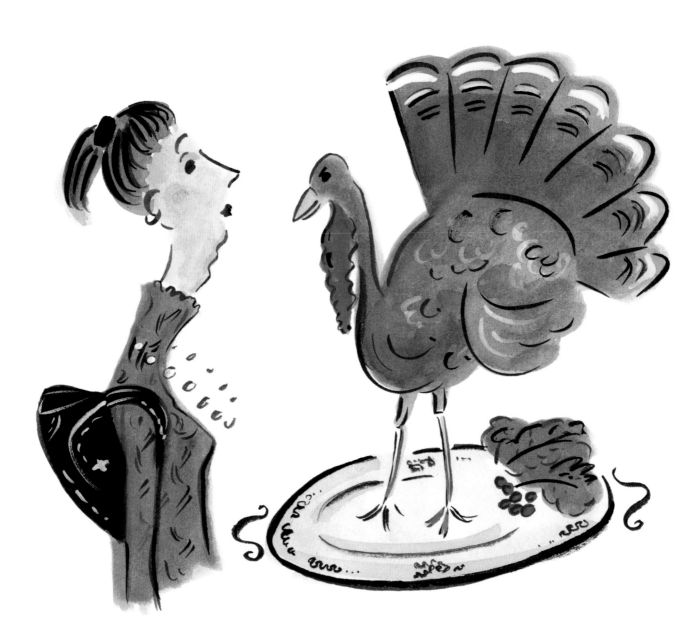

If your neck has taken on the look of Tom Turkey, in all his wattled glory, consider liposuction. Dermatologist Dr. Gervais Gerstner, clinical professor of dermatology at Mount Sinai School of Medicine, recommends this procedure as an effective way of getting rid of a turkey neck, since it's caused by fatty deposits. And no amount of exercise or over the counter neck cream will remedy this. The procedure removes the fat buildup in your neck and under your jaw, producing great results for those afflicted with double chins. Sometimes, liposuction is combined with a laser procedure to simultaneously tighten skin.

Cost: Approximately $5,000.

Quick tip for hands: Don't forget to slather them in sunscreen when you're out and about, especially when you're on the go—literally. When you drive, your hands are vulnerable to sun damage, since they're exposed as they grip the wheel. If you're the "girl" in the convertible with the top down and your hair is blowing in the wind (and I hope you are), be doubly sure to dose your hands.

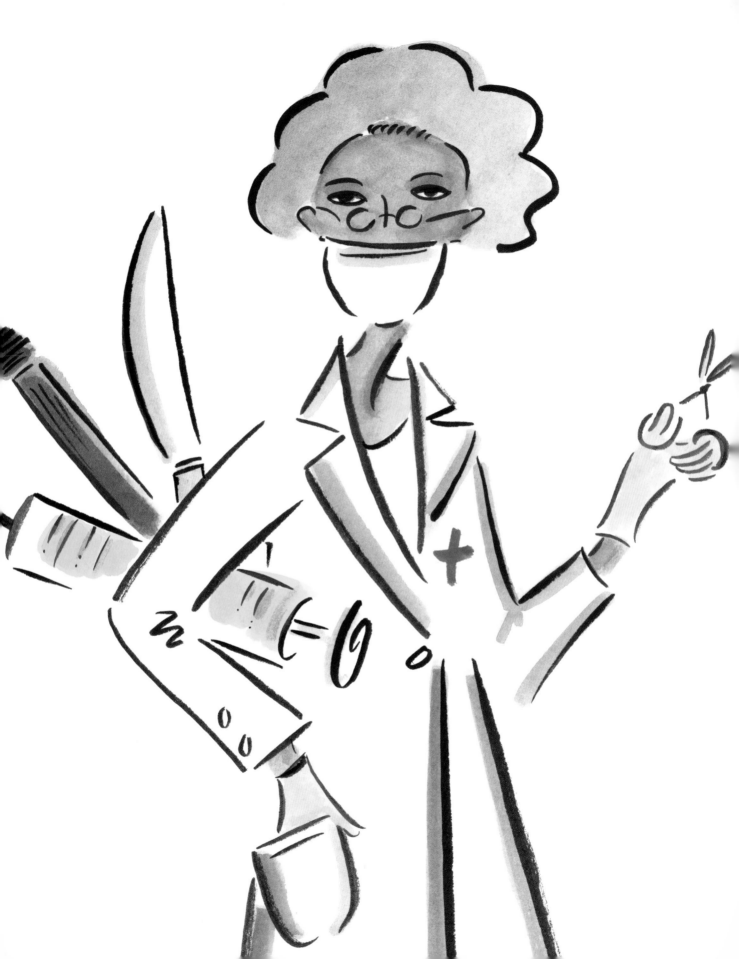

CHAPTER TWELVE

Cosmetic Tweaks

the needle, the knife, the know-how

LET'S BE FRANK: AT THIS POINT IN OUR LIVES IT IS SO VERY OKAY TO BE VAIN. IT TOOK ME YEARS OF PRACTICE, BUT HERE I AM, MRS. VAIN GLORIOUS, BEING KIND OF BOASTFUL ABOUT HOW I'VE LEARNED TO EMBRACE MY VANITY.

If you have, too—welcome to the club. If you haven't—no problem (and most likely, you're not reading this book, anyway).

There are women who've never missed a day of exercise, but rarely (or never) have worn makeup except to their child's wedding. I like to think I have a foot in both camps. Everyday exercise is something I try to accomplish, but I'll admit I still like getting asked about my minimal makeup or hair, or my toenail polish. The feminine ritual of maintaining my appearance makes me feel energetic, youthful, and together. And when others appreciate it, so much the better. It's a little like tending to a garden, weeding and cutting to make it bloom to its most beautiful best, or restoring parts of a house to give a platform to its natural elegance.

I certainly do want to look like myself, only better . . . not for him, not for them . . . for me.

I fully comprehend the fact that confidence and true beauty come from within, but I also embrace the notion that well-being can be enhanced by maintaining a look of health that exudes the energy of youth and vitality. And if you've learned one thing about me from reading this book, I certainly do want to look like myself, only better . . . not for him, not for them . . . for me.

We are, at this stage of our lives, in full control of how we present ourselves to the world. It's kind of fun to feel empowered enough to flip the middle finger at the toll that having a good long life has exacted on our looks. So here's my thought for you: If you believe in going through life looking as good as you can, and keenly feel you want to reclaim some of your physical beauty—stick with me on this one—it may mean using not just what you've learned here about makeup, but also investing in some capital improvements via more involved cosmetic enhancements. And by "enhancements," I mean anything from chemical peels to eye lifts. Taboo territory? *Uh uh*—not any longer.

Chances are, if you look around you, you'll see that "the face of change" is beginning to happen among your peers. Have you been to any thirty- or forty-year college reunions yet? I have. And chances are, a few of your friends have even had some kind of "work," whether it's Botox, lasers, fillers, or possibly the "hard stuff," by which I mean adjustments involving the scalpel—plastic surgery. And chances are, that number is higher than you think.

"Does she or doesn't she?"

Nowadays, it's a little like finding out who lost her virginity in high school. By the time we graduated, there were few who hadn't, and those who had were beginning to kiss and tell.

Perhaps you're realizing that using moisturizers, sun protection, and other skin solutions isn't doing enough to keep your face as fresh as you'd like, and you're now thinking, *Should I or shouldn't I?* If so, you're not alone. According to the American Society of Aesthetic Plastic Surgery, nearly 10 million procedures are done every year. And while 80 percent represent procedures such as Botox, lasers, and fillers, the other 20 percent are surgical (from liposuction to nose jobs).

Sure, in our twenties and thirties, we probably claimed we'd never use fillers, let alone undergo any form of plastic surgery. I certainly said, "Never ever!" But guess what? We've changed, and perhaps more important, so has the technology. The types of treatments available now didn't exist twenty years ago. They're less invasive, less uncomfortable, and more effective than ever. And while I will never be a proponent of face-swapping plastic surgery and over-the-top injections (sorry, Joan, you've gone too far),

I'm totally on board with taking advantage of cosmetic breakthroughs to spring out of the physical rut of age-related doldrums—with one caveat: Be conservative.

surface issues: lasers, fillers, and botox

If you're considering any of these cosmetic procedures, you want to find a good doctor, one who has a long history and rate of success with all of the procedures I am about to discuss. New York–based dermatologist Dr. Gervaise Gerstner (you met her in my chapters on lipstick and necks), who has refinished, refined, and reshaped countless faces, says the average age of her patients is forty-three, but it is skewing younger each year, with women in their twenties and thirties—along with a growing number of men—starting to form a sizable base in her practice as well. Below are some of her more commonly used procedures:

be conservative . . . .

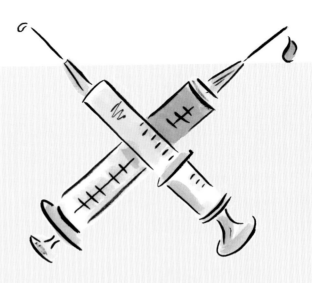

LASER TREATMENTS

Even those with advanced signs of aging can benefit from lasers, which resurface skin, diminishing wrinkles, scars, red spots, and sun damage. The goal of this procedure is to reveal healthy and even skin. Recovery time varies depending on the depth of the treatment. Some of Dr. Gerstner treatments include Lumenis Duet Hair Removal, Candela V Beam, and the lasers from Solta Fraxel Re:store Dual, Clear + Brilliant, and Thermage, which she uses for tightening of the neck.

- RISKS: Discomfort during procedure, temporary redness, skin flaking.
- COST: Approximately $350 to $2,000 per treatment, depending on the type of laser.

BOTOX

This injectable drug revolutionized the beauty industry. Botox is a bacteria called *Clostridium botulinum*, and, when used in small targeted doses, it helps to weaken and relax the nerve impulses, disengaging the muscles that give you that permanent furrow on your forehead, the vertical lines at the top of your nose, and other facial wrinkles. The desired result should make you appear softer and less wrinkled, less angry-looking (despite not feeling that way), and less

worried. And yes, more youthful. The effect lasts three to six months.

- RISKS: Too much Botox will give you a shiny forehead and a frozen, deer-in-the-headlights look (see most of the women from the *Real Housewives* franchise as a cautionary tale). In a small percentage of cases, there can be drooping of the eyelid (ptosis), headache, difficulty swallowing (when injected around the neck), dryness of mouth or eyes, and neck pain. And of course, discomfort at the injection site.
- COST: Approximately $400 to $800.

DERMAL FILLERS

Sometimes referred to as "liquid facelifts," these are procedures that offer some of the benefits of a surgical facelift without the long recovery time. Fillers like Restylane, Juvéderm, and

Belotero give you a youthful fullness, enhance shallow contours, and smooth away facial lines and wrinkles. I used Restylane regularly, which filled in and smoothed out my skin, especially the vertical folds that appear by the side of the nose, and the "puppet" lines around the mouth. It also helped stave off spending the big bucks on a neck lift . . . for a while, anyway. It lasts for six to nine months.

- RISKS: Localized pain or discomfort at injection site, redness, swelling, bruising (in some cases).
- COST: Approximately $600 to $1,000 per vial.

IPL (INTENSE PULSED LIGHT) TREATMENT

This procedure helps the appearance of sun-damaged skin by removing redness caused by broken capillaries, sunspots, freckles, and brown spots. IPL Treatment utilizes intense, broad-spectrum, pulsed light to help erase these particular issues with no downtime and great results within a short period of time. To see full results, it usually requires four or five treatments, depending on the issue. The effect is permanent, providing you stay out of the sun.

- RISKS: Temporary, mild swelling, redness, brown-spot crusting, occasional bruising, and superficial blisters.
- COST: Approximately $300 to $500 per treatment.

CHEMICAL PEELS

These procedures improve the texture and appearance of the skin by using a chemical solution that causes dead skin to slough and peel off, fostering cell renewal and collagen production. Chemical peels are great for addressing issues of aging (fine lines and even deeper wrinkles), acne, sun damage, and hyperpigmentation, and you'll see visible results after one procedure, depending on your particular issues and the chemicals used. Some mild peels that Dr. Gerstner uses are Salicylic, Glycolic, and Melange peels. The downtime involved is none to three weeks, depending on the peel.

- RISKS: Discomfort or pain, redness, swelling, scabbing and crusting, depending on the depth of the chemical peel.
- COST: Approximately $250 to $5,000, depending on the type of peel.

I'm a big proponent of safe and conservative (underscore safe and conservative) cosmetic tweaks for many reasons:

- The results last for several months (three to nine months, depending on where on the face/neck it is used).

- The changes can be dramatic yet not detectable.

- Some procedures can be done before work, after work, or at lunch time (the appointments never take more than an hour).

- There's no long recovery process.

However, fair warning: Any of the above "noninvasive" cosmetic procedures can be performed unwisely in the hands of the wrong doctor, so diligently check your doctor's expertise, and start with small tweaks until you are comfortable with the dermatologist's skill and handling of your face. Understand and know the slippery slope of dermatological fillers so you don't wind up like so many of those "freaky-faced" Hollywood celebrities—beware of big lips, frozen brows, a bulbous forehead, and over-plumped cheeks. Leave those exaggerated looks to Barbie dolls and reality TV stars.

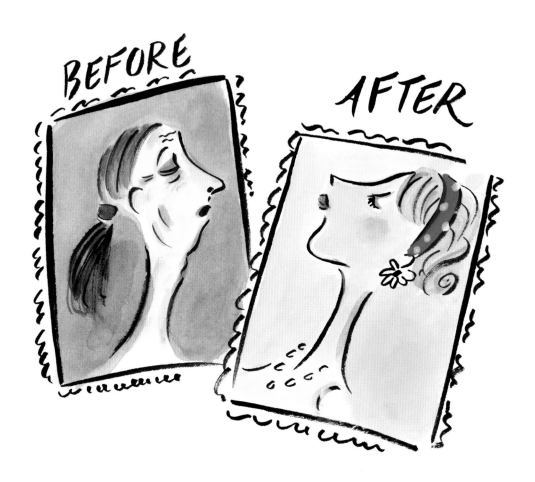

If you're considering visiting a dermatologist for any of these procedures, Dr. Gerstner recommends keeping in mind the following questions:

1 Is the dermatologist board certified?

2 How experienced is the doctor at using the technology/procedure you are considering?

3 Is the doctor interested in your general health (e.g., Does she/he do a melanoma check on first visit and annually after that)?

4 What is the doctor's aesthetic when it comes to fillers and Botox? (Gerstner suggests looking for answers like "less is more," "rested," "healthy," "natural," "soft," and avoid doctors who believe in the "California, celebrity, red carpet, or big cheek" look.)

5 Is the doctor listening to your needs, desires, and bothersome skin issues rather than telling you what you need (the latter comes with time and trust)?

6 Does your doctor discuss all options for treating your particular skin issues?

7 Does the doctor ask you about your history of sun exposure and whether you have a family history of skin cancer?

diligently check your doctor's expertise . . .

the last frontier

I have to admit, there was a time when Botox and fillers were a lunch-time (or after work) maintenance thing with me, on the same schedule as getting my hair highlighted—pretty much every three or four months. But cosmetic surgery required a lot more thought, angst, and, in my case, a good dose of Catholic guilt about spending a boatload of money on this narcissistic pursuit. Facing the reality of getting a face-

Facing the reality of getting a facelift reached deeply into the dark side of my vanity: Was this unmentionable procedure full of deceit?

lift reached deeply into the dark side of my vanity: Was this unmentionable procedure full of deceit? Did it cross the line into my fears about aging and touch the underbelly of my lost youth? Was I in denial and didn't want to acknowledge it? Was I surrendering my notions about aging gracefully? I do know it treaded somehow uncomfortably on the frank territory that overlaps cosmetic products, which I use and believe in, and was perfectly happy to discuss, guilt-free.

When I finally made an appointment with a plastic surgeon, I was hoping the doctor would send me away with, "You don't really need my services." No such luck . . .

A good friend admitted to me that she had a facelift, so she was some help, but her face—which looked great—was not my face. Also, it didn't help that my imagination took flight with all the things that could go wrong. In the spirit of spilling it all, when it got to the point where I couldn't stand my neck anymore (and my dermatologist couldn't stand to hear my complaints any longer), I contacted Dr. Rosenberg, a New York City facial plastic surgeon who is part magician, part artist, part shrink. He talked me through all my fears and questions—I mean, can you imagine having me for a patient?

His brilliant hands have recrafted the face of many people, from politicians to movie stars to women like you and me. I kept telling myself it was only an informational meeting, because I was very nervous. I mean, God forbid something should happen to me on the operating table—what would my kids say when they learned how I'd met my final end? "Rest in peace, Mrs. Robinson. She died trying to get her neck back." No thank you!

Dr. R. got my anguish on this one immediately, and said, "Mrs. Robinson, you're afraid you won't wake up, right? I have never lost a patient and I assure you, you will not be the first." Suddenly, with that simple reassurance addressing the top of my fear list, I felt calmer. Ultimately I made the decision to move forward with the procedure. I'm not minimizing that it was costly and uncomfortable—recovery took about seven days in my case. But think of it this way: IT'S YOUR FACE! It's more expensive to buy a car than to fix your face—and you don't guzzle gas money, require collision insurance, or need a monthly parking space.

Here, some wise observations from Dr. Rosenberg that may ring familiar to those of you considering plastic surgery (even if it's only in secret, in your head). He says, "When women reach an age (usually in their late forties or early fifties) where, typically, their hormones start diminishing, they rapidly notice a change in their facial structure, and, over a very short period of time, they stop recognizing themselves in the mirror. So this vibrant, often fit person who is taking care of herself looks in the mirror, and, despite all her work, she sees a tired face. That starts to affect how she feels about herself . . . no matter how hard a woman works out, and how well she eats, the face ages at a certain point. There is often a dissatisfaction and a disconnect—'who is this person in the mirror?' And that starts to lead to a sense of loss—a loss of who they were physically."

He adds, "What makes people happy after surgery is that they've regained something, and they are able to extend that period in their lives where they feel vibrant and attractive. So there's a sense of well-being that comes from taking care of themselves, and seeing how well they can look again."

But think of it this way: IT'S YOUR FACE! It's more expensive to buy a car than to fix your face—and you don't guzzle gas money, require collision insurance, or need a monthly parking space.

His philosophy? "Youth is not the magic potion. What I'm trying to do is not necessarily make people look younger; I'm trying to make them look beautiful now. So that when they look in the mirror and see a reflection, it feels familiar, and they feel excited about what they see, and comfortable in their own skin" (if you've been following this book's ultimate message of "Look like yourself, only better," you'll recognize this sentiment!).

Don't be afraid to explore plastic surgery when considering your options; it's only a consultation, and the information you will acquire will make a huge difference in how you feel about proceeding—or not.

Dr. Rosenberg describes his consultation methods this way: "I always begin the same way, by asking a patient how I can help her. I hand them a mirror and ask her to identify what bothers her. It's a very big decision to think about having elective surgery, so I listen carefully and very quickly can assess how much surgery the patient can handle.

Most often, this opens a door, and she will ask me what I pick up on, and we 'walk through' her face together. I always underscore that the goal is to make her look as good as possible without a sign of surgery."

There is a case to be made for plastic surgery. It's not for everyone, but it may be for you. Don't be afraid to explore it when considering your options; it's only a consultation, and the information you will acquire will make a huge difference in how you feel about proceeding—or not. The consultation cost is most often deducted from the final bill when moving forward with the procedure, but I recommend getting two so you can compare physicians and approaches. And when you do, be sure to follow this . . .

BEAUTY TRUTH:

Cosmetic surgery is an acceptable option—just be smart about why, when, where, and with whom to choose it.

it's not for everyone . . .

Here are some questions you should always ask your doctor before committing to a plastic surgery procedure.

1 How many procedures like mine have you performed?

2 Can you show me before-and-after photos?

3 What are the risks associated with this procedure?

4 Are there alternative treatments for my issues?

5 What is the recovery like?

6 When will I begin to see results?

7 Where will you perform the surgery?

8 Is there anything that you recommend I do or take before the procedure to ensure better results or a quicker recovery?

9 Is the place accredited?

10 What type of anesthesia will you use?

11 What complications could occur?

12 Are you board certified?

13 What is the total fee, including you, your anesthesiologist, cost of the operating room, and any other assistance required?

And here are some questions that Dr. Rosenberg says you should ask yourself while meeting these doctors:

1 Is the place clean? Assess the atmosphere of the office.

2 Is the staff respectful and discreet?

3 Is there attention to detail? Is it a quiet, low-key, well-maintained environment?

He comments further, "Everything matters. This is about detail. To do surgery on someone, and do it well, you need to be a detail-oriented person. If you don't see an office that's run well, then you have to question the person who will be touching you—how will he or she run his operating room?"

know thyself

True, a few injections can iron out forehead creases and deliver plump cheeks. And while it's safe to assume that furrowed brows will never be in vogue, other issues like jowls and necks can require the scalpel, so choose treatments wisely—and sparingly.

If your motive is to trade in your physical identity for someone else—and if you think looking flawless means any actual flaws in your life will melt away after the surgery—you aren't being fair to yourself.

It's not about seeking perfection, it's about feeling better about yourself—the *Wabi-Sabi* way. And yes, while Angelina Jolie may be beautiful, she hasn't raised your kids or conquered your office issues, so forget about who's on the *Vanity Fair* cover and just do you because you are the best thing about YOU. Recognize that cosmetic surgery is an imperfect art—or, as Dr. Rosenberg puts it, "an individual surgeon performing a craft, working on a person's face within its limitations. The surgeon can only work with what he is given."

WHEN DONE FOR the right reasons and with a skillful surgeon, the results of a cosmetic procedure will be really satisfying. And the beauty of it all is that we can remain attractive at any age, whether it's from good genes, good decisions, good makeup or—when appropriate—good doctors.

we can remain attractive at any age . . .

YOU SHOULD KNOW

Here are a few tips from dermatologist Dr. Gervaise Gerstner about cosmetic enhancements and daily maintenance for treated skin:

If you're considering fillers (such as Restylane, or Juvéderm), she feels two vials of filler, max, should be used per visit.

If you're looking into peels, she favors glycolic peels over traditional facials (for value and results), and believes that the following three rituals help keep skin looking its best:

- Sunscreen daily

- Glycolic peel pads used three times a week

- Retin A (pea-size dose) once a week

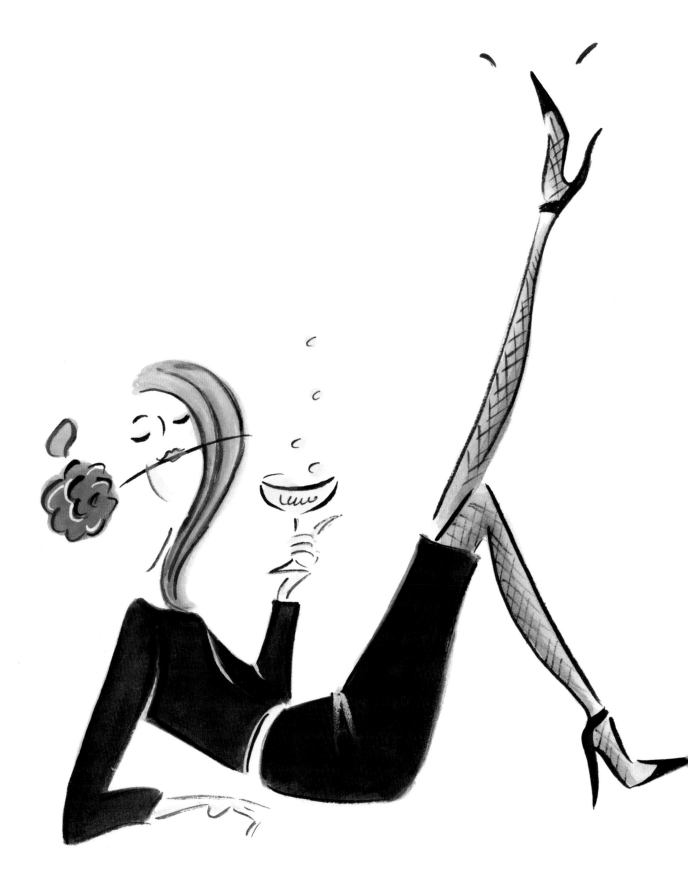

Sexy Doesn't Have an Age

I HAVE TO ADMIT IT . . . I LOOK FORWARD TO WATCHING THE GOLDEN GLOBES AND THE OSCARS TO SEE WHAT THE SCREEN GODDESSES ARE WEARING, AND EACH TIME I ADMIRE THE SMALL MIRACLES IN CELEBRITY MAKE OVERS.

I am always inspired—yes, inspired—when Janet has lost weight or Ellen's gotten a new haircut or Julianne has tried new eye makeup because it moves me to think about self-reinvention. I've watched them all age, with curiosity and appreciation for their transformations from girls to women—some more gracefully and honestly than others.

197

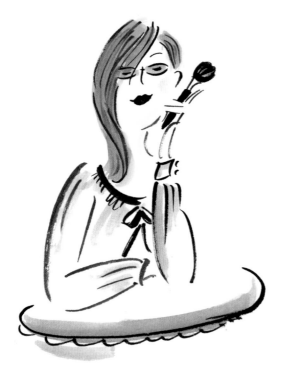

But . . . I've never been someone obsessed— I don't care about their trips to Starbucks or their pet's name, though I do confess to taking special notice of Meryl Streep. I mean, Meryl Streep is ridiculously attractive. Who among us didn't envy her portrayal of a fifty+ divorced woman in the movie *It's Complicated,* as her ex came begging for a second go around, ditching the younger second wife in the process? His slack jaw as Meryl dropped her robe is an image we should tape to our mirrors and embed in our brains, if only to remind ourselves of the last but definitely not least of my . . .

BEAUTY TRUTH:

Sexy doesn't have an age.

What I *do* think is true about sex appeal and beauty is this: Age is an asset that doesn't erase it; we are more confident now, and we are more appreciative of any physical gifts that we may possess. And after reading this book, we recognize that looking great is the only way to honor those gifts. We know that it is up to us to move beyond inertia to create the persona that matches our vision of how we'd like to present ourselves to ourselves, and to others, every day—it doesn't just happen by accident.

At the beginning of this book I challenged you to look in the mirror, sans makeup—and absorb what you see. Now that we're at the end of our journey together, I am going to ask you to do it again. So, put down this book, look in the mirror, and embrace the lines on your face. And damn it, really do it. Those lines are years of pleasure, tears, madness, and happiness. You have lived it and earned them. Do you remember your first wrinkle? I do. I remember getting my very first crow's foot after crying my broken heart out for days over a boyfriend. Ironically, he told a friend who bumped into him recently that I was the love of his life! Can you imagine? I still have that wrinkle, and he made me work hard for it, and it inhabits me daily, along with the rest of the personal history written on my face. Sometimes I ponder that perhaps I've erased part of my physical legacy with the facelift—but no, I don't think so. There are enough wrinkles left to keep that in place.

Personally, I take real pleasure in using the knowledge of cosmetics I have been privileged to acquire through a fantastic career and a good dose of curiosity. I unapologetically embrace and enjoy the feminine ritual of using cosmetics, and I believe that what my mother called "powder and paint" can do more for my face and my soul than any expensive cream. Makeup has real psychic value. On the days when I've made a real effort and someone who loves me tells me I look beautiful, I want to bottle that feeling.

I totally respect that for some women, cosmetics or fillers or plastic surgery have nothing to do with self-expression, but deeply understand how for others of us, a new tube of lipstick can make our day. You, only better . . . that's the mantra . . . think it each time you lift a tube of lipstick or eye pencil or blush compact from your cosmetic pouch. I thoroughly fess up to the notion that I am a very long drawn out makeover in progress, and suspect that if you have finished reading this book you know of what I speak.

Take it from a woman in the know: Some things do get better with age, and *we* are one of them!

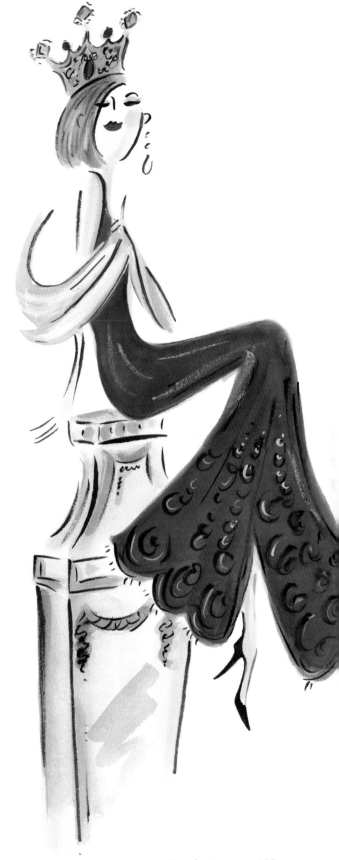

MY THANKS

SINCE THIS BOOK is as much about lessons learned along the winding road of a happy career as it is about the beautiful road ahead for all of us who are fifty and beyond, there are several people I would like to thank for making the path magnificent along the way and seeding it for all the "to comes."

First, not all men are created equal and not all men are "suits." Here are some brilliantly talented men who mentored, supported, and believed in me—I thank you profusely for that: Lindsay Owen-Jones, Alexander Liberman, Irving Penn, Gilles Weil, Ronald Perelman, Bob Nielsen, and Tom Ford, and my deepest gratitude goes to Ralph Lauren and Guy Peyrelongue for providing the happiest eight years of my career.

To some exceptional women who "wore the pants" when it came to creativity, friendship, and encouragement—huge thanks:

To Gloria Appel, my inspiration and cheerleader for so many pages of this book; to my *Mademoiselle* soul mates forever, Nonnie Moore, Sandy Horvitz, Deborah Turbeville, and Edie Locke; to Felicia Milewicz, who supported me on everything; to Midge Richardson, who challenged me

on everything; to my *Vogue* best friends, Grace Mirabella, editor extraordinaire, Jade Hobson, and special thanks to my dear friend and beauty colleague Dorothy Schefer Faux, how would this book have been possible without your encouragement?

To my agent at ICM, Kristyn Keene, who stepped up and stepped in where an agent can make magic and you did, and to Andy Barzvi, my former agent, thank you for believing in this project from the minute you saw it and for steering it through its incubation. Thanks also to Andy's able associate, Lindsay Hemphill.

To the thoughtful and wonderful gang at Seal Press, especially my lovely editor, Laura Mazer, and the talented, patient, and kind Merrik Bush-Pirkle, who improved everything I wrote; and to Brooke Warner, who loved and encouraged this project from the outset. I thank you all and ask you in the same sentence—how did you ever put up with my shenanigans?

If a picture is worth a thousand words, then this book should go into the Guinness Book of World Records. Chesley McLaren, your pictures say volumes, make us laugh, and add endless charm to my book. Thank you for your creative brilliance. And thank you to Amanda Davidson for your artful thoughts, organization, and hard work. To the production team at Seal Press—Jane Musser and Domini Dragoone—thank you for your collaborative spirit and creative book design.

To Ali MacGraw, who "tossed the gloss" long before this book was a concept, thank you for that—and to my readers, I say: You should know Ali's beauty is only trumped—no, scratch that, magnified—by her facile mind, her sense of humor, and the joy she takes in life.

I have the pleasure of knowing the best of the best experts and reaping the bounty of their wisdom, knowledge, and love of their expertise—that's why they are so good. Thank you, Dr. David Rosenberg, Dr. Michelle Warren, Dr. Gervaise Gerstner, Louis Licari, and Gad Cohen—I am honored by your presence in this book.

To Susan Trumpbour, Mary Maclean, Faran Krentcil, Claudia Herr, Fiorella Valdesolo, Kristina Stewart Ward, Dana Wood, Dale Burg, Karen Wilder, Holly Siegel, and Betty Beaument—I am so grateful for your valuable research, edits, suggestions, input, and general turns on a dime that you all made to bring shape to this book.

Last, I firmly assert that it does take a village and words cannot express the deep debt of gratitude to my family and friends, without whom I could not breathe. Thank you particularly to my friends Lara Modjeski, Pamela Pilkonis, Daniela Morera, Geoff Donaldson, and Jack Wiswall; and to my talented and brilliant son, Lucius—even though a mother should never brag, one and all, your gift of time, talent, and instinct helped enormously to bring this project into being.

ABOUT ANDREA Q. ROBINSON

ANDREA ROBINSON IS legendary in the fashion and beauty business.

In a career spanning more than forty years, she's revolutionized the way women look and the way they feel about beauty. From her early days as beauty editor of *Vogue*, fashion editor of *Mademoiselle*, and creative director of *Seventeen* magazine, to more recently managing the Ralph Lauren beauty brand and building the Tom Ford beauty business from scratch, Andrea has earned a reputation for always being an innovator. Andrea's personal mission in the beauty business has been to help women look like themselves, only better. This concept has driven her revolutionary beauty industry trends and fostered her passionate interest in cosmetics for her generation.

Andrea modernized the business of cosmetics by inventing the "naked" (or natural) makeup trend and the longwearing lipstick trend when she was president of Ultima II—both major beauty concepts that continue to engage the interest of women.

Andrea is also a business leader. As president of Ralph Lauren Fragrances, she worked hand-in-hand with Ralph Lauren during an eight-year period of unprecedented growth. She went on to launch the Tom Ford Fragrance and Beauty business for Estée Lauder—in addition to assuming the role of Chief Marketing Officer at Estée Lauder.

Andrea has served on the boards of Cosmetic Executive Women and The Fashion Group International, and has been recognized as an innovative business leader with multiple awards such as Cosmetic Executive Women's Legend and Leaders Award, Women's Wear Daily's Marketing Innovator of the Year Award, and several FIFI awards (the Oscars of the beauty industry) for "Fragrance Star of the Year."

Andrea has two adult children and lives in New York City.

SELECTED TITLES FROM SEAL PRESS

Yogalosophy: 28 Days to the Ultimate Mind-Body Makeover, by Mandy Ingber. $18.00, 978-1-58005-445-4. Celebrity yoga instructor Mandy Ingber offers a realistic, flexible, daily plan that will help readers transform their minds, their bodies, and their lives.

For Keeps: Women Tell the Truth About Their Bodies, Growing Older, and Acceptance, edited by Victoria Zackheim. $15.95, 978-1-58005-204-7. This inspirational collection of personal essays explores the relationship that aging women have with their bodies.

The 3-Day Reset: Restore Your Cravings For Healthy Foods in Three Easy, Empowering Days, by Pooja Mottl. $22.00, 978-1-58005-527-7. These 10 simple resets target and revamp your eating habits in practical, three-day increments.

Rescue Me, He's Wearing a Moose Hat: And 40 Other Dates After 50, by Sherry Halperin. $13.95, 978-1-58005-068-5. The hilarious account of a woman who finds herself back in the dating scene after midlife.

About Face: Women Write about What They See When They Look in the Mirror, edited by Anne Burt and Christina Baker Kline. $15.95, 978-1-58005-246-7. 25 women writers candidly examine their own faces—and each face has a story to tell.

Hot & Heavy: Fierce Fat Girls on Life, Love & Fashion, by Virgie Tovar. $16.00, 978-1-58005-438-6. A fun, fresh anthology that celebrates positive body image, feeling comfortable in one's own skin, and being fabulously fine with being fat.

Find Seal Press Online
www.SealPress.com
www.Facebook.com/SealPress
Twitter: @SealPress

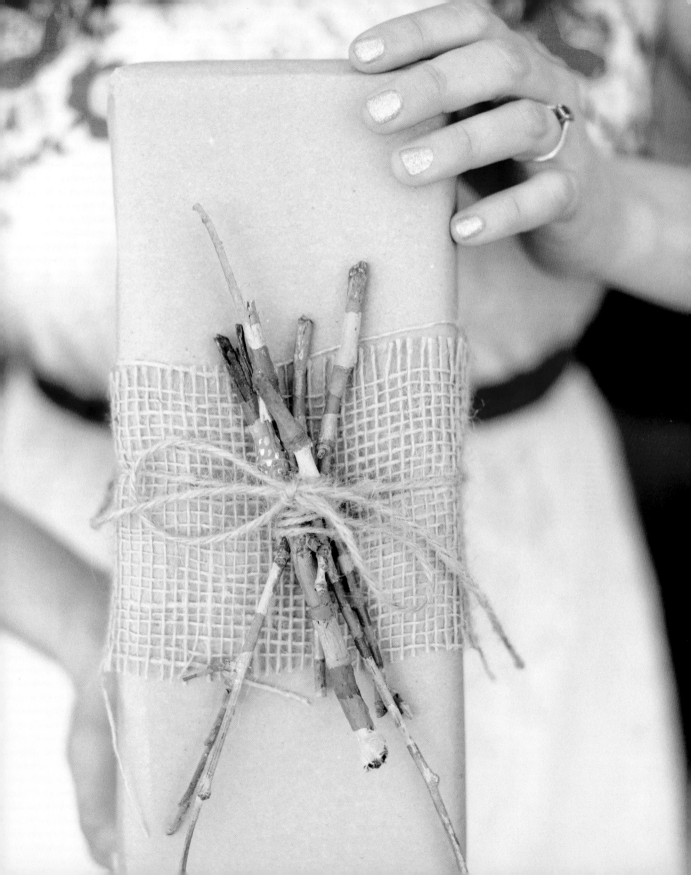

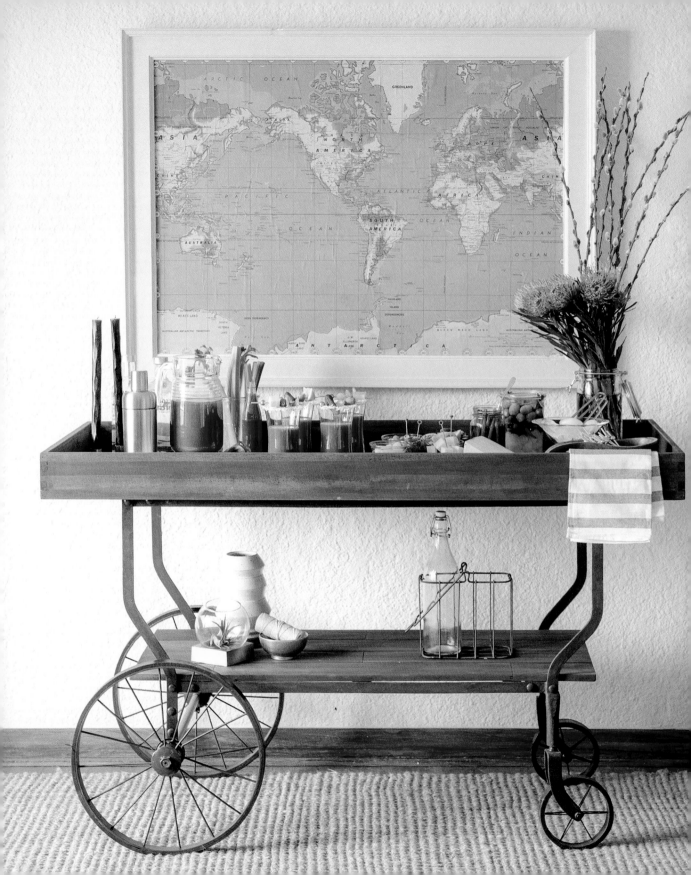

Pretty Prudent
HOME

Your Ultimate Guide to Creating
a Beautiful Family Home

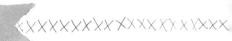

JACINDA BONEAU &
JAIME MORRISON CURTIS

STEWART, TABORI & CHANG | NEW YORK

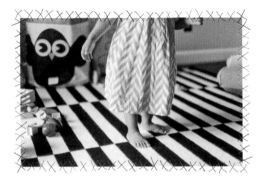

Published in 2015 by Stewart, Tabori & Chang
An imprint of ABRAMS

Text copyright © 2015 Jacinda Boneau and Jaime Morrison Curtis
Photographs copyright © Ainsley / Carlisle, unless otherwise noted on page 223.
Illustrations ©2015 Sonya Lee Benham

Library of Congress Control Number: 2014942989
ISBN: 978-1-61769-154-6

Editor: Rebecca Kaplan
Designer: Sarah Gifford
Production Manager: True Sims

The text of this book was composed in Fournier, Balance, and Bryant.

Printed and bound in the United States
10 9 8 7 6 5 4 3 2 1

Stewart, Tabori & Chang books are available at special discounts when purchased in quantity
for premiums and promotions as well as fundraising or educational use. Special editions can also be
created to specification. For details, contact specialsales@abramsbooks.com or the address below.

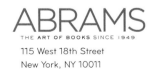

ABRAMS
THE ART OF BOOKS SINCE 1949

115 West 18th Street
New York, NY 10011
www.abramsbooks.com

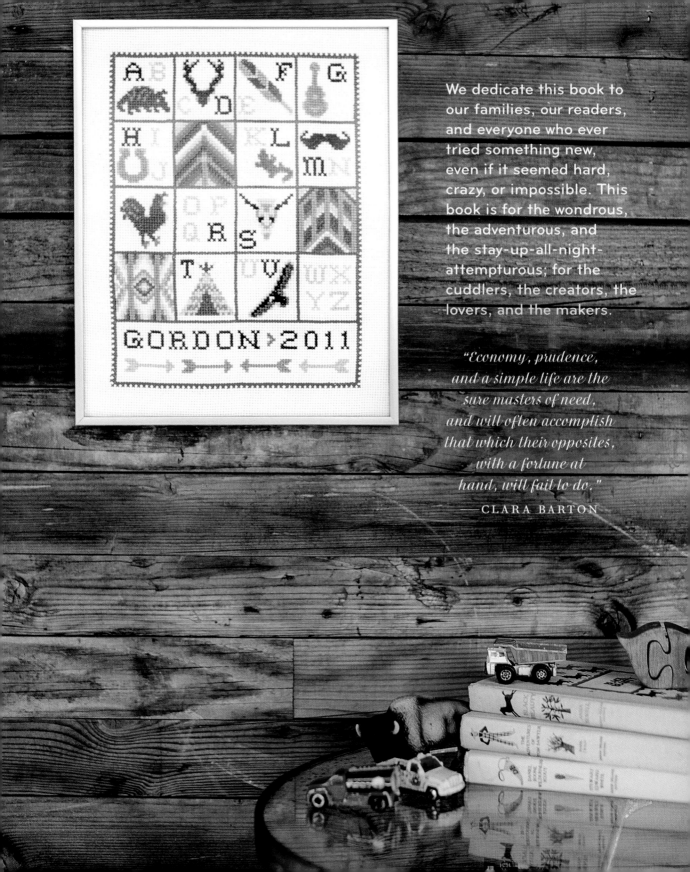

We dedicate this book to our families, our readers, and everyone who ever tried something new, even if it seemed hard, crazy, or impossible. This book is for the wondrous, the adventurous, and the stay-up-all-night-attempturous; for the cuddlers, the creators, the lovers, and the makers.

"Economy, prudence, and a simple life are the sure masters of need, and will often accomplish that which their opposites, with a fortune at hand, will fail to do."
—CLARA BARTON

contents

INTRODUCTION WHAT IS A PRUDENT HOME? 9

the prudent home

Peek into Prudent Homes 12
Finding Your Style 24
Planning Your Space 28
Defining Your Palette 36

pretty prudent décor

Vintage Finds & Thrift Store DIYs 42
Decorating from the Hardware Store 70
Walls, Floors & Windows 78
Pillows & Linens 96
The Details 112

prudent entertaining

134 Party Planning
138 Tabletop Design
152 Wall Décor
160 Around-the-Clock Entertaining
175 For the Host
182 That's a Wrap

a prudent family

190 Creating Special Spaces for Kids
204 Making Family Time

PATTERNS & TEMPLATES 220

CONTRIBUTORS & PHOTO CREDITS 223

ACKNOWLEDGMENTS 224

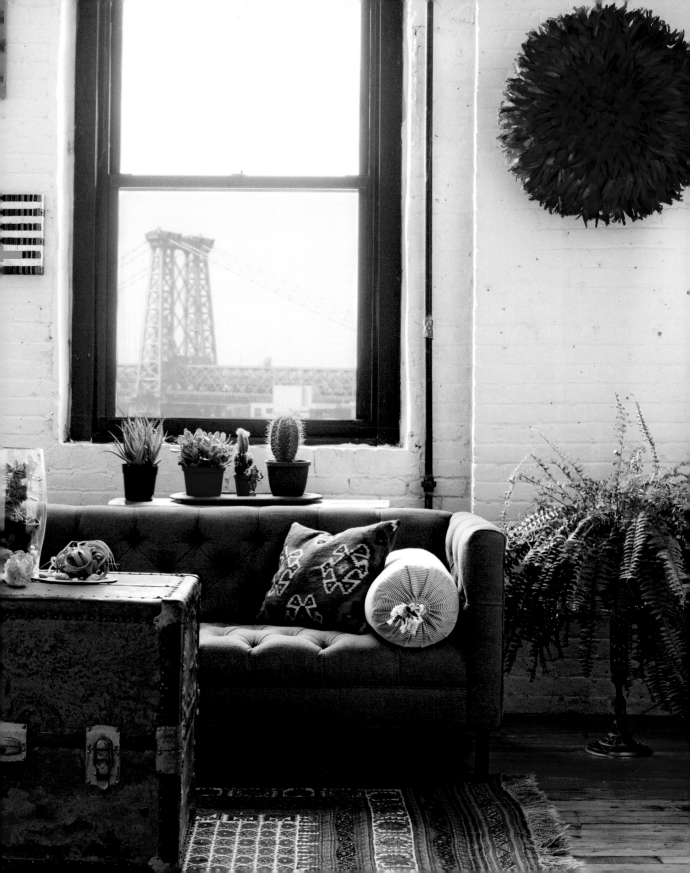

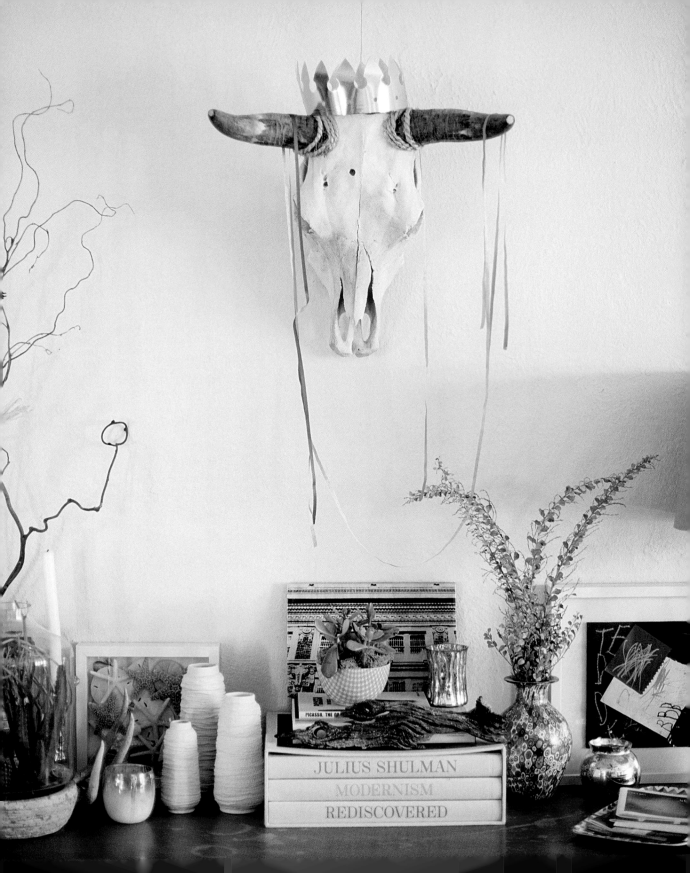

WHAT IS A PRUDENT HOME?

A prudent home is lovingly handmade with attention to detail and care for the future. It is a family place that is beautiful, comfortable, and functional: rich in everything that matters.

Prudence, as an ideal, is about more than the simple pinching of pennies. It's a way of living in which we consciously invest ourselves wisely toward future returns. When it comes to shaping our homes, families, and lives, we can't help but contribute more than just money. We invest our time, sweat, attention, and love. And while the returns we generate don't come in the form of dividends, they are the most meaningful rewards, both tangible and immeasurable.

When we devote ourselves to designing our family homes and creating household occasions, we believe that what we're really doing is building our ideal life itself, bit by bit, stitch by stitch, and moment by moment. For the prudent, a do-it-yourself project is not only a means to an end. The time spent creating is a meditation, and the final result is a reflection of who we believe ourselves to be and a contemplation of the family we think we can become. We are the creators of our own prudent worlds. We are not just making things, we are making memories.

1

the prudent *home*

You live in a place. Maybe it's a house you own, maybe it's an apartment you rent, maybe it's a loft or a tent or a tree house. To you (and to us, if you would just invite us over already), it feels like home. Your family is with you, your routine is established, and all is well in the world. You have everything that you need. Your life is good; it's actually so good that when you stop to think about it, you can't help but feel grateful for everything that you have. It's all so fortuitous, and you are so fortunate. We agree.

Still, sometimes, you think about home improvements or redecorating or making stuff—because it looks like fun, and you need a hobby, and you think your kids might benefit from a new desk on which to do their homework (so why not make them the perfect desk in their favorite shade of aqua?). It's just a seed of an idea that spills out while searching and pinning in your off-hours, borne of your desire to make actual things and your unspoken, but ever-present, desire to make everything even better for your family in every way possible. But how do you start on that path? And once you open that door, how do you avoid getting swallowed up by all the things you might want and narrow your focus to the things you can really do?

We're here to help. To begin, we suggest you first take a step back and paint a personal picture of your prudent home. Find practical points and inspirational exercises to focus your planning, and have some fun figuring out where house design and home life intersect in your heart.

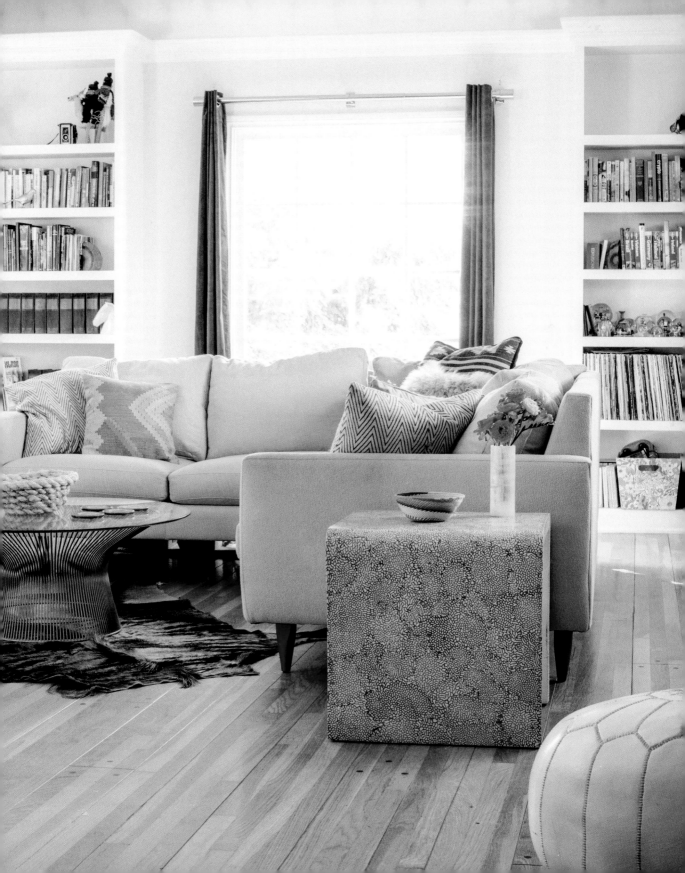

peek into prudent homes

It's so fun to sneak a peek inside the homes of people who inspire you—real people who have given great thought to the elegance and function of their family living spaces. We've gathered some of our favorites here. Ranging from sleek modern spaces to cozy antique-filled abodes, these intriguing homes exemplify the principles of prudent decorating.

See FINDING YOUR STYLE quiz on page 24 to discover your own style profile.

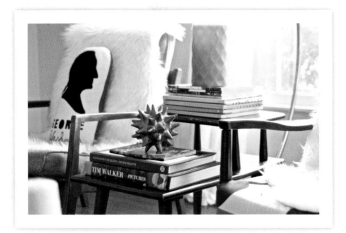

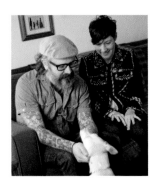

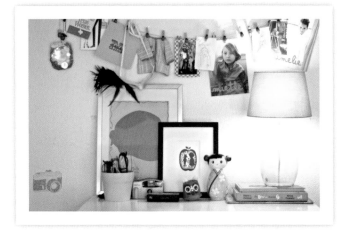

CHRISTINE & STEVEN VISNEAU

Christine and Steven Visneau are the owners of VEE CARAVAN, a shop for unique, organized living (veecaravan.com). She's a stylist and he's a fashion photographer, and together they share a cozy mid-century-inspired home in Dallas, Texas, with their two young daughters. Creative and eclectic choices in décor mix with everyday necessities presented in a clean and organized way to make their home a comfortable and inspiring space to raise a family in style.

★ MODERNIST + ECLECTIC ENTHUSIAST

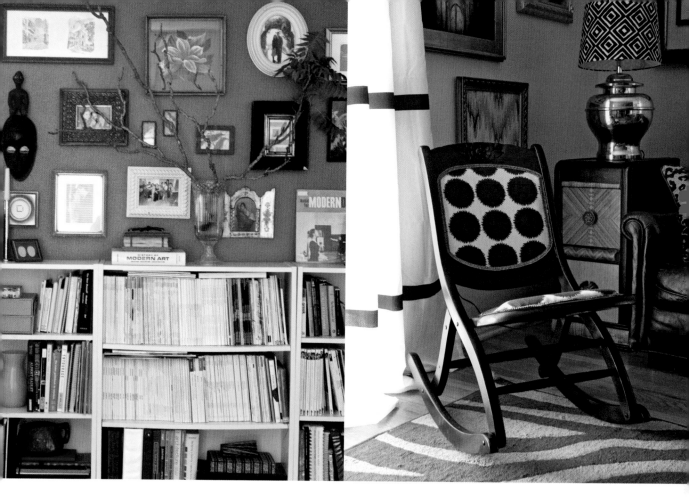

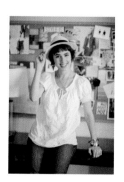

HILARY & DAVID WALKER

Fort Worth, Texas–based photo stylists and bloggers Hilary and David Walker (ourstylestories.com) have built a home brimming with vintage finds, travel treasures, and exquisite fine art. We love how photographer Hilary brings her displays together with casual organization.

★ THRIFTER + ECLECTIC ENTHUSIAST

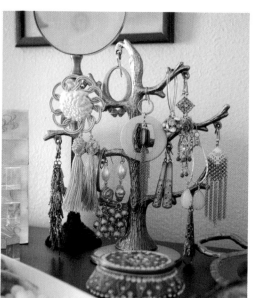

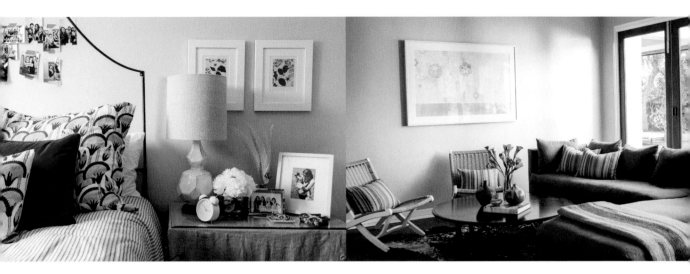

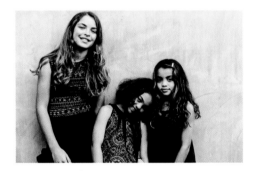

ANDREA & STEVE STANFORD

Artisanal touches, from hand-carved beams to curved built-ins, make the home of Andrea Stanford a stunner. She and her husband, Steve, have complemented the architecture of their Beverly Hills, California, abode with a carefully curated selection of antiques, family heirlooms, and rich textures. Their space feels opulent, yet clean and uncluttered. The couple's furniture selections reflect their modern sensibilities while referencing a sense of history that surely makes their three daughters, Ryan, Brooke, and Jade, feel grounded.

★ TRADITIONALIST + MODERNIST

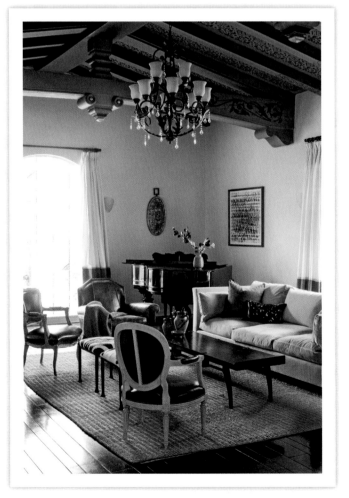

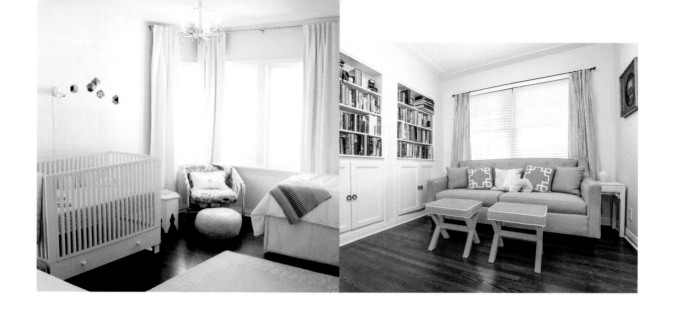

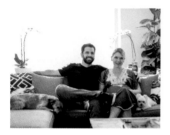

NINA & DARYL BERG

Touches of Hollywood Regency style including metallic wallpaper and high-lacquer furniture make this California bungalow a stunning space for entertaining both indoors and out. And no-nonsense elements like a farmhouse sink and bare hardwood floors make Nina and Daryl's first home family-friendly for their pets and first child, newborn daughter Lennox.

★ GLAMOURIST + TRADITIONALIST

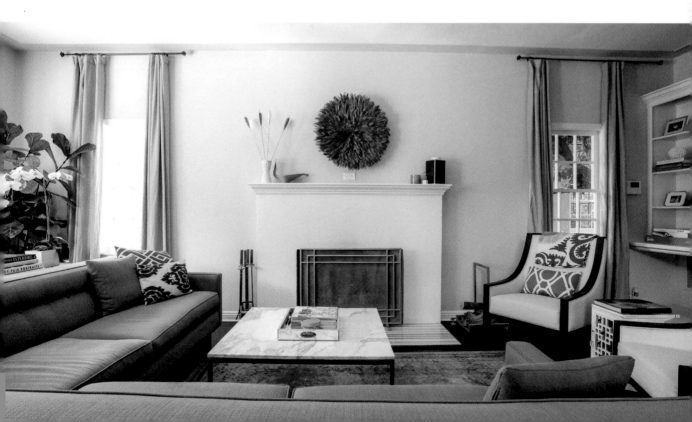

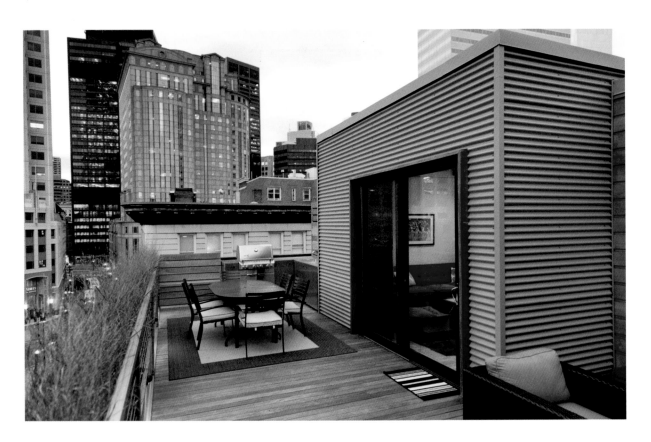

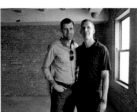

BRAD BLAKE & ALAN GOVE

When the top story of the renovated mill in Boston, Massachusetts, they call home went up for sale, Brad and Alan made a bold move. The couple purchased the penthouse and busted through its roof to create a two-story dwelling and rooftop deck overlooking the city.

★ MODERNIST

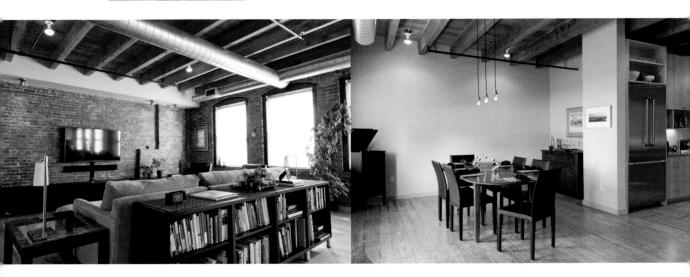

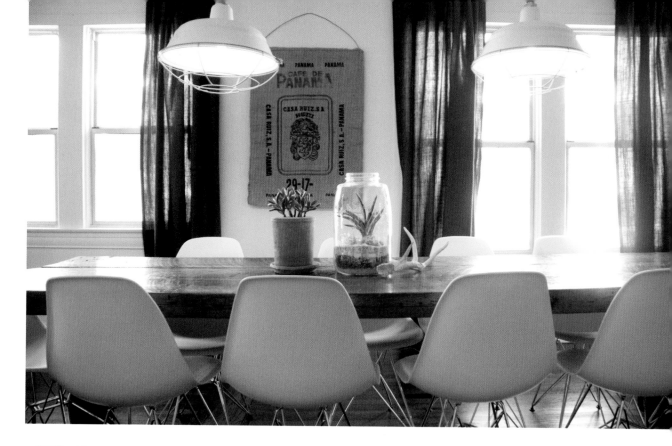

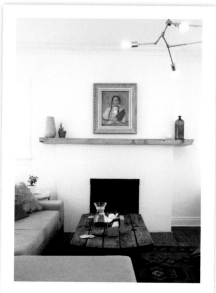

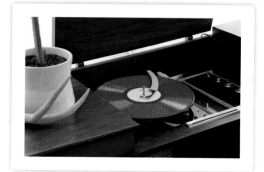

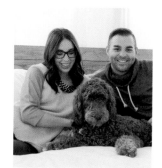

SARA & ROCKY GARZA

Beautiful sunlight fills the home of photographers Sara and Rocky Garza (saraandrocky.com; ourcozycasa.com). White walls unify the rooms of their Dallas, Texas, bungalow and create the perfect modern base for their carefully curated collection of artisanal finds, iconic furniture, and rustic touches.

★ MODERNIST + RANCHIST

ÝR KÁRADÓTTIR & ANTHONY BACIGALUPO

Overlooking the forest on one side and the harbor of Hafnarfjörður, Iceland, on the other, this 1896 cottage features original exposed oak beams and beautiful natural light. Ýr and Anthony, owners of Reykjavík Trading Co. (reykjaviktrading.com), also share a small home studio where they can spend some work days away from their workshop and closer to their young daughter. This minimalist home, decorated with a mixture of Scandinavian design and vintage American elements found on trips to Anthony's native California, makes us want to toss everything we own and start fresh.

★ MODERNIST + ECLECTIC ENTHUSIAST

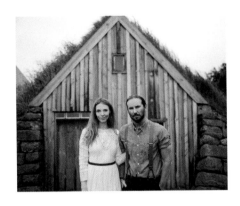

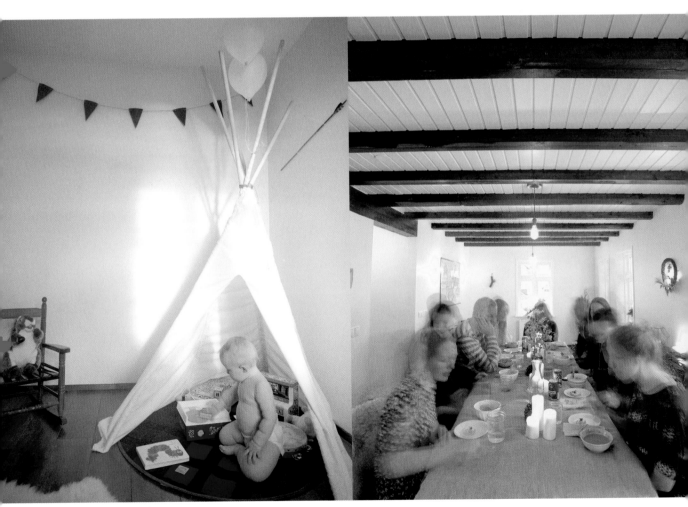

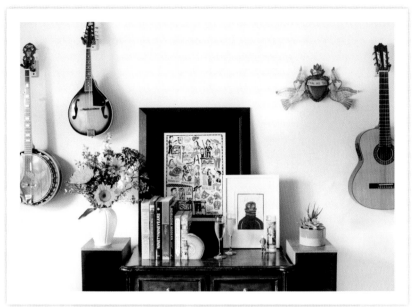

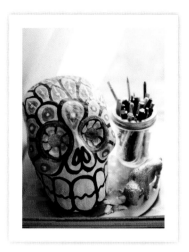

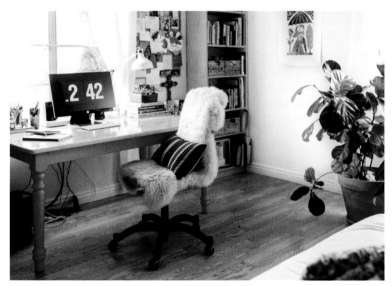

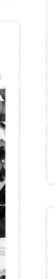

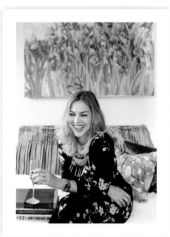

LAUREN KELP

The Phoenix, Arizona, home of stylist Lauren Kelp (laurenkelp
.com) is dappled with southwestern- and Mexican-inspired treasures,
making this otherwise clean space lively and fun. Lauren grew up
with two artists as parents, and it shows in her ability to craft a space
filled with art, beautiful books, and creative inspiration.

★ RANCHIST + THRIFTER

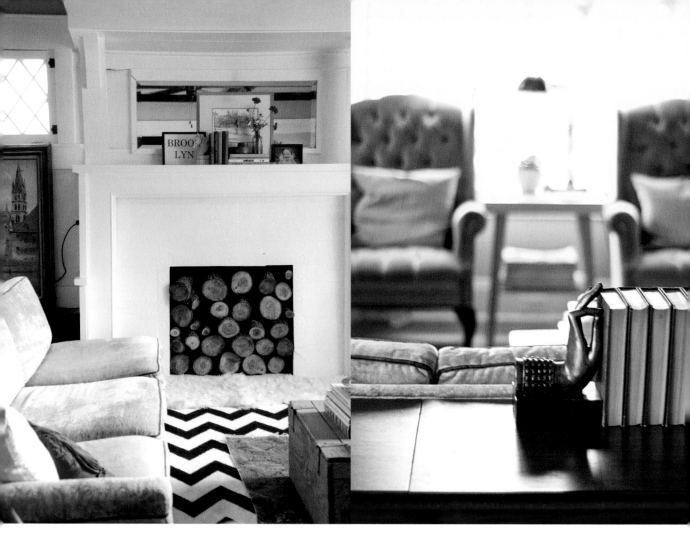

MISTY SPENCER

Misty Spencer's beautiful abode proves that you don't
have to give up sophisticated style when you have
kids. Touches like rich navy walls, glamorous lighting,
and vintage furniture in rich luxurious fabrics give
this home an elegant, yet comfortable, style. We love
how Misty uses black and white stripes as a repeating
design element throughout the house.

★ TRADITIONALIST + GLAMOURIST

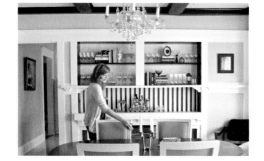

Seven Principles of Prudent Decorating

The prudent aesthetic is about investing in the right items and projects to make your vision come to life. We've found these seven principles can be universally applied to any household on any budget. Use these guidelines as a jumping-off point to decide what to keep, what to buy, and what to DIY.

1 WORK WITH WHAT YOU HAVE

Perhaps it's a family heirloom like your great-grandfather's clock, or maybe it's a couch you don't love but can't afford to replace. Take a look at what you have to start with and build up from there. There's no piece you can't incorporate into your current style with a little creative thinking.

2 SHUFFLE IT UP

Often a simple re-imagining of a room's layout is all you need. Sometimes you'll find that one object (a bar cart) can serve a whole new purpose (voilà, an end table!), or that an area rug from the bedroom can give your living room new life.

3 SELECT INVESTMENT PIECES

Every now and then you need to go all-out for that one item you love—say a vintage kilim rug, a statement chandelier, or a piece of quality artwork. Save your pennies for those pieces you know you and your family will treasure for lifetimes to come.

LEFT: This blue couch had been lived in and loved, but once a kid came into the picture, it proved too small for the whole family to snuggle on. In fact, with the whole house feeling too small, they transformed their breakfast nook into a guest room. When the priorities for this family's space changed, they shuffled the furniture as well, ending up with a room both useful and comfortable.

CENTER: For those lucky enough to live in a warm climate year-round, outdoor space acts as an extra room in a home; albeit a more finicky one. For families that spend a significant amount of time outdoors, investing in patio furniture that is both beautiful and sturdy against the elements (even if it's just wind, dust, and the occasional sprinkle) is a logical choice. These handwoven rattan chairs may have cost more up front, but they've proven worthy of the investment years later.

RIGHT: This painting was paid for over the course of seven years through the Los Angeles County Museum of Art's rental and sales gallery, where artworks are professionally curated and then offered on a rent-to-own basis. For a young couple just starting out, this painting, which cost thousands of dollars and took years to purchase, deserves a perch in the heart of their home.

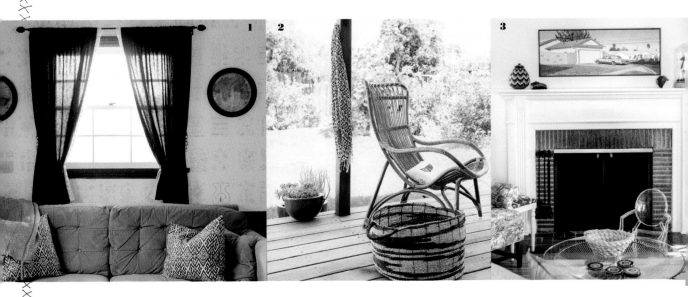

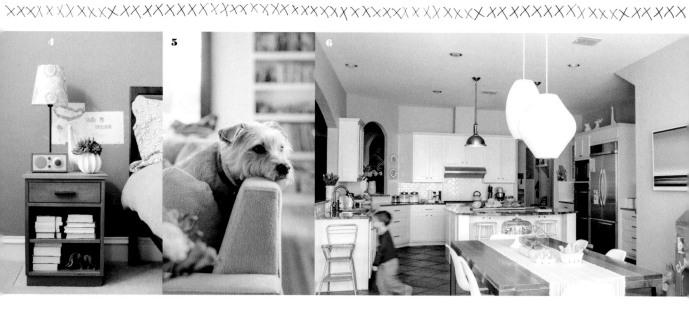

4 CHOOSE BUDGET PIECES

There are great deals to be had on high-design items. The trick is mixing and matching, so your home doesn't look like the store catalog. When you choose the right inexpensive pieces to complement your thrifts, gifts, and splurges, no one will ever know the difference.

An Ikea lampshade and nightstand look positively in-place when complemented with hand-sewn pillow shams and handmade children's drawings. Keep everything full yet coordinated (turning mismatched books so the white pages face out is a great designer trick for un-cluttering a space).

5 LOOK FOR COMFORT AND DURABILITY

The prudent home is meant to be lived in, which means comfort is key. A family doesn't want a couch so stiff it prevents snuggles, or a tablecloth so delicate no one is allowed to eat on it. Know which items your family will use frequently—which rugs will get the most wear, which bedspread will be jumped on, which tables will get covered in crayon—and choose pieces that can withstand the wear.

Princess Cheese may be a rugged street nugget, but she still needs a soft place to lay her head. This sturdy couch gives her a perfect view of any potential intruders with upholstery that handle dirty paws.

6 READY FOR ANY OCCASION

Think about how your family celebrates special moments and every day occasions throughout the year and design your home to adjust easily and inexpensively for those events. If you like to cook and throw dinner parties, your kitchen and dining area are a spending priority. Indulge in extra seating areas and stock up on serving platters. What kind of family are you—do you cozy up on the couch and watch movies? Do you have a collection you love to share with guests? Do you need a quiet spot to paint? Arrange your furniture around the way that you live with purpose and prudence.

A dining room is often the one space that manages to stay orderly and welcoming (unless the table doubles as your desk), while the kitchen usually manages to stay a mess. Make an effort to keep one clear surface, while adding a few well-thought out accents like extra seating means you will always be ready to entertain a group of friends or gather for an intimate family meal.

7 SOMETHING FOR EVERYONE

Sometimes it feels like it's their world, and you just live in it. Now you are out to build a home that meets everyone's needs. Agreeing with your partner on décor you both are comfortable with, or agreeing to create separate spaces within your home to express yourselves are equally good solutions. Then there's making sure the kids have room to grow too . . . combining the two.

This loft living room/dining room is masculine enough for Grant, but whimsical enough for our managing editor, Colleen. The dark walls, vibrant couch, and romantic touches (like black-and-white photography and hanging dried florals) reveal the blend of hearts and styles that make this space a home.

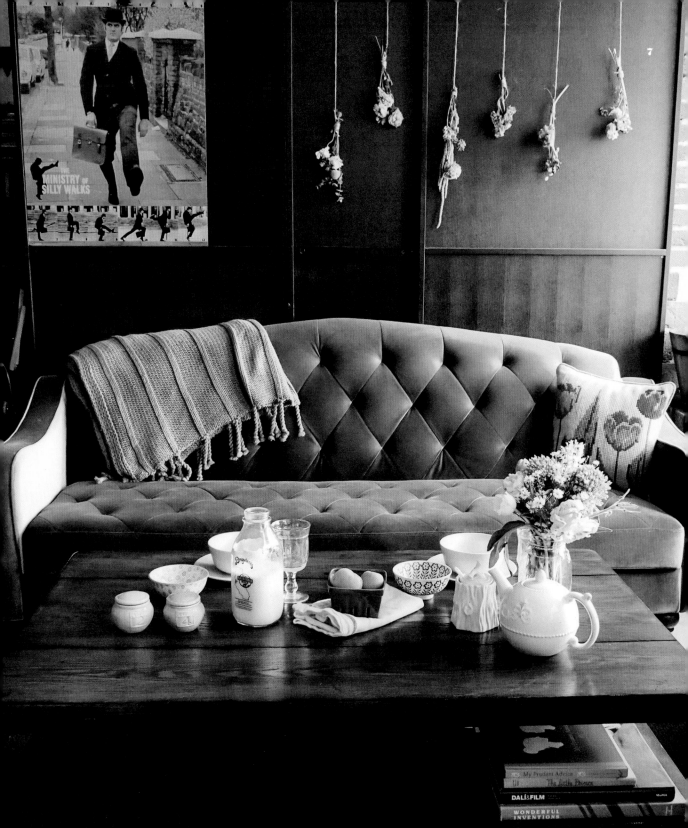

finding your style

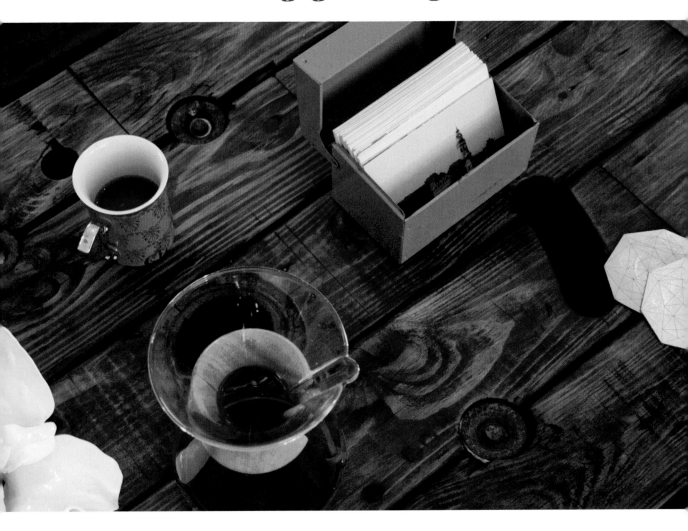

Although we resist the urge to categorize homes and those who curate them into style profiles, we believe that understanding what attracts you, inspires you, and makes you most comfortable can help you confidently move ahead with building a beautiful and functional family home.

Here are eight mood boards created to represent the décor styles we see most often. Take our completely unscientific quiz and find out which team you play for—there are no winners or losers in this game; it's merely an exercise in decorating self-awareness.

HOW TO PLAY:

1 For each item on pages 25–26, give yourself a score of 0 for "no," 1 for "maybe," and 2 for "yes."
2 Add up your scores from each quadrant.
3 Based on your totals, read about your style profile on page 27. You might be a mixture of several different styles.
4 Contemplate what it all means.
5 Take a nap.

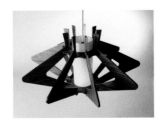

0 1 2

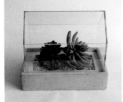

0 1 2

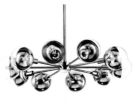

0 1 2

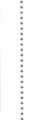

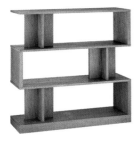

0 1 2

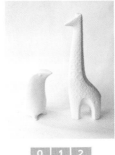

0 1 2

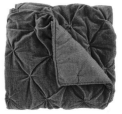

0 1 2

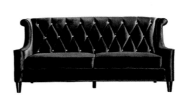

0 1 2

1

2

3

4

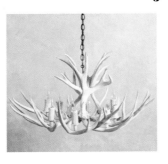

0 1 2

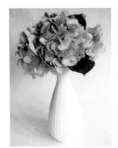

0 1 2

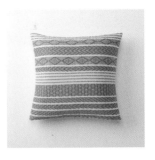

0 1 2

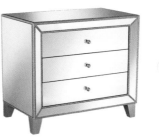

0 1 2

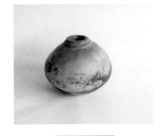

0 1 2

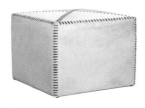

0 1 2

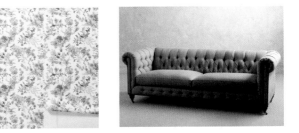

0 1 2

THE PRUDENT HOME

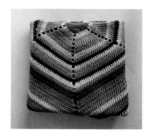

0 1 2

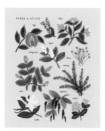

0 1 2

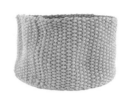

0 1 2

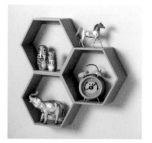

0 1 2

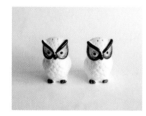

0 1 2

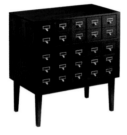

0 1 2

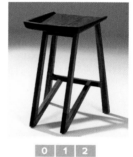

0 1 2

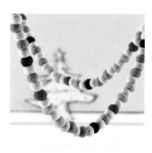

0 1 2

5 **6**

7 **8**

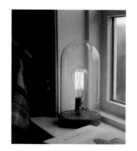

0 1 2

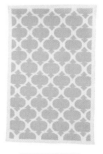

0 1 2

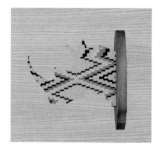

0 1 2

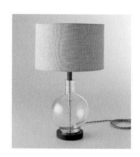

0 1 2

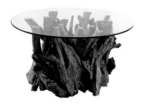

0 1 2

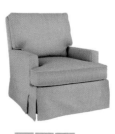

0 1 2

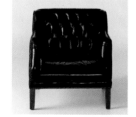

0 1 2

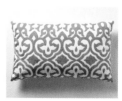

0 1 2

1 MODERNIST

You are a purist. A blank white wall is worth a thousand words. If you had cats, they would be named Nelson and Eames, but you don't have cats because they haven't designed a litter box that works with your laundry room aesthetic. Marble and leather are considered texture. A *former* friend once gave your daughter a talking princess mirror for her birthday.

2 GLAMOURIST

There is never a bad spot for a chandelier, and animal prints never go out of style. When you build your dream house, your closet will have a shoe island and flocked velvet wallpaper. When your girlfriends come over for brunch, they can expect that you have pulled out your gold-plated Jonathan Adler napkin rings and arranged an amazing display of roses and peonies. Not only do said friends present hostess gifts, you present guest gifts. Your dog wears cashmere.

3 RANCHIST

If your heart is too tender for a full-on deer mount, you have scattered shed antlers on several horizontal surfaces. Pendleton is your friendleton. Birch isn't just a tree, it's a wallpaper, a vase, and generally your surface pattern of choice. Tree stumps are end tables, and you use a piece of driftwood as a jewelry holder. Speaking of which, your jewelry collection is made entirely of bone, feathers, and animal teeth. You have a teepee in your backyard, next to your chicken coop.

4 TRADITIONALIST

You have furniture that requires polish. Your adult bed is the same brass bed that you used as a child, and the same brass bed your mother used as a child, except with a new mattress. You are patiently awaiting the inevitable resurgence of Laura Ashley. There is no wiser investment piece than a Persian rug, and TVs are meant to hide in armoires, not be seen or heard. Watercolor landscapes adorn your walls, as do photos of several long-deceased relatives. In fact, they might be complete strangers to which you have no relation.

5 THRIFTER

Milk glass is your white whale. There is no better way to spend a Saturday than at an estate sale, rummaging through the pristine linens that some ungrateful nephew has recently inherited. You don't feel guilty—you are giving them a good home. Your friends and family have finally accepted that "Wait, back up!" means that someone has abandoned an amazing nightstand curbside. You start collections of globes and thermoses just to have an excuse to hunt. You have a paint-by-number, which was painted by a stranger, hanging in your house. You were probably the first of your friends to get bangs and have strongly considered stealing bowling shoes.

6 MAKER

"I could totally make that!" will be engraved on your tombstone. Heck, why not buy the granite now and do it yourself?! You are the reason stores have "No Photography" signs. Bedding is home sewn, birthday invitations are assembled with washi tape, birthday cakes are made exclusively at 3 A.M., and you have either spray paint or Mod Podge under one of your fingernails as you are reading this. People are constantly asking you to do everything from make them an Easter wreath to hem their pants. Don't they know that you have three baby afghans to crochet by June and a half-whittled toy walrus to carve? If you were to get a tattoo, it would involve scissors, a spool of thread, or the name of your blog in cross-stitch.

7 ECLECTIC ENTHUSIAST

You don't need no stinking mood board. Your home is a reflection of your own personal life. A weaving from your honeymoon in Mexico hangs next to a velvet painting of Dolly Parton. It works because it's all about the people who live there. There is no master plan, you just add things as you go and move them around on a whim. Your perplexed husband is staring at your newly painted orange coffee table at this very moment. Sometimes it works, sometimes it doesn't, but that's OK because nothing is permanent.

8 IMPRESSIONIST

You do not care about decorating, making junk, or thread count. Someone gave you this book as a gift because they assumed you love to decorate when they noticed that your house looks like a beautiful page from a catalog. That is because one day you had five minutes on your lunch break and quickly ordered everything shown on a spread in a catalog titled *U-Taupe-ia*. You are only reading this book right now because you are hiding from your kids in the bathroom. You have better things to do than match the rug with the drapes. Let's have a drink.

planning your space

Even the most confident interior design mavericks like to have a plan. Typically that starts with a mood or inspiration board. Mood boards can be used to share your vision with clients/cohabitators, they can help keep you on track, and most importantly, they give you an idea of what an area will look like as a finished space. Here are some of the ways we have seen skilled amateurs and professional decorators collect and organize their ideas and inspiration into a visual representation of a space.

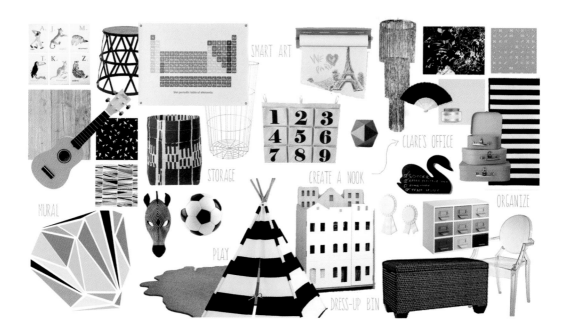

CURATION WEBSITES

The easiest and most flexible inspiration board tool is a free online curation website. Pinterest (pinterest.com) or Keep (keep.com) users can build inspiring boards for each room in their house and fill them with beautiful ideas and objects for designing their space.

pros: Easy to use; portable on a smartphone; linked to purchasing destination.

cons: Colors and textures are not accurate, making it more difficult to visualize a finished space; limited flexibility in reorganizing items and controlling scale; all inspiration must exist digitally.

MOOD BOARD APPLICATIONS

Online mood board tools like SampleBoard (sampleboard. com) are so great that even the professionals are using them to collect, organize, and share their boards. Not only does SampleBoard let you publish a portfolio of your boards, but the site also collects all of the product links and prices in addition to providing a place for you to keep notes. Its capabilities rival those of Photoshop except that SampleBoard is simple to use and requires no training. You can remove backgrounds, correct images, add text, and resize and crop images with ease.

pros: Easy to use; portable, professional-looking boards with total visual control; ability to easily share online via social networks or by email.

cons: Monthly fees starting at $25; colors and textures are not accurate.

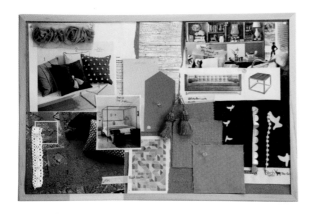

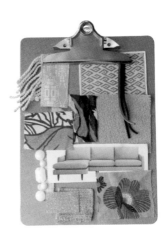

THE CLASSIC CORKBOARD

If you are inspired by a tactical experience and a mood board just won't do without swatches of upholstery fabric and paint chips, you might not be ready to go digital. A corkboard allows you to tear pages from magazines and catalogs and it gives you an excuse to use those cute fabric-covered thumbtacks you couldn't live without. With your new space on display, you will have the opportunity to see how it feels long-term.

pros: A break from the screen; true color swatches; easy to revise and revisit.

cons: You will probably end up taking a digital photo of your analog mood board to post online.

THE CLIPBOARD

Like the corkboard but more portable, the clipboard has the added features of a no-fuss clip and a convenient hole for hanging. They look pretty displayed in a row on the wall.

pros: You will look like you mean business (if your business is coaching a basketball team) with a clipboard. They are a no-fuss way to collect and replace inspiring photos in a portable format that can also be put on display.

cons: They can easily become overrun and disorganized; also you may look like a basketball coach.

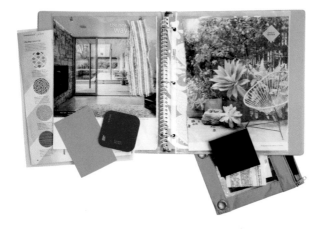

THE BINDER

For hardcore decorating projects like building or redecorating an entire home, the three-ring binder is still king. Create a tab for every room. Add photos of the space, receipts, and budget spreadsheets. Plastic sleeves can hold fabric swatches, paint chips, and carpet samples. You will not go anywhere without the binder. Five years from now when you want to retouch the paint in the mudroom, you will have an entire reference guide to everything in your house.

pros: An organization nerd's fantasy, the binder will put your fancy label maker to work. It gives you everything at your fingertips and is totally portable. You will have a complete record of all home-related products. The binder can be a stunning visual scrapbook of your decorating journey that you can leave on the coffee table and share with unsuspecting visitors or a bare-bones workhorse for your eyes only.

cons: Don't lose the binder.

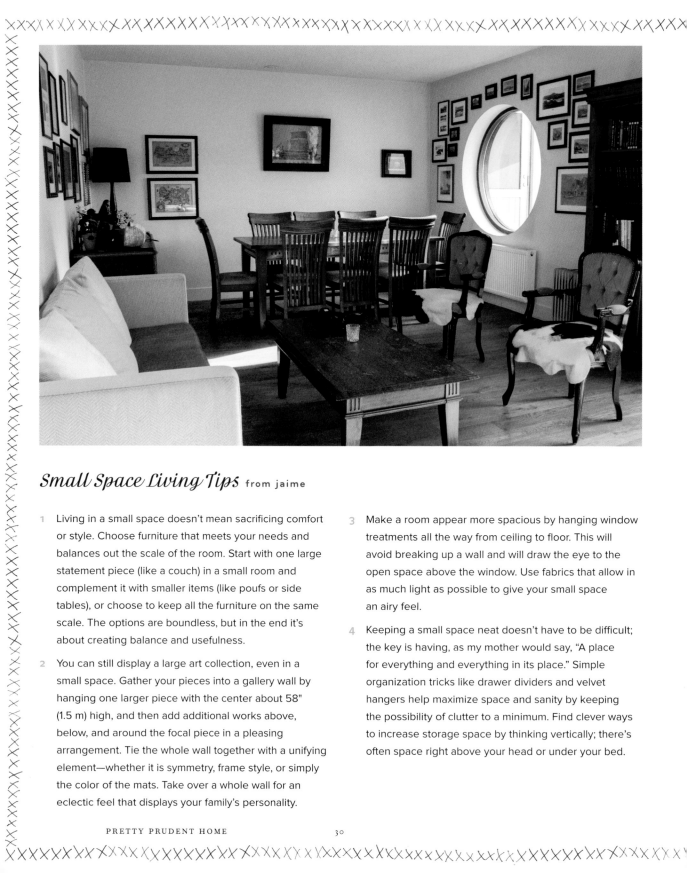

Small Space Living Tips from jaime

1 Living in a small space doesn't mean sacrificing comfort or style. Choose furniture that meets your needs and balances out the scale of the room. Start with one large statement piece (like a couch) in a small room and complement it with smaller items (like poufs or side tables), or choose to keep all the furniture on the same scale. The options are boundless, but in the end it's about creating balance and usefulness.

2 You can still display a large art collection, even in a small space. Gather your pieces into a gallery wall by hanging one larger piece with the center about 58" (1.5 m) high, and then add additional works above, below, and around the focal piece in a pleasing arrangement. Tie the whole wall together with a unifying element—whether it is symmetry, frame style, or simply the color of the mats. Take over a whole wall for an eclectic feel that displays your family's personality.

3 Make a room appear more spacious by hanging window treatments all the way from ceiling to floor. This will avoid breaking up a wall and will draw the eye to the open space above the window. Use fabrics that allow in as much light as possible to give your small space an airy feel.

4 Keeping a small space neat doesn't have to be difficult; the key is having, as my mother would say, "A place for everything and everything in its place." Simple organization tricks like drawer dividers and velvet hangers help maximize space and sanity by keeping the possibility of clutter to a minimum. Find clever ways to increase storage space by thinking vertically; there's often space right above your head or under your bed.

5   The idea that a small home needs to be painted in a unifying light color is a myth—you can add splashes of color and still give the illusion of more space. The key is avoiding dull colors in favor of strong, clear colors and tying the rooms together with varying shades in the same family. You don't want to hop from bright color to bright color as you move around the home, but a brightly painted door, focal wall, or even radiator can break up a home into pleasing vignettes. Just go with a light color for the ceiling to open the space up.

6   Place decorative hooks in useful places. A hook by the desk for your laptop bag; a series of hooks by the front door for purses, keys, and jackets; hooks along the inside walls of closets for hats, umbrellas, and backpacks. Beautiful hooks add a little touch of class and create space in places that were formerly just walls. They also allow some of your more beautiful items like handbags, hats, and jewelry to act as décor when not in use. Investing in attractive cleaning supplies and placing them on hooks does double duty in keeping a small space looking crisp and neat.

7   A small home can still offer opportunities to create special spaces. Find space under the stairs for a playroom, turn a closet into an office, or fill a tray with bath products and candles to set next to the tub when you get a quite moment alone.

8   Add a mirror to open a space up. Above a fireplace is traditional, but we also like a large mirror in a small bedroom that faces out the door or an entryway mirror for last minute touch-ups as you head out the door.

9   A big floral arrangement can create a beautiful statement in a small space, but you can save your tabletops for more useful items while still enjoying the beauty and scent of flowers. Try placing single blooms in bud vases, teacups, and shot glasses and displaying them in little nooks and crannies.

10 While utilizing a small space well does require some paring down of knickknacks and decorative items, it doesn't mean your home has to lose all of its charisma. Grouping your decorative items and collections into vignettes creates the illusion of more individual spaces while retaining your personal charm.

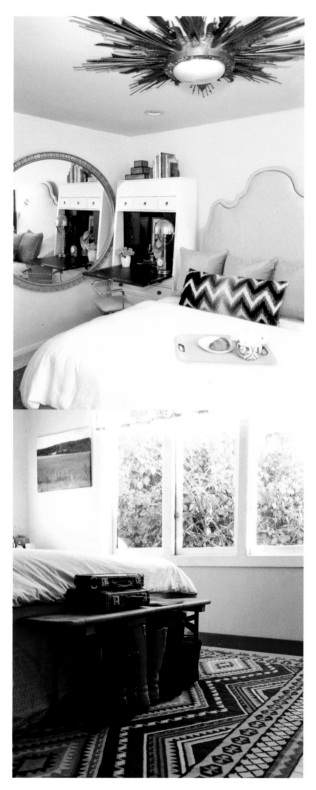

THE PRUDENT HOME

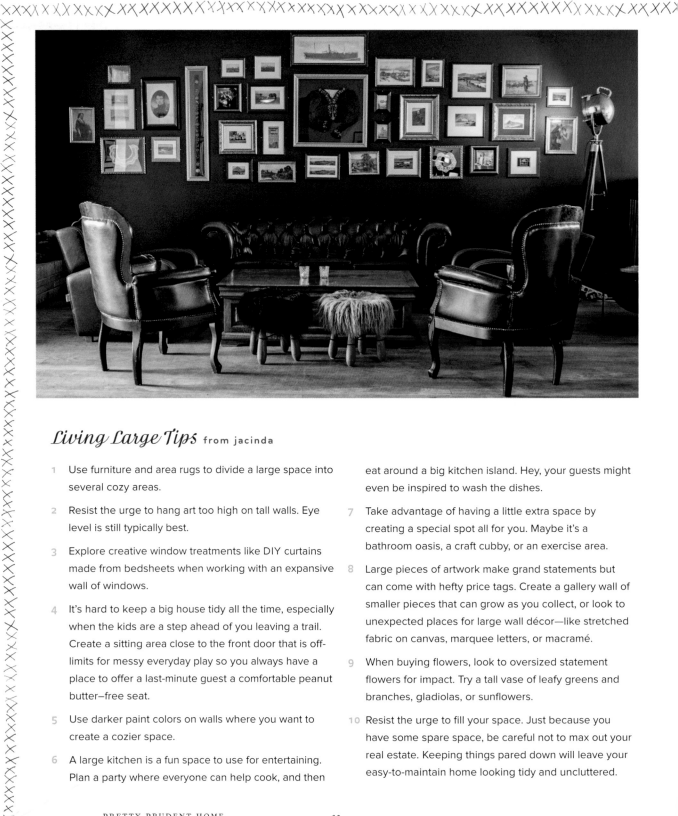

Living Large Tips from jacinda

1. Use furniture and area rugs to divide a large space into several cozy areas.

2. Resist the urge to hang art too high on tall walls. Eye level is still typically best.

3. Explore creative window treatments like DIY curtains made from bedsheets when working with an expansive wall of windows.

4. It's hard to keep a big house tidy all the time, especially when the kids are a step ahead of you leaving a trail. Create a sitting area close to the front door that is off-limits for messy everyday play so you always have a place to offer a last-minute guest a comfortable peanut butter–free seat.

5. Use darker paint colors on walls where you want to create a cozier space.

6. A large kitchen is a fun space to use for entertaining. Plan a party where everyone can help cook, and then eat around a big kitchen island. Hey, your guests might even be inspired to wash the dishes.

7. Take advantage of having a little extra space by creating a special spot all for you. Maybe it's a bathroom oasis, a craft cubby, or an exercise area.

8. Large pieces of artwork make grand statements but can come with hefty price tags. Create a gallery wall of smaller pieces that can grow as you collect, or look to unexpected places for large wall décor—like stretched fabric on canvas, marquee letters, or macramé.

9. When buying flowers, look to oversized statement flowers for impact. Try a tall vase of leafy greens and branches, gladiolas, or sunflowers.

10. Resist the urge to fill your space. Just because you have some spare space, be careful not to max out your real estate. Keeping things pared down will leave your easy-to-maintain home looking tidy and uncluttered.

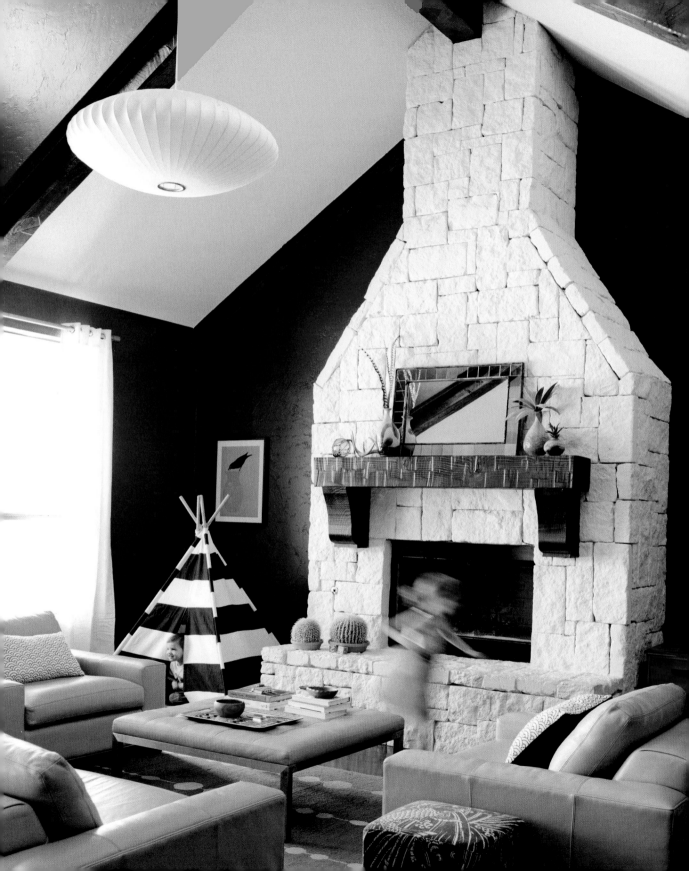

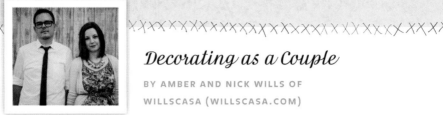

Decorating as a Couple

BY AMBER AND NICK WILLS OF
WILLSCASA (WILLSCASA.COM)

1 When we first started decorating our home, Nick was more into it than I was. We are odd that way. I made some terrible choices, and he let me. Not that his choices were amazing either, but we had to give ourselves time to find our style and figure out what worked for both of us.

2 Your tastes will change, and that's OK. Sometimes your best option is to tell your settee, "I think it's time we see other people." You should allow yourself to part with things that no longer work with your space.

3 It's you two against the world. Even if it's a world of paint chips and pattern mixing, you both have to support your decisions. You are a united front against all the perils in design. This is especially true when dealing with contractors.

4 Always be on the lookout for design cues. Great design is everywhere. We get a ton of ideas from coffee shops, restaurants, and hotels. The inspiration for our garage doors came from an old fire station we drove by.

5 Keep something neutral—either the walls or your furniture. More skilled designers can pull off everything colorful or completely minimalist, but we're always happier with the end result when there's a neutral base somewhere in the room.

6 It may take one of you longer to come around on an idea. Give your spouse the chance to convince you that it will work. We've found that inspiration images are the most effective way for this to happen. If it doesn't work, move on. Your next moment of genius will hit before you know it.

7 Each of you should have your own space in the house. He needs a place for all his mismatched coffee mugs that have great sentimental value (no joke). She needs a place to hoard fabric for projects she's never going to make. Get your crazy out all over that space so you can compromise on other areas.

8 Splurges are great and can really make a room, but be smart about them. You don't want to be the couple that has nowhere for your friends to sit because you spent five grand on a rug.

9 Blending your two styles together makes your house unique. You play off each other and create something unexpected and fun. Nick likes things clean and simple, while I tend to want more color and pattern. His house would be pretty boring without me while mine would be straight from the pages of Dr. Seuss.

10 Stop working on a project when you and your spouse hit the boiling point. Take a break. Home design isn't worth getting into a knock-down, drag-out fight over.

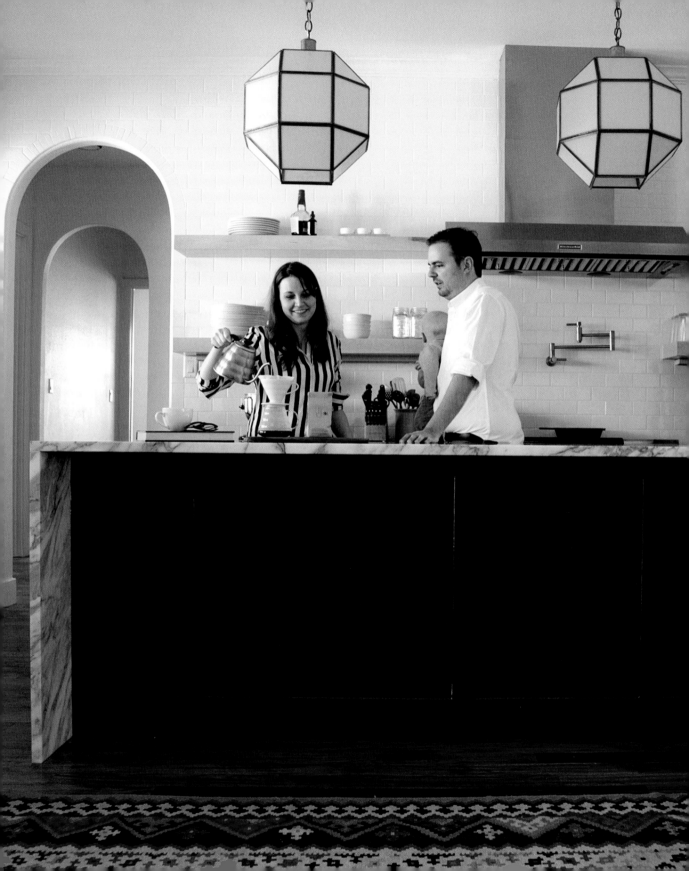

defining your palette

Jumping into a room or home makeover involving color can be intimidating—
even paralyzing. Where do you start? Which decision is the most important and
where do you go from there? Do you really like Wolfbrow Gray or is it just the name?
Jaime once selected a paint color because the name included the word
"scarlet" (her daughter's name). True story.

SOME TIPS AND EXERCISES FOR JUMPING INTO COLOR
(OR LACK THEREOF) IN YOUR HOME PROJECTS

PICK A FOCAL POINT: I was once having difficulty selecting a palette for my guestroom because it was a completely blank palette. There were too many options! Amber Wills from Wills Casa (willscasa.com) suggested that bedding was a great place to start in a bedroom. Find bedding that you love and work from there. It is much more difficult to retrofit bedding to coordinate with a random wall color that appealed to you on its own. If you start with one item that makes your eyeballs sing, you will be that much more excited about the space, and the rest of the room will easily fall into place.

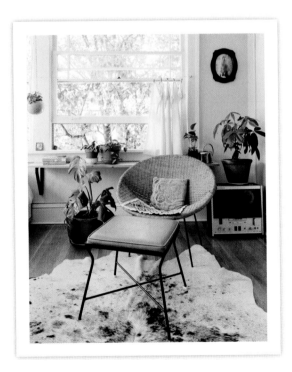

THAT HUE IS YOU: Make a mental note of spaces that appeal to you. A hotel lobby that makes you happy or a swanky lounge that puts you at ease might feature colors that speak to you personally. Keep a record of all the color combinations that catch your eye and think about why. Of course a room doesn't have to evoke a strong emotional reaction, but you will find that you are consistently attracted to a certain palette of colors. Don't miss the opportunity to look for color inspiration outside of the four walls. Look for inspiration in nature, fashion, and art.

LIGHT THOUGHTS: You've decided that your living room must be navy but there are hundreds of tints, shades, and hues. The trickiest part is that they are all going to appear different at various hours of the day and in natural versus artificial lighting. The ideal way to test the colors and make the right decision is to paint large patches of each color on each wall of the room and then study them throughout the day. Be conscious of the fact that the existing wall color can also create a shift in the color you're testing.

A SIZE THAT FITS: Typically a dark color will make a room appear smaller and light colors will make a space feel roomier. Is your intention to maximize a small space by filling it with white or to give a cavernous space a more intimate vibe?

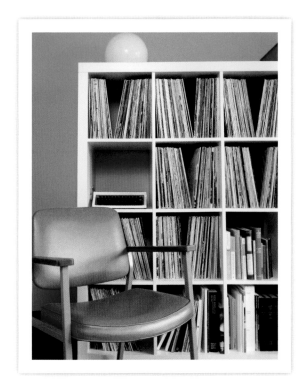

RENT OR OWN: Some renters feel it's worth the work to make a unit a home for the time they are there and proceed with painting despite the inevitable late-night white coats of paint they will be applying before they leave. Others feel it saves money and unnecessary burden to leave the walls alone and use their decorating budget on items they can take with them, like art instead of wallpaper, lamps instead of fixtures, and rugs instead of flooring. Luckily there are many new products such as decals, temporary wallpaper, and carpet tiles—and DIY solutions like those featured in the next chapter of this book—that can help renters personalize their space temporarily and fabulously.

BUILDING A THEMATIC APPROACH: Incorporating a theme into your space can be a slippery slope to roadside attraction. It's very tempting to latch onto one idea such as nautical and quickly go overboard. The most tempting spaces to overdo a theme are children's rooms and play areas. An Alice in Wonderland or superhero bedroom is guaranteed to thrill but will be quickly outgrown as the child moves on to a new passion.

COMMITMENT AND TRENDS: If you're a daring decorator who doesn't mind a biannual redo, proceed with painting your ceiling the hot color for spring. If you want your hard work to last until the kids go to college, consider using flexible, classic colors and accenting with pillows and décor that can be swapped out each year or even rotated with the seasons.

WALL TO WALL: Think about how the colors in your home flow from room to room. Picking a completely new color scheme for each room in the house might work better in a larger home where neutral halls and connecting spaces can "cleanse the palate." Most homes benefit from harmonious color transitions from room to room. That is not to say that you should paint your entire home Almond Butter or Crème Brûlée, simply consider how the spaces work together as you travel through the house.

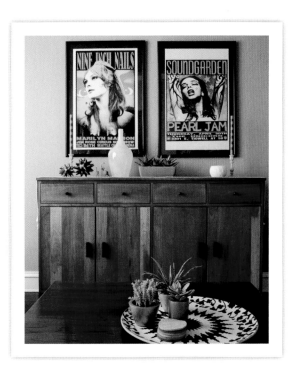

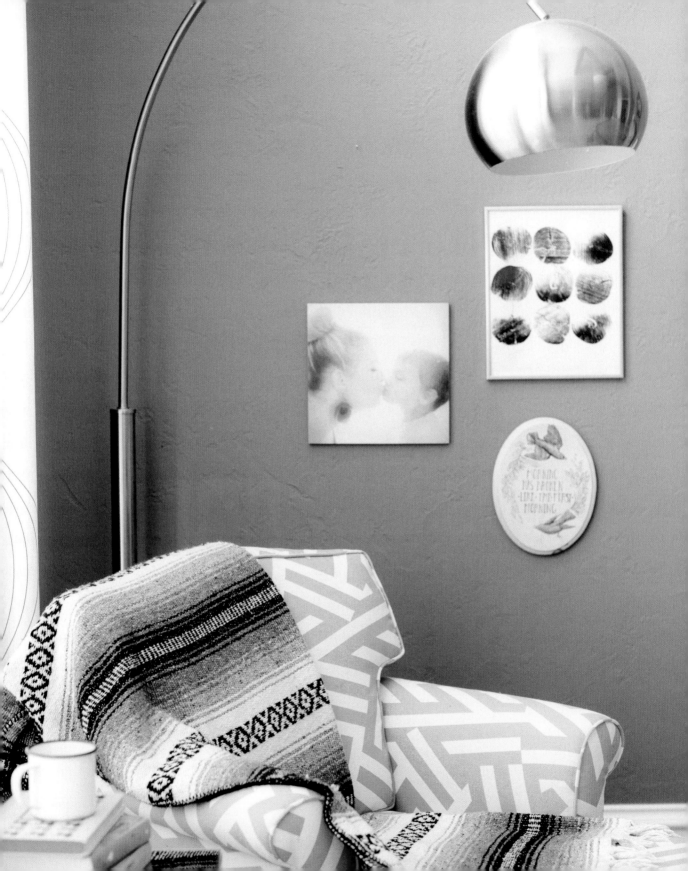

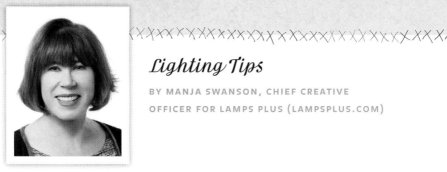

Lighting Tips

BY MANJA SWANSON, CHIEF CREATIVE
OFFICER FOR LAMPS PLUS (LAMPSPLUS.COM)

1   For a one-step room makeover, update your lamp shades. The right lamp shades can provide an instant new look, and they will help freshen up any room with a pop of color.

2   When designing with lighting, remember the rule of three, which is the three types of lighting: general/ambient (chandeliers and floor lamps), task (recessed lighting and desk lamps), and accent (picture lights and uplights).

3   If replacing the bathroom lighting, place sconces on either side of the mirror, and then install an overhead light. This adds essential lighting for personal grooming.

4   Dimmers are not just for overhead lights. Placing the whole room lighting on a central dimmer switch allows you to set the atmosphere for anything—from a romantic dinner to playing video games.

5   Swap out builder's basic light fixtures. If you live in a new home, chances are that many of your ceiling fixtures are inexpensive builder's basics. Close-to-ceiling lights, which are typically found in hallways, kitchens, and bathrooms, can be easily changed out with more stylish options. You can do this even if you're a renter— just keep the original fixtures and make sure to re-install them when you move.

6   To highlight your artwork, add a picture light. You can mount these above the frame, stand back, and accept the compliments.

7   LED stands for light-emitting diode. While LEDs have been around since the 1960s, their use in household lighting is relatively new. Today's LED lightbulbs are more efficient, radiate little heat, are dimmable, and have a life of 35,000 to 50,000+ hours. (For reference, the life span of an incandescent bulb is 1,000 to 2,000 hours.)

8   Lasting up to ten times longer than a regular lightbulb, a compact fluorescent lamp (CFL) lightbulb can save you lots of annoying bulb changes, and over the lifetime of a CFL bulb will save enough energy to pay for itself ten times over.

9   When selecting new lighting to go by the front door, remember this general rule: The light fixture should be about one-third the size of your door height.

10 Selecting the perfect-sized dining room chandelier is a breeze when you remember that the size of the fixture should be one-third the length of the table. When hanging the chandelier, it should be 30"–34" (76–86 cm) from the top of the table.

2

pretty prudent
décor

Create a home your family will remember—not just
for its clever use of color or artistically arranged
décor, but also for the comfort, inspiration, and joy it
inspires. Fond recollections of feeling quiet breezes
through gauze curtains, curling up with snuggly-
soft blankets, or winning epic pillow fights are what
will stay with your loved ones forever. Experiences
like these rest in that particular place in the heart
where the five senses coalesce to create memories.
Every time your crew laughs through a late-night
conversation at a cozy kitchen table or runs their bare
toes across a cushy carpet, they will feel at home.

The act of building, decorating, and sewing for your family home fills the space
between each of you with pleasing things and attractive individuality. At the
same time, your creations surround all of you with gratifying warmth, leaving
a legacy of craftsmanship and affection that will glow far beyond your family's
four walls.

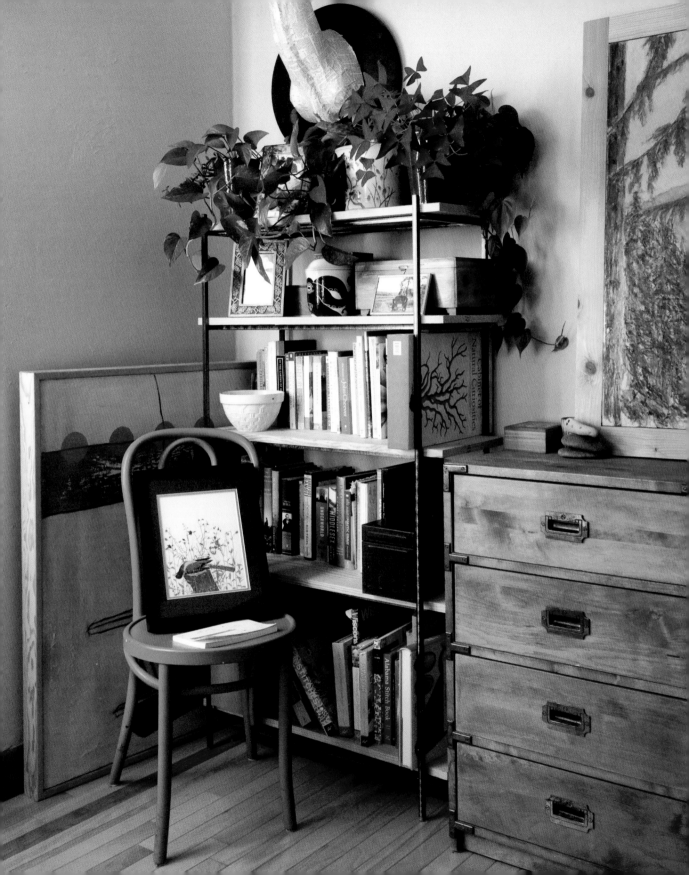

vintage finds & thrift store DIYs

Learn the secrets of hunting flea markets, thrift stores, and yard sales
to track down the perfect vintage finds and then discover the best ways to make them
your own with our hints, tricks, and detailed D I Y instructions. Happy hunting!

OUR FAVORITE VINTAGE FINDS

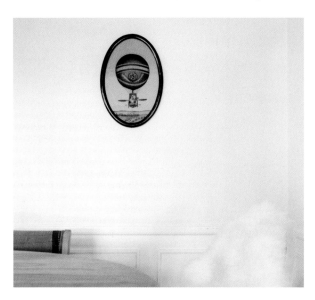

I first spotted these beautiful reverse-glass paintings at an antique shop on Sutter Street in Folsom, California. They each depict a crew of ragtag misfits embarking on a hot air balloon journey, but this one is my favorite.

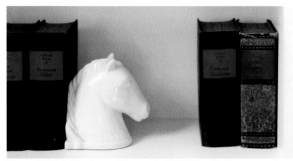

When my husband's beloved Grandma Jane passed away we were gifted a few of her simple but beautiful possessions; these horse head bookends now live on our daughter's bookshelf, a reminder of her namesake.

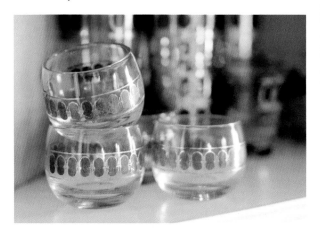

These blue-and-gold glasses graced my mother's brass bar cart in the kids-were-not-allowed-to-enter living room as long as I can remember. The day she moved away and gave them to me was bittersweet.

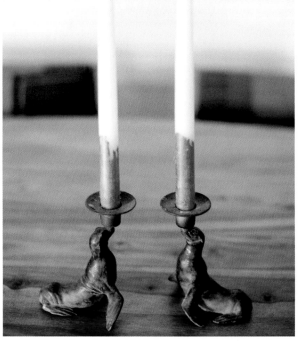

I found these sea lion candlesticks in a vintage mall in Northern California just days after my daughter, husband, and I had seen these playful animals in the wild while road tripping up the California coast.

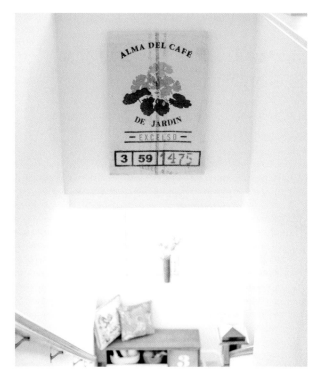

This burlap sack cost only two dollars at my local trade days. (Some coffee shops will even give them away for free, although I've never seen any this pretty.) I stretched it over a basic canvas from the craft store and stapled around the edges to create this large piece of rustic artwork.

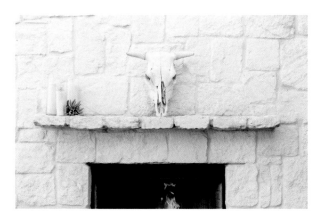

Living in Texas, there is never a shortage of animal skulls and antlers gracing the shelves of trade days and antique shops, and the folks selling them are as interesting as their collections. Bartering for a few shed antlers or a stuffed armadillo will inevitably give you a fun story to take home, along with some beautiful home décor. This bleached cow skull is my one outdoor decoration that can withstand the elements of the Texas seasons, and it reminds me of Georgia O'Keefe every time I pass by.

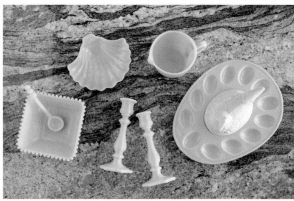

Before I was married or even had a place of my own I fell in love with jadeite. I found a few pieces on my own, my mom added to my collection, and now I only splurge on truly irresistible pieces both vintage and brand-new. My most recent addition is the pair of candlestick holders, which I found at Watson Kennedy in Seattle on a recent birthday trip with my husband.

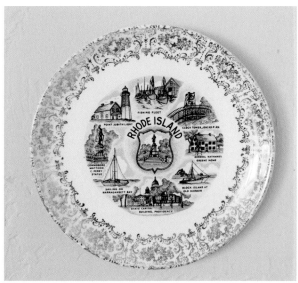

When I married into my husband's family I was leery of their tradition of sending out detailed Christmas wish lists. Doesn't that take away some of the thoughtfulness and surprise of gift giving? Ten years later, I gleefully fantasize about and itemize my frivolous desires—vintage souvenir plates, specifically from Texas, New Mexico, California, and Rhode Island. My mother-in-law found them all for me and left them tied with a bow under the tree. Sometimes the most thoughtful gift is just exactly what you asked for.

PRETTY PRUDENT DÉCOR

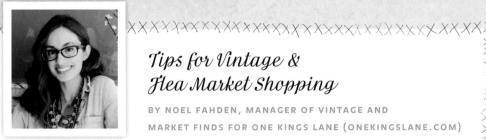

Tips for Vintage & Flea Market Shopping

BY NOEL FAHDEN, MANAGER OF VINTAGE AND
MARKET FINDS FOR ONE KINGS LANE (ONEKINGSLANE.COM)

1   Vintage hunting takes practice. The more you can look at what's out there, the more you'll build your confidence in determining bargains and truly unique finds. After you've been to a few flea markets, you'll be surprised how often you see the same types of items. When you eventually come across something you've never seen before, you'll know it's time to pounce!

2   Start a collection. Some inexpensive, relatively easy-to-find examples include: vintage brass (animals, candlesticks, vases); silver trays and bowls; vintage art glass; and handmade pottery from the 1970s.

3   Ask vendors about their recommendations for other flea markets, antique emporiums, or thrift stores. They may sometimes be reluctant to give away their sources, but if you express a genuine interest in collecting vintage, they'll be more likely to share their tips.

4   Look beyond eye level—especially in crowded vintage booths or shops. Sometimes the best treasures are still available because no one else has noticed them.

5   Ask questions. It's always helpful to know the story behind an item. Asking, "Do you know when or where this is from?" is an open-ended and polite way to find out more

information. Even if vendors don't know the correct era, they'll still be able to tell you if the piece came from an interesting estate or has a compelling story.

6   Start low risk. If you're new to flea markets, limit your budget to five to ten dollars per item. As you get more comfortable, increase your budget per item until you feel confident determining when something is worth five or fifty dollars.

7   Timing is everything. The best flea market finds are available first thing in the morning. The best deals can be had at the end of the day when vendors want to pack up as little as possible.

8   Buy in bulk (and always bring cash!). If you find a lot of items you like from the same vendor, they'll be more likely to give you a better price on everything.

9   Make a wish list. Going in with an agenda can actually make flea markets more manageable. Flea markets can be overwhelming, but knowing what you're looking for can help you stay focused— and you'll actually find what you want!

10 Vintage or antique books with unique covers can make great decorative accents and add a much-needed pop of color.

PAINT MAKEOVERS

On occasion, searching flea markets or your mom's basement will present you with the perfect treasure— one that's just sitting there waiting for you to scoop it up, bring it home, and arrange it in the perfect spot (without chipping a nail!). But sometimes a find requires a little bit of imagination and a fresh coat of paint. Let these simple paint makeovers inspire you to easily upgrade your thrift store find with a fresh hue.

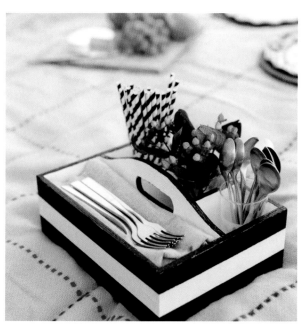

High-contrast black and white stripes turned this rustic-looking Thanksgiving silverware caddy into a stylish, modern showpiece worthy of your next party or picnic.

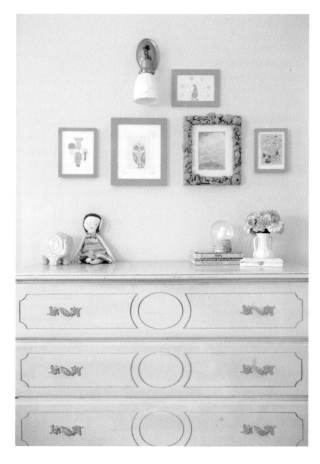

A kitschy shell frame turns monochrome-modern with the addition of coral-colored spray paint. I gave this vintage dresser a quick update by removing the handles and coating them in spray paint designed for metals.

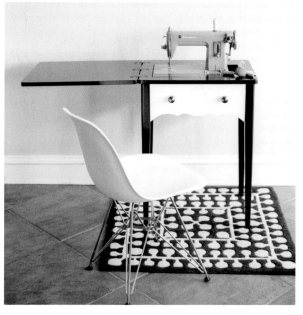

This vintage sewing table was rescued from the trash heap and turned into a classy entryway table with a combo of black and cream paint and new drawer pulls. Getting the sewing machine working is a task for another day.

HOW TO PAINT ANYTHING

"Should I cover that knotty pine wainscoting?" "Do I paint that cedar rocking horse?" "Would that pickled white dresser look better with a shiny new coat of paint?" These are the sorts of questions that have tormented DIYers since the dawn of spray paint. We say go for it. Consult our nifty guide to the supplies and techniques you'll use to prep, paint, and finish different surfaces.

MATERIAL	ABOUT	CLEAN	PREP	PRIME	PAINT	FINISH
WOOD	From beautiful hardwood dressers to ornate picture frames, wood is a common vintage and thrift store find. For beginners, re-painting wood is a less-stressful and more-likely-to-succeed first-time re-haul project. So grab your sandpaper and get to work.	Wipe clean with damp cloth and let dry. For stained or smelly items, use household detergent or mineral spirits to clean. Let dry. If the wood is glossy, use a sander/deglosser to remove the finish.	Sand with 80 grit, then 150 grit, then 220 grit, wiping away dust with tack cloth or cheesecloth after each coat. If necessary, fill scratches or holes with wood filler and sand until smooth.	Spray or brush with primer. Let dry and sand with a super-fine grit in between coats for a smooth surface. Completely remove dust by wiping with a tack cloth.	Spray paint or brush on thin layers. We like Montana Black spray paint.	Seal with a clear acrylic or polyurethane sealant.
MELAMINE	Most IKEA furniture, and that of other less-expensive brands, is made from particle board with a veneer of melamine. Knowing how to update the standard white and birch offerings will open up a whole new world of design possibilities.	Scrub clean using a rag or sponge and a liquid tri-sodium phosphate detergent. To dull glossy finishes apply a commercial sander/deglosser. Wipe clean and allow to dry completely, for several hours or overnight.	Sand with a sanding block (to avoid creating dings) to rough up the surface—we suggest 150 grit. Melamine is too smooth to accept paint, so be sure to uniformly create texture across the entire surface. Completely remove dust by wiping with a tack cloth.	Apply an oil- or shellac- based primer or, ideally, a melamine-specific primer (latex primer will not allow your paint to adhere to melamine). Apply several even coats, scuffing gently with 220 or higher grit sandpaper on a sanding block between coats. Completely remove dust by wiping with a tack cloth.	Use a paint roller or sprayer to apply a very thin coat of melamine-specific paint (available at your local hardware store). Allow to dry completely and repeat twice for a total of three thin coats. You may use a regular eggshell or gloss finish house paint, but you will not have the same adhesion or durability you would get from a melamine-specific paint.	Allow your item to cure for a minimum of 48 hours before use.
METAL	Flea markets are filled with worn-down brass light fixtures, rusty step stools and ladders, ornate plant stands, and rickety bicycles. Give them new life in a few simple steps.	Remove rust with a wire brush, steel wool, or a chemical rust-removal product. Remove oil with dish soap or a chemical degreaser. Let dry.	Sand until all surfaces are smooth.	Spray with a rust-proof primer to prevent future corrosion.	Spray with a metal-adherent or all-purpose spray paint.	Seal with a clear acrylic or polyurethane sealant.
PLASTIC	You may not think of plastic as a super-exciting "find," until you spot the perfect set of vintage sign letters or that mod molded chair. Know that you can bring back the former glossy glory of vintage plastics with paint.	Cleanse with dish soap. Clean with mineral spirits to remove old paint. Let dry.	If previously painted, lightly sand with 220 or 320 grit. Remove dust with tack cloth.	Priming is not absolutely necessary, but if desired use a paint designed specifically to adhere to plastics.	Spray with paint specifically designed to adhere to plastics.	If desired, seal with a clear acrylic or polyurethane sealant.

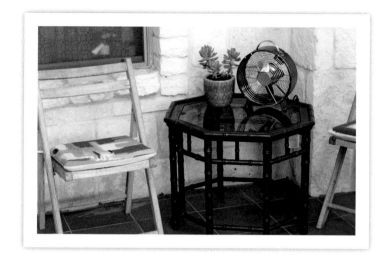

MATERIAL	ABOUT	CLEAN	PREP	PRIME	PAINT	FINISH
WICKER	From decorative baskets to statement-making peacock chairs, natural woven wicker designs are totally on-trend. Because wicker ages quickly without proper cleaning and care, it often gets dumped by those who have yet to take our wicker wisdom to heart. Great finds are abundant at thrift stores and flea markets, so grab your grandma and start combing garage sales.	Vacuum, then wipe or brush with an ammonia-based cleaner. If mildew is present, wash with 50/50 water-bleach solution.	If previously painted, lightly sand by hand with 220-grit sandpaper. Remove dust with tack cloth.	Prime with an all-purpose spray primer.	Paint with all-purpose spray paint.	Seal with a clear acrylic or polyurethane sealant.
GLASS & CERAMIC	Glass and tile usually only require a good cleaning to bring back their original sparkle and shine, but sometimes the perfect planter needs a punch of color, or a boring clear vase needs to transform into a transparent fuchsia centerpiece. A little attention to detail and the right set of tools can re-invigorate these delicate cast-offs into timeless treasures.	Clean with water and/or glass cleaner.	Lightly sand with fine-grit sandpaper to improve paint adherence.	Prime with an all-purpose spray primer if an opaque finish is desired. Otherwise, use lead (either strip or squeeze-on variety) to lay out a design. A stencil or transfer can be helpful.	Sponge or brush with a resin-based paint, an enamel paint designed for glass, or an acrylic paint mixed with glass and tile medium.	Depending on the paint you've selected, you may want to bake the item for a long-lasting finish. Follow the instructions on your chosen paint.
OUR FAVORITE MULTI-PURPOSE PRODUCTS TO HAVE ON HAND	We keep a stash of latex gloves, drop cloths, tack cloths, and sandpaper in 80, 150, 220, and 320 grit on hand for any sweet projects that find their way to us.	We like Klean-Strip Easy Liquid Sander Deglosser for tough jobs removing old paint, stain, and varnishes for its simple application and fast results.	We love Minwax Hi-Performance wood filler, especially to spiff up our more "rustic" finds.	We adore all KILZ Brand Primers. KILZ Original Aerosol Primer is multi-purpose and blocks odors while allowing for a smooth finish.	We like Montana Black spray paints for most surfaces. They come with a variety of tips and in a wide range of gorgeous colors.	We like Krylon Crystal Clear Acrylic in spray form. It won't yellow with age and gives a beautiful glow to any project.

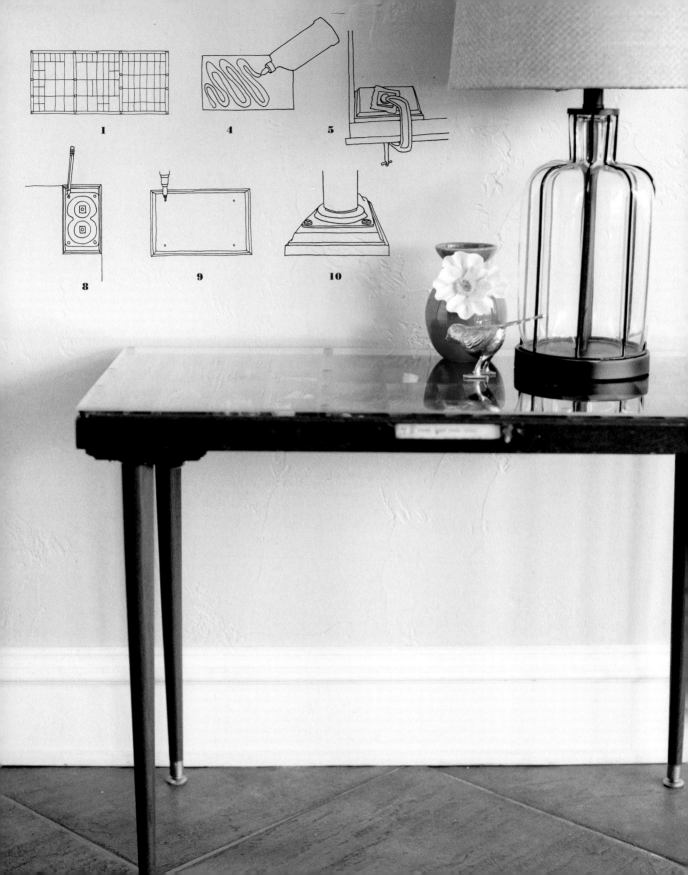

1

4

5

8

9

10

Letterpress Tray Table

A vintage letterpress tray is a common flea market find that can easily be turned into an eye-catching, conversation-starting piece of furniture. In fact, any sturdy and flat object can be transformed into a table following these simple steps.

MATERIALS

24 (approximately) strong magnets, each ½" (12 mm) diameter × ⅛" (3 mm) thick (we used rare-earth magnets)

Letterpress tray

All-purpose quick-bonding gel glue (we used Krazy Glue)

⅜"- (1-cm-) thick acrylic glass (such as Plexiglas), cut to same length and width as the tray

4 oz. (59 ml) acrylic paint in a coordinating color to your letterpress tray (we used Martha Stewart's Multi-Surface Paint in Vanilla Bean)

Four 22" (56-cm) tapered table legs (we used Waddell's Hardwood Round Taper Legs available at The Home Depot)

Four 3" × 5" × ¾" (7.5 cm × 12 cm × 2 cm) wooden plaques (found in the wood aisle of most hobby stores), or 4 blocks of wood similar in size

Two paintbrushes

One quart (1 L) polyurethane (optional)

Wood glue (we used Elmers ProBond Advanced)

Four C-clamps

Wax paper

Small wood scraps or cardboard

Spray paint for metal, in a coordinating color to the acrylic paint (optional)

Four dual top plate hardware pieces, for table assembly (you can use straight or angled top plate hardware)

Pencil

Drill with ⁷⁄₆₄" (2.8-mm) drill bit

Screwdriver

note: For end tables and night stands 22" (56-cm) legs are best. Use 16" (41-cm) legs for a coffee table.

INSTRUCTIONS

1   Stack two magnets, one on top of the other, at all four corners of the letterpress tray and at additional key points where the dividers will allow. (See illustration.) Use the gel glue to adhere only the bottom magnets to the tray. Let the glue dry completely.

2   Place a drop of gel glue on the top side of each top magnet. Then carefully position the acrylic glass, edges even with the tray, on top of the magnets. Let the glue dry completely.

3   Paint the table legs and wooden plaques with the acrylic paint. Let the paint dry. Then, if desired, seal with polyurethane and let dry.

4   Remove the acrylic glass and set aside. Place the tray, wrong side up, on a protected work surface. Completely cover the bottom of one wooden plaque with a thin coat of wood glue.

5   Adhere the wooden plaque to one corner of the tray, aligning the two edges. Secure them with a C-clamp. (Note: Place wax paper and a small piece of wood or a few layers of cardboard between the C-clamps and the plaques to prevent the clamps from sticking to them and leaving marks.) Repeat these steps to glue the remaining three wooden plaques to the bottom of the tray. Wait 24 hours before removing the clamps to allow the glue to dry.

6   While the glue is setting up, spray paint the dual top plate hardware, if you desire.

7   Once everything is dry, remove the clamps and position your hardware on the wooden plaques. (The dual top plate hardware lets you select whether you want angled or straight legs. We used straight.)

8   Mark the holes for the screws using a pencil. Repeat this step at all four corners.

9   Temporarily remove the dual top plate hardware to pre-drill holes for the screws at the marked points at all four corners. (Be sure to not drill through the front of the tray.)

10 Replace the hardware and secure them with the screws. When finished, screw the legs into the hardware at all four corners. Turn the table right side up and fill with your tiniest treasures and keepsakes. Place the acrylic glass back on the table tray over the magnets.

PRETTY PRUDENT DÉCOR

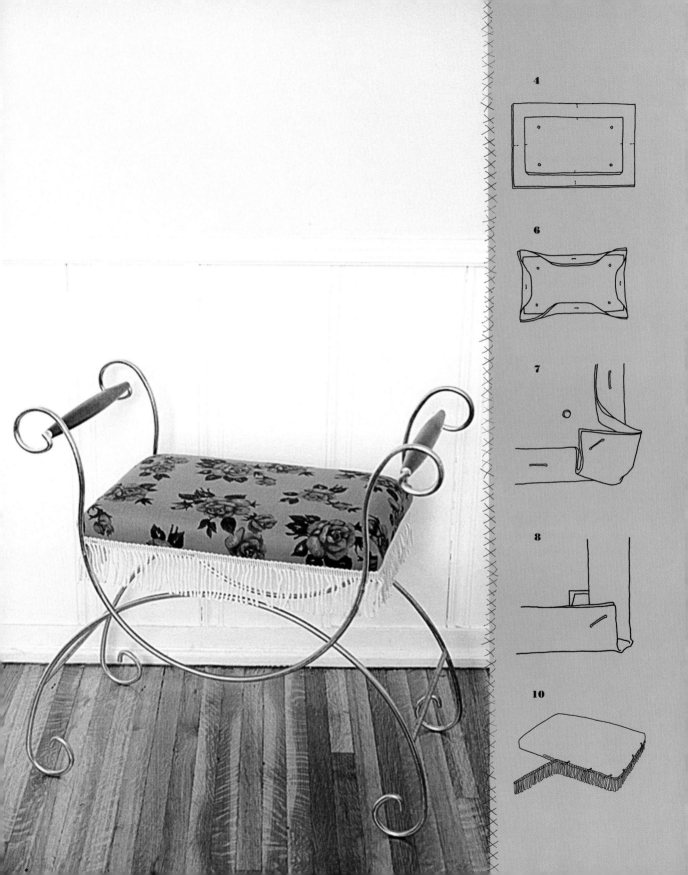

4

6

7

8

10

Beginner's Basic
Upholstered Footstool

Footstools are crazy useful (vanity pouf, chair to scoot under a desk in a small space, footrest, end table), and they are so easy to find at thrift shops. They also make for the perfect introduction to upholstering—all by yourself!

MATERIALS

Footstool
Screwdriver
Scissors
Foam, only if the original foam needs replacing
  (search "foam" in your local yellow pages or on Yelp.com)
Serrated knife (electric or bread knife)
Spray adhesive
Measuring tape
Home-décor or medium-weight cotton fabric
  (see step 3 for amount)
High-loft polyester batting (see step 3 for amount)
Pencil
Staple gun with staples
Fringe
Fabric glue
Straight pins

INSTRUCTIONS

1   Disassemble the footstool by removing the screws that hold the seat and base together.

2   Inspect the upholstered seat. If the fabric is in good shape, you can place your new fabric right on top of the old material. If the fabric has deteriorated or if it smells, use the scissors to cut it off. Removing the fabric should reveal a foam piece attached to a wooden base. If your foam is moldy or otherwise gross, peel it off. Use a serrated knife and the spray adhesive to cut and glue a new piece of foam to the wooden base.

3   Measure the width, length, and depth of the seat with the foam. Add two times the depth to the width. Add two times the depth to the length. Then add an extra 2" (5 cm) to each of these measurements to determine the size you'll need to cut your fabric and batting. (For example, if your seat is 12" × 18" × 2" [30.5 cm × 46 cm × 5 cm], you will need 18" × 24" [46 cm × 61 cm] of fabric.) Place your fabric wrong side up, and then place the batting on top of the fabric. Now center your seat, foam side down, on top of the batting.

4   On all four outside edges of the seat, measure and mark the center points with a pencil. On all four outside edges of the fabric, measure and mark the center points by snipping them with your scissors. This will help you to keep your pattern aligned.

5   Fold over the fabric and batting on one long side of the seat, aligning the center marks on the seat and fabric, and staple the material to the seat at that point. Repeat on the opposite long side, making sure to pull the fabric and batting taut before stapling the material to the seat.

6   Repeat step 5 to staple the short sides of the fabric to the seat.

7   Secure the rest of the fabric to the seat. Start at the center of each side, pull the fabric taut, and place staples every 1"–1½" (2.5–4 cm) apart, stopping approximately 2" (5 cm) from each corner. At each corner pull the fabric in, diagonally, and staple it to the seat.

8   To create a nice, neat, notched corner, tightly fold over one corner flap piece and then the other. Smooth the fabric flat and staple in place. Repeat to finish the remaining three corners.

9   Trim the edges of your fabric. Use the original screws to re-install your seat to the base of your footstool with a screwdriver.

10   To add fringe to your footstool, you'll first need to measure and cut the appropriate length of trim. To determine the length, measure the perimeter of your seat and add 2" (5 cm) (2× the width + 2× the length + 2 inches). Apply fabric glue around the bottom edge of the seat. Press the fringe against the glue and pin in place as you go. The pins will secure the fringe until the glue dries. If you are using a very heavy fringe, you may want to add a few staples.

11   When the fabric glue is dry, remove the pins and put your feet up.

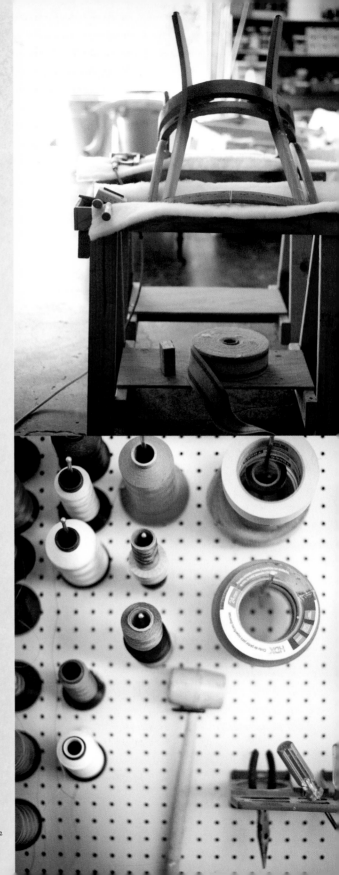

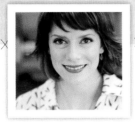

Ten Tips for DIY Beginner Upholstery

BY AMANDA BROWN OF SPRUCE UPHOLSTERY (SPRUCEAUSTIN.COM)

1   Start with a small project and work your way up to that three-seater sofa.

2   Do your work in a space that you don't mind getting dirty.

3   Invest in sharp scissors, a good pair of sawhorses, and a pneumatic stapler.

4   Take plenty of photos before deconstructing your project to avoid confusion later.

5   While stripping, wear gloves, protective eyewear, and a dust mask.

6   Keep old padding and fabric to reference later.

7   Refinish or paint the frame after stripping and before re-upholstering.

8   For spring tying, prevent blisters by wrapping your fingers with medical tape.

9   Test your skills on scrap fabric before cutting or stapling good fabric.

10 Keep a notebook handy for jotting down fabric dimensions or lessons learned along the way.

MULTI-MEDIUM MAKEOVERS

Sometimes found treasures require more than a simple spritz of spray paint before they are ready for their big debut. Once you master the repaint, don't be afraid to take on a multi-medium makeover. A coat of stain or paint and some fresh fabric can bring an item from the curbside to your foyer. And, yes, that was us loading your neighbor's trash into our hatchback.

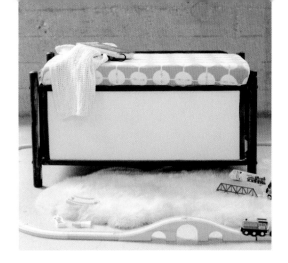

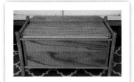

This water-damaged toy chest was brought back to life by refinishing and staining the pine, spray painting the plywood, and adding foam and fabric to the lid. Now this cast-off is a comfy storage bench.

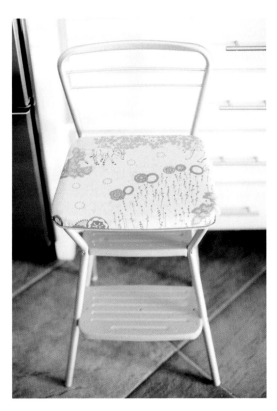

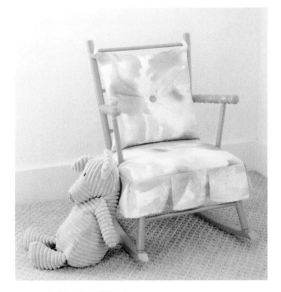

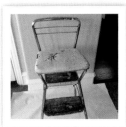

The state of this vintage stepstool was comical when we found it, but a fresh coat of paint and a new oilcloth seat cover gave it a whole new life and an updated look.

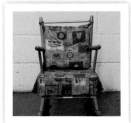

A ten-dollar score at Canton Trade Days in Texas, this tiny rocker had pretty bones but the polyester bicentennial print fabric needed to go. Spruce Upholstery in Austin painted the wood this stunning coral then used my own watercolor fabric (available on Spoonflower .com) to update the upholstery.

Vintage Linen Transformations

Finding a stall of pristine vintage linens while antiquing is a beautiful experience. Who were these people who kept their whites so white and their brights so bright? Were these stunning textiles tucked away for special occasions, or were folks just better at laundering fifty years ago? It's most likely a combination of the two. If you are lucky enough to happen upon beautiful vintage linens, the price is usually right for picking out a treasured piece to use for its original purpose or to display.

While immaculate linens are a fabulous find, the piles of worn printed sheets, torn quilts, and tea-stained towels can really make a crafter's heart sing. Often yards and yards of vintage linens sit crumpled in boxes, for just pennies a piece. With a little digging and a little bartering, those beauties will be headed home with endless upcycle possibilities.

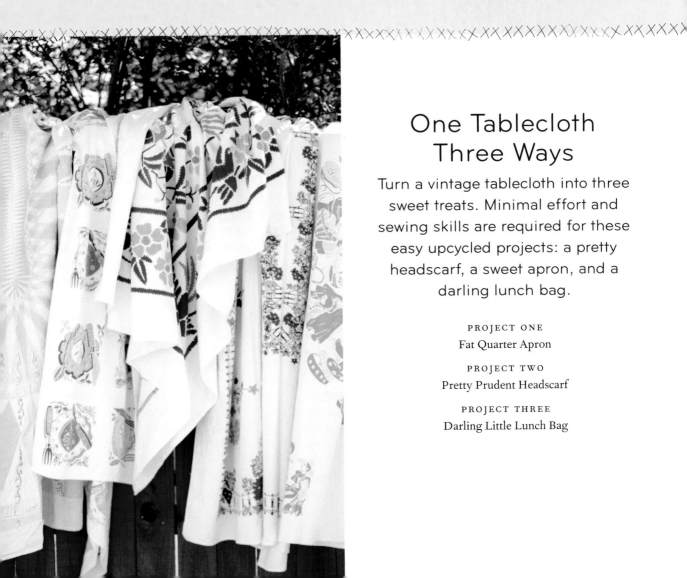

One Tablecloth Three Ways

Turn a vintage tablecloth into three sweet treats. Minimal effort and sewing skills are required for these easy upcycled projects: a pretty headscarf, a sweet apron, and a darling lunch bag.

PROJECT ONE
Fat Quarter Apron

PROJECT TWO
Pretty Prudent Headscarf

PROJECT THREE
Darling Little Lunch Bag

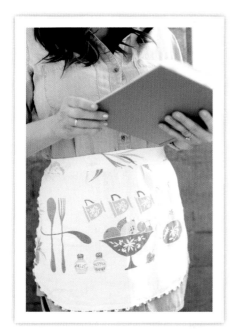

Fat Quarter Apron

First in line is our famous fat quarter apron. All you need is a fat quarter, some trim, and thirty minutes to make this adorable half-apron. Wear it while cooking up a feast, or select vintage linen with a pattern sure to tickle your hostess's fancy when you deliver it to her at the door.

MATERIALS

Iron and ironing board
One 18" × 22" (46 cm × 56 cm) piece of fabric cut from vintage linen, or one fat quarter of another pretty fabric
Scissors
Ruler
Lampshade or plate (something with a rounded edge)
Fabric marker
Straight pins
Three pieces of trim, one cut 52" (132 cm) and two cut 27" (69 cm)
Sewing machine
Coordinating thread

INSTRUCTIONS

1 Pre-wash and iron your fabric.

2 To make the waistband cut a 4"- (10-cm-) wide strip off one long side of your fat quarter.

3 Place the cut fabric strip wrong side up. Fold over both short ends of the strip ¼" (6 mm) and iron flat. Now fold over both long sides of the strip ¼" (6 mm) and iron flat.

4 Fold the strip in half lengthwise with wrong sides together and press. Set this piece aside.

5 To make the apron body, take your remaining fat quarter of fabric and lay it, wrong side up, with the long length of fabric running from left to right. Place the lampshade on the bottom right-hand corner of the fabric and trace along the edge of the lampshade with a fabric marker.

6 Fold your fabric in half with short sides together and right sides facing. The traced line should be facing up. Cut along your line, through both layers of fabric, to form what will be the two rounded bottom corners of the apron.

7 Open the fabric and lay it right side up. Pin the 52" (132-cm) piece of trim along the sides and bottom of the

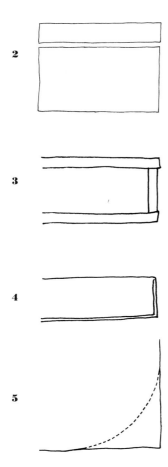

apron, with right sides facing (you want the pretty part of the trim face down on the apron) and raw edges even.

8   Sew the trim to the apron with a ⅛" (3-mm) seam, removing pins as you sew.

9   Turn the fabric over to the wrong side and press the trim out and away from the apron. Press the seam allowances to the fabric side. Turn the fabric over and top stitch through all the layers a scant ⅛" (3 mm) from the seam line.

10 With the apron body right side up, create a pleat in the center top of the fabric by pinching it with your fingers. Pin the pleat in place.

11 Lay your waistband, right side up, above your apron body. (You choose which side of the waistband you want showing on the front side of the apron.) If the apron body is longer or shorter than the waistband, adjust the size of the pleat; they should be the same length. Next, open up the flap on the waistband.

12 Place the unfinished edge of the apron body inside the flap, ½" (12 mm) down from the top fold; then fold down the waistband.

13 Secure the waistband to the apron with pins. Remove your pinch-pleat pin and reposition it on the outside of the waistband, keeping the pleat intact.

14 To add the apron ties, open the flap on one end of the waistband. Insert 1" (2.5 cm) of the 27" (69-cm) piece of trim inside and along the top fold of the waistband (the trim should be right side up.) Pin the trim in place. Repeat these steps on the opposite side of the waistband with the remaining piece of trim for the second apron tie.

15 Secure the waistband and apron ties to the apron with a ¼" (6-mm) seam. Begin sewing at one short edge of the waistband, continue across the bottom, and then sew up the second short edge. Backstitch at the beginning and end of the seam to secure your stitches. To securely hold the apron ties in place, reinforce both short sides with a second row of stitches.

16 To finish the ends of your apron ties, simply tie them with a knot.

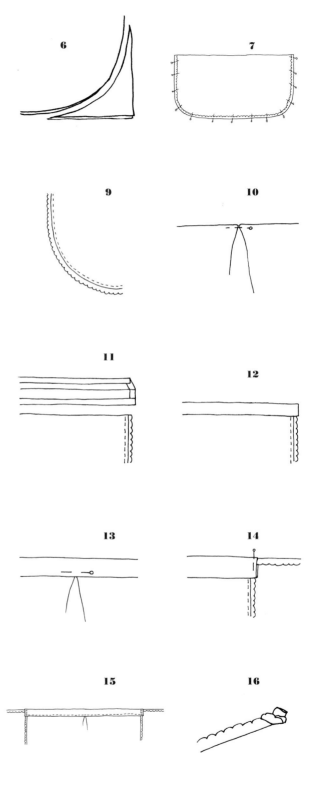

Pretty Prudent Headscarf

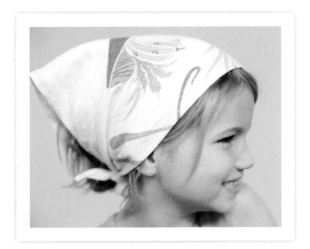

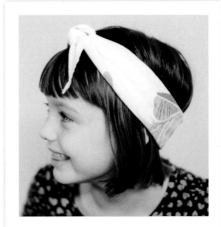

Vintage tablecloth fabric is so soft that even these sensitive-skinned little beauties loved tying one on in a cutie babushka or cheeky topknot. This is a simple way to put the prettiest graphic from a tablecloth on display. Grab your convertible and a picnic basket and cruise through the countryside in kitschy style.

MATERIALS

Fabric, at least a 21"- (53-cm-) square cut from vintage linen or another pretty fabric
Ruler
Air-erasable fabric marker (or chalk)
Scissors
Iron and ironing board
Straight pins
Sewing machine
Coordinating thread

INSTRUCTIONS

1   Place the fabric right side up on your work surface. Use the ruler and fabric marker to make a mark on the bottom edge of the fabric 21" (53 cm) in from the bottom right-hand corner of the fabric. Make a second mark on the right-hand edge of the fabric 21" (53 cm) up from the bottom right-hand corner of the fabric. Draw a line between these two marks to create a triangle. Cut along this line.

2   Place the fabric triangle, wrong side up, with the triangle's long side along the top. Fold over the long raw edge by ¼" (6 mm) and iron flat.

3   Fold this edge over again by another ¼" (6 mm) and iron flat. Trim away the excess folded fabric on each end.

4   Pin the hem in place.

5   Sew the hem with a ⅛" (3-mm) seam.

6   Wrap the headscarf around your tousled bed head and look fab.

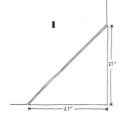

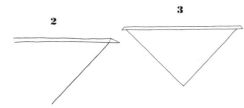

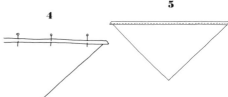

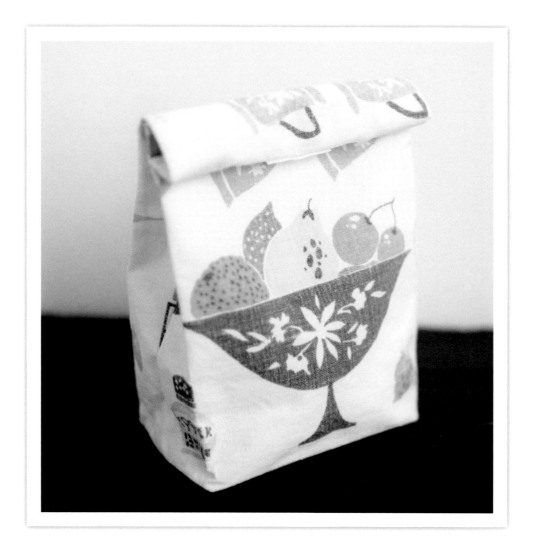

Darling Little Lunch Bag

Often adorned with sweet fruits and veggies, a vintage tablecloth transforms adorably into a fabric lunch bag. This one sews up so quickly that you'll want to make one for yourself and another for someone you love who appreciates a little style with their PB&J. Skip the paper and plastic and go for panache with this sweet and simple lunch (or treasure) bag.

MATERIALS

9" × 26" (23 cm × 66 cm) piece of fabric, cut from vintage linen, or canvas or home-décor weight fabric

Sewing machine

Coordinating thread

Iron and ironing board

Ruler

Scissors

Point turner or chopstick

One 2" (5-cm) length of ¾"- (2-cm-) wide hook and loop tape (such as Velcro) that's not adhesive backed

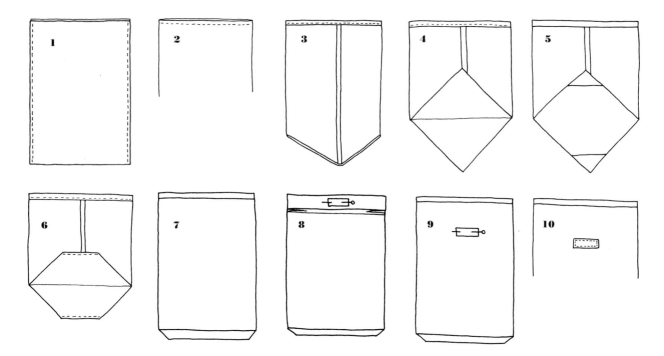

INSTRUCTIONS

1   Fold your piece of fabric in half with the short sides together and right sides facing. Sew both long edges with a ⅜" (1-cm) seam. Leave the short end (which will be the top of the lunch bag) open.

2   To hem the bag's opening, fold and press the top edge of the fabric to the wrong side by ¼" (6 mm). Then fold and press the top edge again by an additional ¼" (6 mm). Sew the hem at the inside folded edge.

3   Create the gussets. With the bag inside out, rotate it so that one of the side seams is front and center. (The bottom will fold in on itself, creating two matching triangles.) Smooth everything flat. Make sure that the seam on the front lines up exactly with the seam on the back, and then iron flat.

4   On the side facing you, fold one triangle up to create a diamond shape; iron flat.

5   Measure 2" (6 cm) in from the tips of both triangles and draw perpendicular lines using the fabric marker. (Make sure each line is even.)

6   Sew along each drawn line, backstitching at the beginning and end of each seam to secure your stitching. Trim the excess fabric at the tips of the triangles, cutting ¼" (6 mm) away from the seams.

7   Turn the bag right side out and gently poke out the corners using a point turner or chopstick. Fold the sack into a lunch bag shape. Use the steam setting on your iron to create crisp seams.

8   To make the closure, separate the hook and loop tape into two parts. Determine which side of the bag will be the front. Fold down the top of the bag 1½" (4 cm) toward the front side. Center and pin the hook part of the tape to the middle of the folded portion. (If you were to unfold the flap, the tape would be positioned on the back side of the bag.) Make sure to pin the tape through only one layer of fabric.

9   Fold the top of the bag over again by 1½" (4 cm). Lift the folded portion up slightly to position the loop part of the tape so that it will match the hook part of the tape. (The loop tape should be positioned on the front side of the bag.) Pin the loop tape in place, making sure to pin through just one layer of fabric.

10 Sew the hook and loop tape onto the bag with a ⅛" (3-mm) seam.

11 Fill the bag with delicious treats and head out to face the day.

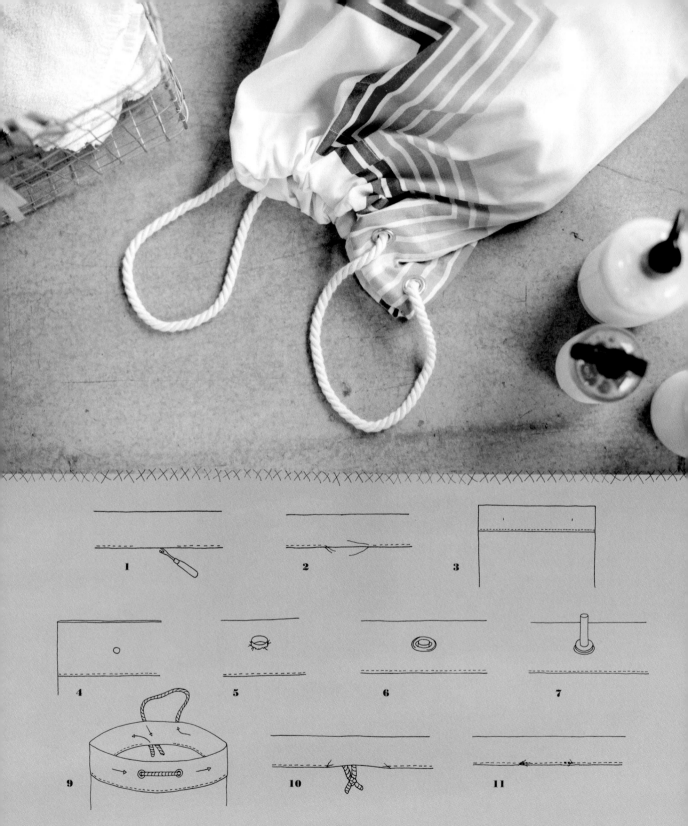

No-Sew Drawstring Pillowcase Bag

A favorite vintage pillowcase can take on a second life as a handy oversized
drawstring bag, perfect for laundry, beach gear, or even to use as reusable gift wrap.

MATERIALS

Pillowcase

Seam ripper

Ruler

Pencil

Small scissors

4 grommets, ⅝" (16 mm) diameter, with grommet installation kit

Hammer or mallet

1–2 yd (1–1.8 m) cotton rope, ½" (12 mm) wide

Iron-on adhesive (we used Therm O Web

Heat n Bond® Ultrahold iron-on adhesive)

Iron and ironing board

INSTRUCTIONS

1   Turn the pillowcase inside out and place it on your work surface vertically. Rotate it so that the side seam runs down the center. At the point where the side seam meets the cuff, remove 2" (5 cm) of stitches from the cuff using the seam ripper.

2   To prevent the opening in the cuff from accidentally getting wider as you work, tie the seam threads at the beginning and at the end of the opening into double knots.

3   Turn the pillowcase right side out and place it flat on your work surface as shown. Using the ruler and pencil, measure and mark 4" (10 cm) in from the right side, half way between the top and bottom edges of the cuff. Repeat these steps to mark the pillowcase on the left side. Then turn the pillowcase over and repeat on this side.

4   Follow the manufacturer's instructions to attach the grommets. Begin by cutting a small hole through only the outside layer of the cuff (leave the inside layer intact) at each 4" (10 cm) mark.

5   Insert 1 "male" half of a grommet (with raised center) through the 2" (5 cm) opening in the cuff and position it in one hole.

6   Place 1 "female" half of a grommet (like a washer) over the "male" half sticking out through the hole.

7   On a sturdy work surface, place the anvil (the cup-shaped tool) inside the pillowcase, directly below the grommet. Place the setter (the long rod) through the holes in the two halves of the grommet and into the anvil.

8   Using a hammer or mallet, hit the setter several times to secure the grommet. Repeat steps 5–8 to attach the 3 remaining grommets.

9   Insert one end of the rope through the opening in the cuff. Working counter-clockwise, push the end through the cuff and out the first grommet. Insert it into the second grommet and continue to move it along the cuff, exiting at the next grommet on the opposite side. Insert it into the following grommet and out the opening in the cuff. The two rope ends should both be at the opening in the cuff.

10 Tie the rope ends together to secure them. Trim away any excess, if necessary. Tuck the tied rope back into the cuff.

11 Cut a strip of iron-on adhesive and position it at the opening in the cuff. Iron to secure. (You can also sew it closed, if you want.)

Oil Painting Shopping Tote

A beautiful painting from a garage sale might not go with your décor
but that doesn't mean it can't have a second life. Scoop up pretty paintings for a few bucks
and turn them into shopping totes for friends and for yourself.

MATERIALS

Oil painting on stretched canvas

Flat-head screwdriver

Pliers

Measuring tape

Scissors

Two pieces of natural cotton canvas, each 2" (5 cm) wider
on all sides than the size of the painting

16 oz. (473 ml) oilcloth medium (we used Martha Stewart Crafts
Decoupage Fabric-to-Fabric Durable Oilcloth Finish)

Squeegee

1"- or 2"- (2.5-cm- or 5-cm-) wide paintbrush

Air-erasable fabric marker

Straight pins

Sewing machine

Coordinating thread

Iron and ironing board

Two yards (1.8 m) of 1½"- (4-cm-) wide cotton webbing
(for the handles)

INSTRUCTIONS

1   Carefully remove the painting from the wooden
stretcher bars (the frame) by pulling out the staples
using a flat-head screwdriver and pliers. Keep as much
of the painting intact as possible. Set it aside.

2   Measure and cut two pieces of canvas, each 2" (5 cm)
wider on all sides than the painting. Set one piece of
canvas aside. Place the second piece on your work
surface. Apply a coat of oilcloth medium by pouring the
medium directly on the top edge of the canvas, and then
spread it using the squeegee for even, solid coverage.

3   Promptly apply the oilcloth medium to the wrong side
of the painting, including the edges. Turn the painting
to the right side and center it on the wet canvas you
prepared in step 2. Smooth the two pieces together to
adhere; let dry.

4   Apply a coat of oilcloth medium to one side of the
remaining piece of canvas; let it dry.

5   Once both pieces are dry, use the paintbrush to apply
a second and then a third coat of medium to the right
sides of both the canvas and the painting; let them dry
between coats.

6   Place the second piece of canvas (the back panel of
the bag) on your work surface wrong side up. Draw
a rectangle on the wrong side of the canvas that's the
same size as the painting with the fabric marker.

7   With the fabrics' right sides together, align and pin the
edges of the painting to the canvas with the marked
rectangle that you prepared in step 6. Sew along the
marked rectangle on three sides, leaving the top open.
Backstitch at the beginning and end of the seam to
secure your stitching.

8   Trim the excess fabric on the three sewn sides to ½"
(12 mm). If needed, trim the top opening, leaving a
2" (5-cm) border of canvas above the painting. Snip
the bottom corners at a 45-degree angle. (Optional:
To prevent fraying, finish the edges with pinking shears
or a serger.)

9   Create a cuff. Fold and press the top edge of the bag to
the wrong side by ½" (12 mm). Then fold and press the
top edge again by 1½" (4 cm). To add the handles to the
bag, cut the cotton webbing into two 18" (46-cm) straps.
Slip both ends of one strap under the cuff on one side
of the bag, in the position you desire, and pin the ends
of the strap in place. Repeat on the opposite side of the
bag with the second strap. Sew all the way around the
bottom edge of the cuff to secure the straps with a ⅛"
(3-mm) seam.

10 To further secure the straps and to create a crisp,
finished-look, sew around the top edge of the cuff with
a ⅛" (3-mm) seam. Turn the bag right side out.

11 Show off your work of art everywhere from the gym to
the farmers' market.

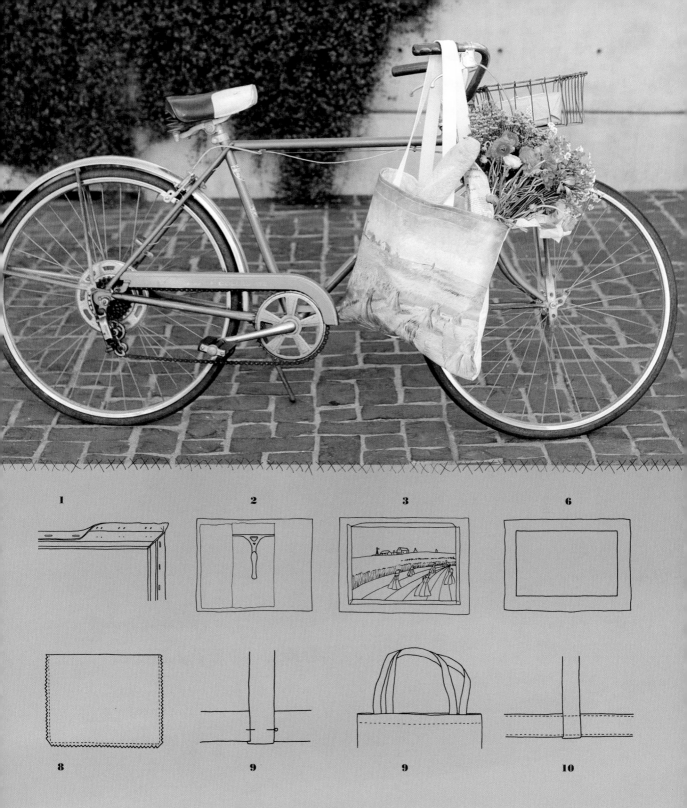

1   2   3   6

8   9   9   10

One Leather Jacket Three Ways

Leather jackets are easy to find, and for just five to ten dollars they provide generous vintage material for crafting. This one jacket made a rustic key holder, clever beanbag bookends, and a pretty sleeve for a glass vase. Here's how to make all three projects from just one vintage leather jacket. No sewing required!

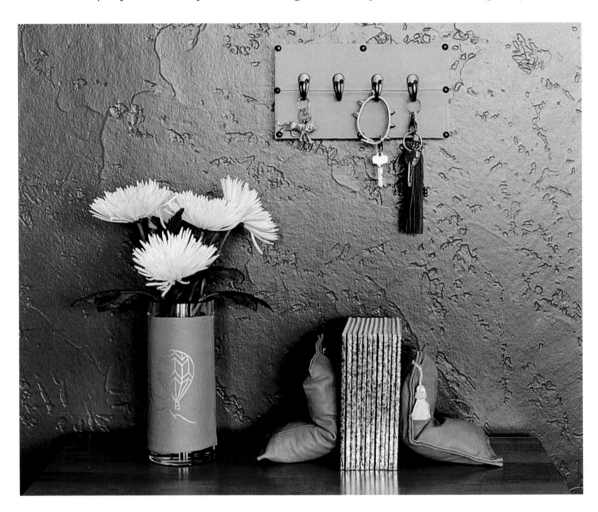

PROJECT ONE
Key Holder with Hooks

PROJECT TWO
Beanbag Book Ends

PROJECT THREE
Leather Vase Wrap

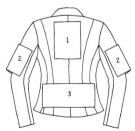

Key Holder with Hooks

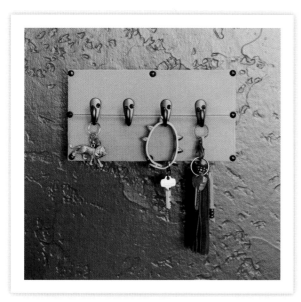

MATERIALS

One 6" × 11" × 2" (15 cm × 28 cm × 5 cm) scrap piece of wood
(most local hardware stores will cut wood to order)

Sandpaper (medium or fine grit)

One 6" × 11" (15 cm × 28 cm) piece of leather cut from a
vintage jacket

Spray adhesive

Eight ⁷⁄₁₆"- (11-mm-) diameter brown hammered upholstery nails
(we used Dritz Home brand)

Needle-nose pliers

Hammer or mallet

Four ¾" × 2" (2 cm × 5 cm) single-prong hooks with screws (we
used bronze-colored Threshold hooks from Target)

Pencil

Electric screwdriver

Sawtooth picture hanger with nails (look in the framing
department of your local hardware store)

We cut our jacket so the seam that ran down the back of the
jacket runs horizontally across the center of our key holder.
It's a nice detail to add without actually sewing!

INSTRUCTIONS

1 Smooth the edges of the wood with the sandpaper.

2 Place the leather on the wood to ensure that the sizes
match. If necessary, trim the leather.

3 Place the wood on a covered work surface. Apply a
light coat of spray adhesive to the front side of the
wood. Position the leather on the wood with the edges
even. Working from the center out, use your hands to
smooth the leather, making sure the front side of the
wood is completely covered. Let it dry completely.

4 Arrange your upholstery tacks as shown in the
illustration, or as desired. To secure them, hold the
stem of one tack with the needle-nose pliers and use a
hammer or mallet to tap the tack into place. Remove the
pliers and use several strong, fluid hits to drive the tack
into the wood. Repeat this step for the remaining tacks.

5 Arrange the hooks as shown in the illustration, or as
desired. Mark the holes for the screws using a pencil.

6 Secure the hooks to the wood using the screws and the
electric screwdriver.

7 Attach a sawtooth picture hanger to the center back of
the wood using the hammer and nails. Now you can
hang it on the wall.

6

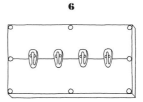

Beanbag Book Ends

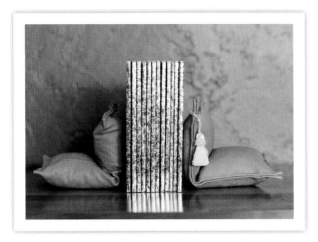

MATERIALS

Two 12" (30.5-cm) squares of leather cut from a vintage jacket

Liquid stitch fabric glue (we used Dritz brand)

Handful of clothespins

Two 2-lb. (907-g) bags dry beans (we used pinto beans that came in a 5" × 10" [12 cm × 25 cm] bag), see note

Two 1"- (2.5-cm-) diameter grommets, with grommet installation kit

Two tassels

Small scissors (needed when adding the grommets)

note: If you're using a bigger bag of beans, use a larger piece of leather. Just be sure it can handle the bulk and remember to add ½" (12 mm) for the seam allowance.

INSTRUCTIONS

1   Place one piece of leather wrong side up. To hem the edges, apply a thin line of liquid stitch fabric glue along the edges on two opposite sides. Fold over both of the glued sides by ¼" (6 mm) and secure with clothespins. Repeat these steps with the remaining two sides until all four sides are hemmed. Now hem the second piece of leather. (As an alternative, you can skip this step and leave the edges raw.)

2   Once the glue is dry, remove the clothespins. Place one piece of hemmed leather wrong side up. Place one bag of beans (still in the bag!) horizontally on the bottom half of the leather. Apply a thin line of liquid stitch fabric glue on the bottom edge of the leather and halfway up the two sides. Fold the leather in half, bringing the top edge down to meet the bottom, keeping the edges even and trapping the beans inside. Secure the edges with the clothespins. Set aside to dry thoroughly. Once dry, remove the clothespins. Repeat these steps to make the second bookend.

3   To finish one bookend, select a corner with less bulk and follow the manufacturer's instructions to install one grommet in the corner, as shown. Repeat this step to add a grommet to the second bookend.

4   Insert the loop end of one tassel through a grommet hole and bring the loop back around to the front. Push the tassel through the loop. Pull on the tassel to secure it. Repeat this step to add the other tassel to the remaining bookend.

5   Find time to sit down and read a book.

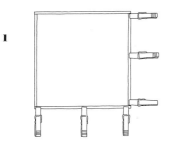

1

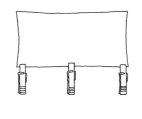

2

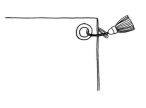

4

Leather Vase Wrap

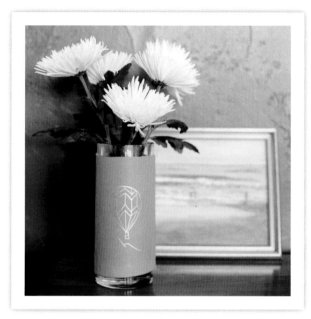

MATERIALS

8" × 14½" (20 cm × 37 cm) piece of leather cut from a vintage jacket

10½" (26.5 cm) glass cylinder vase with a 4" (10-cm) diameter, see note

Masking tape (or any low-tack tape that won't leave marks on the leather)

Four pearl snap fasteners with snap tool (we used ⁷/₁₆"- (11-mm-) diameter Dritz brand snaps)

Pencil

Hammer or mallet

A line drawing of your choice (we used a hot air balloon)

Scissors

Gold leafing pen

note: This project can easily be customized to fit any size glass cylinder vase. Simply cut your leather approximately 2½" (6 cm) shorter than the vase and add an extra 1" (2.5 cm) for the overlap in the back.

INSTRUCTIONS

1   Wrap the leather piece around the vase, overlapping the leather where the ends meet. Secure the leather ends with a piece of tape.

2   Lay the vase down with the overlapping ends face up. Evenly space the pearl snaps vertically along the outer piece of overlapping leather. When you are happy with the snap placement, mark their positions on the leather with a pencil.

3   Move or remove the tape and carefully fold back the outer piece of leather to mark the corresponding snap placement positions on the inner piece of leather.

4   Remove the leather piece from the vase and place it flat on your work surface with the snap placement markings facing up. (Make note of which side is the outer end and which side is the inner end.) Follow the pearl snap manufacturer's instructions to affix the snaps.

5   Photocopy the hot air balloon (or your chosen drawing) to your desired size. Trim away the excess paper. On the backside of the trimmed photocopy, use the side of a pencil tip to shade the entire balloon graphic with graphite.

6   Tape the balloon graphic, right side up, in the desired position on the leather. To transfer the image to the leather, trace over all of the lines with the pencil.

7   Remove the balloon graphic and use a gold leafing pen to trace over the pencil design.

note: When working with vintage leather, stretching and pulling can occur. Always double-check your measurements and alignment for straightness.

2

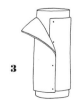
3

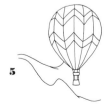
5

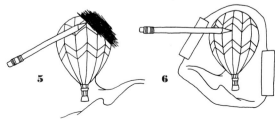
5   **6**

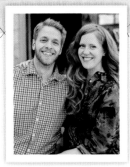

Ten Tips for Working with Leather

BY SAM AND LESLEY GRAHAM OF MAGNOLIALEATHERWORKS.COM AND LESLEYWGRAHAM.COM.

1. Invest in quality tools. Your workmanship and overall satisfaction will suffer if inferior tools hold you back. If you have to, save up and buy them one by one. You'll thank yourself later.

2. A great pair of heavy-duty Gingher shears is my go-to tool for cutting leather. A razor blade or round knife works too.

3. None of the skiving tools you buy at a big box store are any good. Save your money and buy a leatherhead knife. This is a great tool for cutting out leather and for skiving (thinning the leather). Keep it sharp, and be careful when you're using it.

4. Clean and sharpen your tools at the conclusion of each project. It's amazing what a dab of jeweler's rouge, a strop, and some elbow grease can accomplish.

5. Spend some time trolling the internet for good forums related to your craft. It always amazes me how much knowledge is out there. It's so easy to access, and it's free!

6. My favorite leather to work with is full-grain vegetable-tanned leather. It comes in various thicknesses, which are measured in ounces.

7. I recommend Fiebing's oil dye for dyeing your leather. Apply liberally with a wool dauber and let it soak in. Multiple coats are likely necessary.

8. Al Stohlman and his wife, Ann, put together several books regarding just about every discipline of leatherworking. You'll learn more in any one of their books than you could ever teach yourself.

9. Never get leather completely wet unless you plan on permanently altering its shape.

10. Use a leather needle in a sewing machine to sew through thin leather or suede; otherwise, sewing by hand is a skill that you can use for all sorts of projects. The saddle stitch is my go-to stitch.

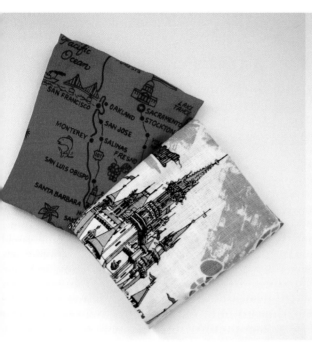

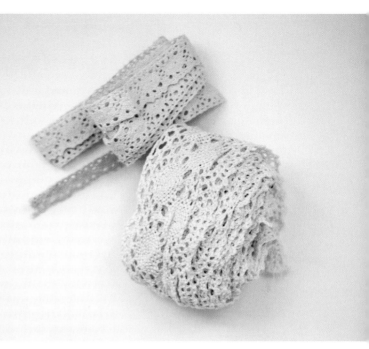

BEST VINTAGE LINEN SCORES

1 Chenille
bedspreads

2 Quilt tops

3 Tablecloths

4 Kitschy sheets

5 Handkerchiefs

6 Doilies

7 Army blankets

8 Tea towels

9 Flocked velvet
curtains

10 Lace curtains

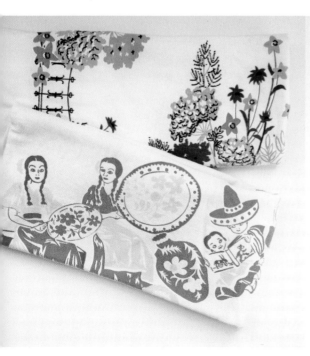

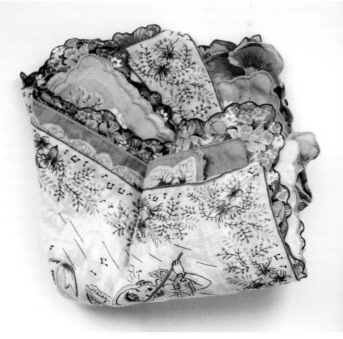

decorating from the hardware store

The hardware store can be a DIY one-stop-shop for unexpectedly beautiful home décor projects. Materials like rope, acrylic glass, tile, and even plumbing hardware can be used to create unique and beautiful home décor items. Plus, for a fraction of the craft-store cost, finishing touches like decorative nail heads, river stones, and chain sold by the yard abound.

PALLET DAYBED

Repurpose pallets and rustproof pipe rod into a cozy, outdoor bed with waterproof tarp cushions. Find the full instructions to make your own on prettyprudent.com.

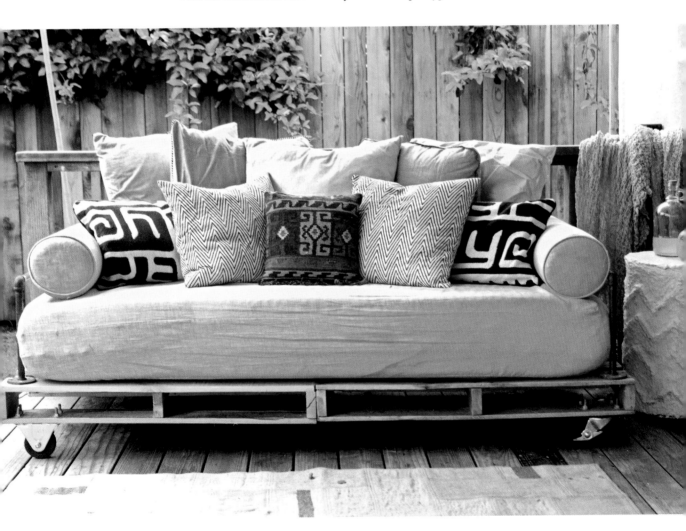

Industrial Curtain Rods

In the plumbing aisle of your local hardware store, you can find everything you need to make these industrial curtain rods (which normally sell for more than 100 dollars at chic home stores). Here's how to recreate the look and all the charm, for one-third the price!

MATERIALS

Two galvanized metal flanges

Two galvanized metal nipples

Two galvanized metal elbows

One galvanized metal pipe cut to the desired rod length (many hardware stores will cut pipe for you and add threads to the end)

Masking tape

Drop cloth

Spray paint for metal in a hammered finish (see note)

Hardware (like screws and wall anchors) and tools appropriate to your particular wall surface

A friend to help you hang it

Level

note: Painting galvanized metal can be tricky. Using paint with a hammered finish helps camouflage possible errors.

We used a 1"- (2.5-cm-) diameter rod and then found flanges, nipples, and elbows that fit accordingly. If you have curtains with existing rings, measure them before heading to the hardware store to ensure your new rod will fit them.

INSTRUCTIONS

1   Clean off any grease or dirt on the flanges, nipples, elbows and the rod.

2   Assemble the flanges, nipples, and elbows as shown in the illustration but don't insert the rod just yet. Use masking tape to cover the threads on both ends of the rod.

3   Place the three parts of the partially assembled curtain rod on a drop cloth and paint them. Add additional coats as needed, allowing for drying time between each coat. Remove the masking tape from the rod.

4   Screw one end of the rod into an elbow. Slide the curtains onto the opposite end of the rod. Attach the remaining elbow.

5   Gather the hardware you need to install the rod, and find a friend to help you! Attach the curtain rod to the wall at the flanges, making sure the curtain rod is level and centered.

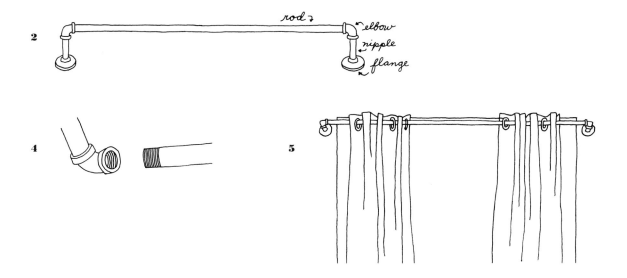

Rope Tassels

These simple tassels help transform basic rope from the hardware store into something decorative and, we think, quite adorable. Use a single tassel as a pull chain for a fan, or bundle a bunch and dangle them from curtain tiebacks. Make smaller tassels to use for gift toppers, or string several across a room as a textural garland.

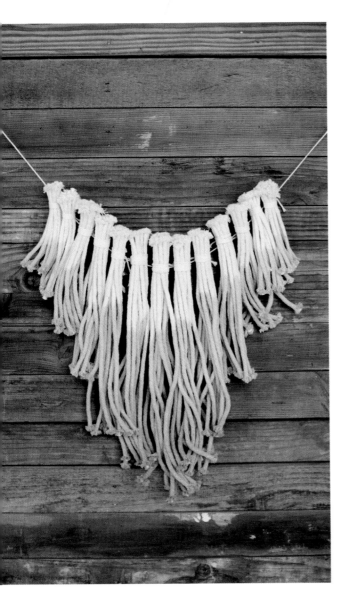

MATERIALS

Cotton rope (we used ½"- [12-mm-] diameter rope)
Twine (we used 3-ply twisted jute twine)
Scissors
Fabric dye (optional)

INSTRUCTIONS

1   Cut lengths of rope into equal-size strips—you'll want about ten strips per tassel.
2   Bundle the cut rope lengths together. Starting 1" (2.5 cm) from the top, wrap a 9"- (23-cm-) long piece of twine around the bundle several times. Tie a knot in the twine to secure the bundle; cut off any excess twine.
3   If necessary, trim the rope lengths on both ends to even them out.
4   Fray the rope bottoms for added interest.
5   For extra fun, dip-dye the ends in bright colors. (Use cotton rope if you intend to dye them!)

Hardware Store Headboard

You're all grown up and it's time for a real headboard. This handsome wooden one costs less than 100 dollars to make (*way* less!) and is actually just three individual boards nailed directly to the wall. You can go with a traditional, rustic, or modern look, depending on your choice of wood stain and bedding.

MATERIALS

Three wooden boards of high-quality pine, oak or cedar (the type of wood depends on your budget and preference), see note for wood dimensions

Sandpaper (medium and fine grit)

Block of wood (optional, for sanding)

Drop cloth

8 oz. (237 ml) wood stain (we used Varathane brand in dark walnut)

Paintbrush

Clean rags or soft cloths

Cardboard

Measuring tape

Pencil

Stud finder

Speed square

Drill and a drill bit smaller than the diameter of the nail

18 lost head nails (we used 2¼" [5.7-cm] nails; you'll need nails long enough to go through the board plus 1" [2.5 cm] of the wall stud)

Level

A friend to help you secure the headboard to the wall

Hammer

note: For a queen or full-sized bed, you'll need three 11½" × 65" × 1" (29 cm × 165 cm × 2.5 cm) boards. The boards can be cut to size at the hardware store or at home if you're comfortable with this task. No matter what size headboard you're making, the final height will be 34½" (88 cm)—the height of each board will always be 11½" (29 cm). To help you determine your width, standard headboard widths are: Twin 39"–43" (99 cm–109 cm); Full/queen 61"–66" (155 cm–168 cm); King: 78"–82" (198 cm–208 cm).

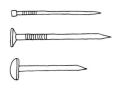

Instead of using lost nails or finishing nails, both which have small heads and are meant to be minimally visible, try using decorative nails.

INSTRUCTIONS

1   Sand the short ends of the boards and the long ends of what will be the top and bottom of your headboard, rounding any sharp edges and smoothing away rough patches. (Fold the sandpaper into thirds or wrap it around a block of wood, as we did, to avoid friction burns.)

2   Cover your work area with a drop cloth. Stain the boards using the wood stain, paintbrush, and rags (see Tips for Staining Wood on page 75). Let your boards completely dry.

3   Place the boards on a protected work surface, wrong side up, in the same position you want them to appear on the wall. (A large piece of cardboard on the floor will prevent your boards from getting scratched.)

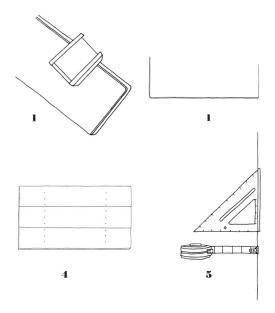

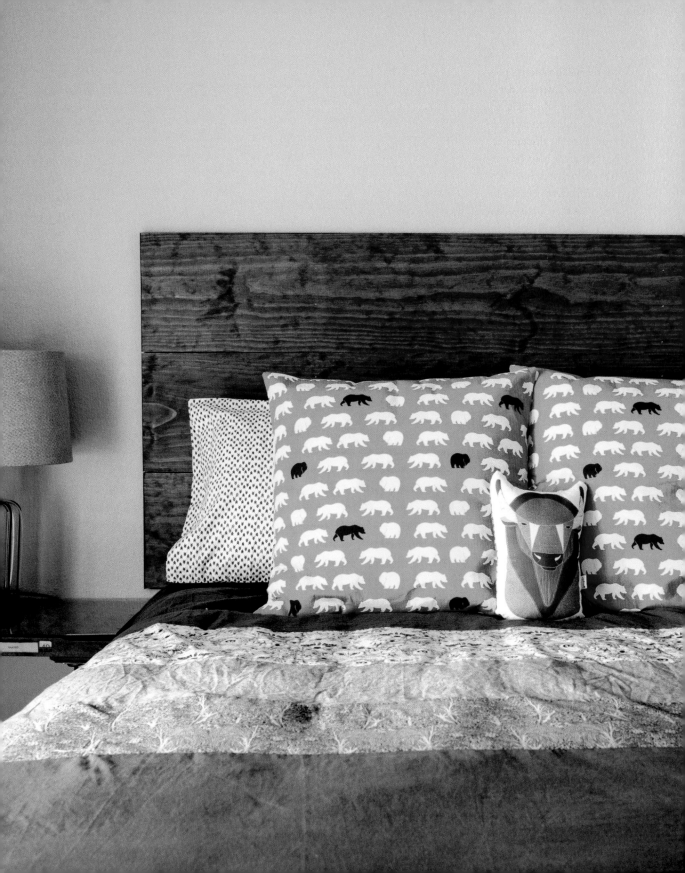

4   Mark the nail positions. To secure the headboard to the wall, you'll need to drive the nails through the boards and into the studs in your wall. Once you locate the wall studs using the stud finder, you'll need to determine the distance between them (because this is how far apart your two rows of nails need to be). Next, you'll determine the vertical positioning of the nails. Each board requires three nails spaced evenly apart. (Our nails were each 2⅜" [3.5 cm] apart.) Unless you're really good with math and fractions, it's best to figure out the spacing on the backs of the boards like we did. Once you've figured it out, jot it down because you'll need to mark the front sides of the boards.

5   Flip the boards back over, right sides facing up, in the same position you want them to appear on the wall. Use a speed square, measuring tape, and pencil to mark each nail position with a "+" mark. (This helps you to see the mark better through the wood stain, but it won't be visible when on the wall.) Double-check your work often to make sure the spacing is correct.

6   Drill a hole through each of the marks on your boards. You'll want to drill from front (the finished side of the board), that way any wood that "blows out" or chips will be on the backside of the board.

7   Make several marks along the wall where the bottom edge of bottom board will sit. (We suggest placing the bottom board a few inches below the top of the mattress.) Use the level to make sure that all of your marks are level.

8   With the help of a friend, align the bottom board with the pencil marks on the wall and hammer one nail into the wall. (If you bend the nail, carefully pull it out, grab a new one, and try again.) Now drive a nail into the same board on the opposite side. Slide the level along the top edge of the board to double-check your work. If it passes the test, nail that baby in!

9   Line up the next board and do the same. (You shouldn't need to use the level after the first board.) Repeat again to attach the last board.

10 Tada—headboard!

Tips for Staining Wood

BY MARIELLE BONEAU

1   With stain, you will want to wear latex/vinyl gloves and be sure that your boards are set out somewhere that you don't mind getting messy.

2   Stir the stain with a stir stick until the color tone is even and there is no goo on the bottom of the can. It is best to apply the stain with a brush and then buff it with a soft cloth. Both of these items will be thrown away after you are done.

3   Test stain out on a scrap piece of wood if you are uncertain how the stain will behave. The scrap piece of wood should be the same type of wood as the wood you plan on using for your project.

4   Brush the stain on the pieces and let it sit for about a minute or two and then rub it in and spread it around a bit with the cloth. This action will remove any hard edges. Do this in sections until the entire piece is stained.

5   Don't forget about the ends and edges of your boards—even the ones that will butt together need some color.

6   End grain is more absorbent than the body of the board. You'll need to use more stain on the ends to get complete coverage.

7   Let the stain dry completely before moving on—information about dry times will be on the container of stain.

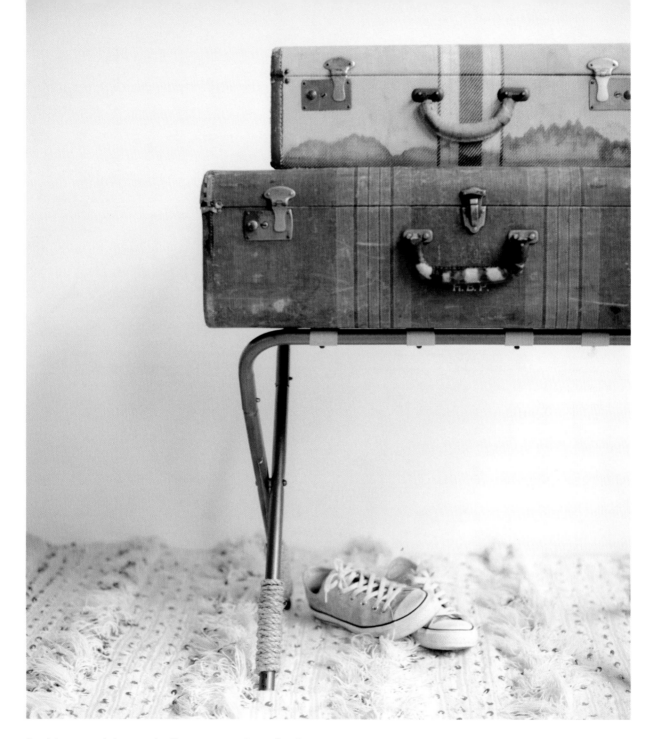

A metal garage-sale luggage stand becomes a guest room favorite
with a few hardware store staples. A coat of copper spray paint lends
modern appeal, while lengths of rope hot glued around each leg add
texture, creating a unique and appealing accent to any guest room.

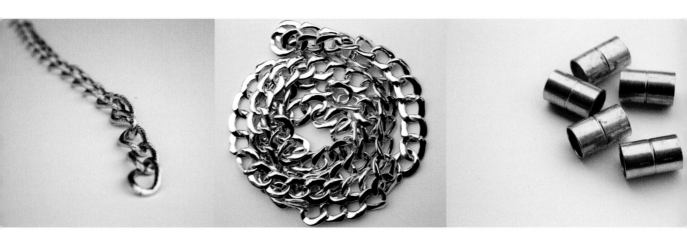

10 BEST THINGS TO SCORE
AT THE HARDWARE STORE

1 Pipe fittings
2 Chain links
3 Parachute cord

4 Rope, rope, rope
5 Twine
6 Canvas tarps

7 Letter stencils
8 Sampler size
paint

9 Furniture legs
10 Parking lot
hot dog

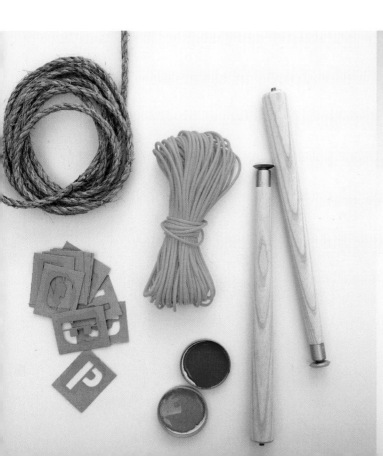

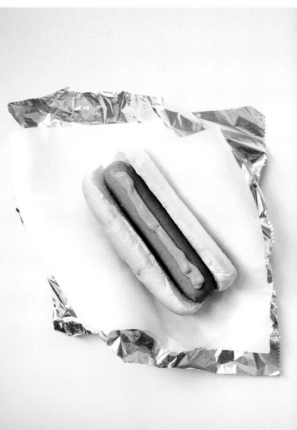

walls, floors & windows

In any old house, a wall is just a wall. In a prudent home, walls, floors, and windows are canvases, each textured with the details of life as seen through one family's eyes. When deciding how to adorn your home we say be whimsical yet forever mindful of your roots. Honor your life's stage by building upon the foundation of your home. Think of the walls as days, the floors as years, and the windows as lifetimes. Decorate your walls to reflect how you feel at any moment; they can and will change, just like you and your children. Choose floors that meet your demands now but will remain sturdy and strong longer than you can fathom. See windows as portals to the future: They create visions that last forever.

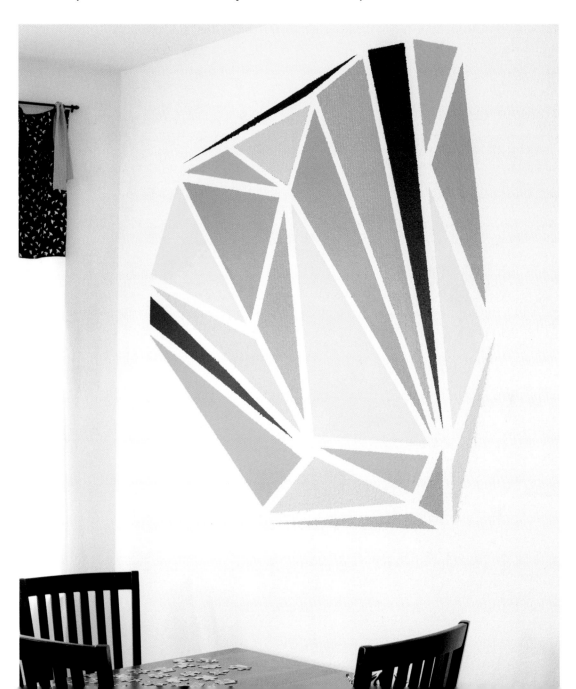

Modern Mural

This bold, geometric mural makes a statement and requires nothing more than a few paint samples, a level, painter's tape, paintbrushes, and a pencil. Note that there was no mention of artistic skills! Choose from your favorite color family or glam it up with some metallic paint.

MATERIALS

Yardstick (meter stick)

Level

Pencil

Modern Mural template (below)

Two rolls of painter's tape, one 1" (2.5 cm) wide and one 1½" (4 cm) wide

4 oz. (118 ml) paint samples (we used black, brown, gold, tangerine, pink, and maize)

Foam brushes, one for each color

Small paintbrush (for touch-ups)

Projector (optional), see note

note: You can scan and project the Modern Mural template onto the wall instead of drawing a grid. If you choose this option, then you can skip step 1.

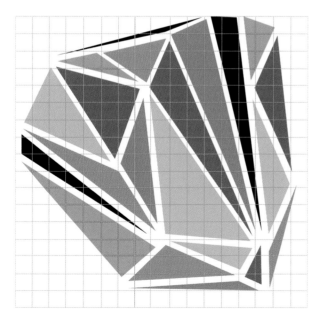

INSTRUCTIONS

1. To paint a mural that's 8' × 8' (2.4 m × 2.4 m) in size, use a yardstick (meter stick), level, and pencil to very lightly draw a grid on the wall. Each box on the grid should be 6" × 6" (15 cm × 15 cm).

2. Following the Modern Mural template, mark off the shapes on your wall using both widths of painter's tape. You may find it easiest to tape off your outside border first using the wider tape. (Taping first lets you visualize how big the finished mural will be and allows you to adjust it, if necessary.)

3. Paint the areas between the lines of tape as shown on the template or as desired.

4. Wait until the paint has dried slightly but is still wet. Then, carefully peel off the tape; this way you get a crisper edge.

5. Use the paintbrush to touch up lines and drips as needed.

Temporary Wallpaper Panel

If you love the textures and interesting patterns that wallpaper offers but have a fear of commitment, why not create a temporary wallpaper panel? This treatment is ideal for dressing a nook (like this one pictured here from Jacinda's home). If your home is nook-free, consider using the very same technique to create a headboard or simply hang the panel on the wall as a piece of art. If you have wallpaper paste and tools, feel free to put them to use. If not, follow these directions using decoupage medium for a similar effect at a lower price.

MATERIALS

Tape

Freezer paper

Scissors

Foam core, large enough to fit the space

Pencil

Craft knife

Ruler

Foam brush

32 oz. (946 ml) decoupage medium, matte finish

Wallpaper (you can use decorative paper too)

One 8' (2.4-m) roll of ½"- (12-mm-) wide hook and loop tape (such as Velcro) with adhesive backing

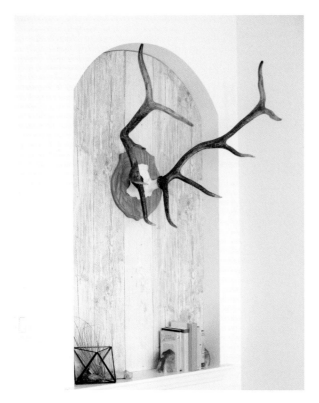

INSTRUCTIONS

1   Use tape to piece together sheets of freezer paper to create a pattern of the area you'd like to temporarily wallpaper. Trim away any excess.

2   Place the pattern on the foam core and trace around the edges with a pencil. Cut out the foam core panel using a craft knife and ruler.

3   Check that the foam core panel fits the intended location. If it's a tight squeeze, add a few tape "tabs" around the edges so you can easily pull the foam core out of the space when you need to.

4   Use the foam brush to apply a layer of decoupage medium to the front of the foam core, at least as thick as the wallpaper.

5   Carefully place the wallpaper on the foam core. Smooth it down, starting at the top of the panel and working your way down to the bottom, releasing any bubbles as you go. Add additional rows of wallpaper as needed to cover the panel. Let the wallpaper dry for several hours or overnight.

6   Optional: To seal the wallpaper, brush on a layer of decoupage medium and let it dry. (You can also change the finish by brushing on a layer of glossy decoupage medium, if you want.)

7   Turn the panel over and trim away any excess wallpaper using the craft knife.

8   Cut several 6" (15-cm) strips of hook and loop tape. Keep the hook sides together with their corresponding loop sides; do not separate them. Beginning with one strip, remove the backing paper from either side and adhere it to the backside of the panel. Continue to remove the backing papers from one side of the remaining strips and adhere them to the panel. Now remove the remaining backing papers and press the panel against the wall to adhere it.

How to Wallpaper with Anything

Working with even the most modest of budgets, you can use this DIY technique to turn virtually any type of paper into a high-end wall covering. Old travel photos, childhood baseball card collections, or the pages of a vintage botanist's guide will allow any room in your home to tell its own unique story. If our walls—adorned with hand-illustrated pages from a nautical knot-tying guide—*could* talk, they would tell captivating tales of sailing the high seas.

INSTRUCTIONS

1. Carefully cut the pages from your book by placing the ruler (held firmly in place) along the gutter of the book. Then run a sharp craft knife along the edge of the ruler.

2. Repeat step 1 until you have as many pages as you need to cover your wall. (This may take a little measuring and math to figure out.)

3. Protect all floors and furniture with drop cloths. Choose which wall you want to wallpaper first, and begin in the center of that space. Apply wallpaper paste directly to the wall with a clean paintbrush and then smooth one book page on top of it. (You have a few seconds to adjust the position of your page after applying it, so quickly check it with a level.) Apply another thin coat of wallpaper paste on top of the page.

4. Remove away any wrinkles or bubbles using a wallpaper smoother. Begin in the center and smooth the page outward in all directions until no bubbles appear.

5. Continue adding book pages to create rows and columns, overlapping their edges for a slightly imperfect charm. (We love this look!) When the paper is dry, use the ruler and craft knife to trim away any overhang.

6. Tip: To negotiate a corner, position the page on the wall before adding the paste. Push the page into the corner and crease it. Trim away any excess and then adhere it to the wall. Use this same technique to apply pages when you come to wall edges.

7. Continue wallpapering until your entire wall, room, or house tells a story.

MATERIALS

Book (one you'd like to cut pages from)
Ruler
Craft knife
Drop cloths
Wallpaper paste
Paintbrush
Level
Wallpaper smoother or old credit card
  (we used an expired driver's license)

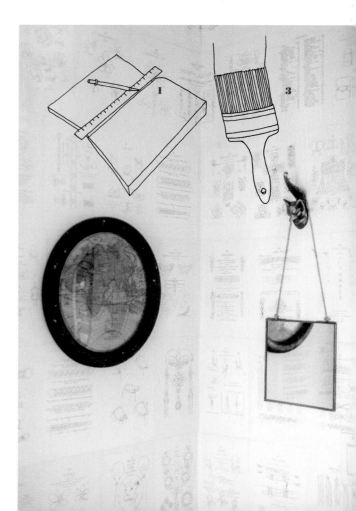

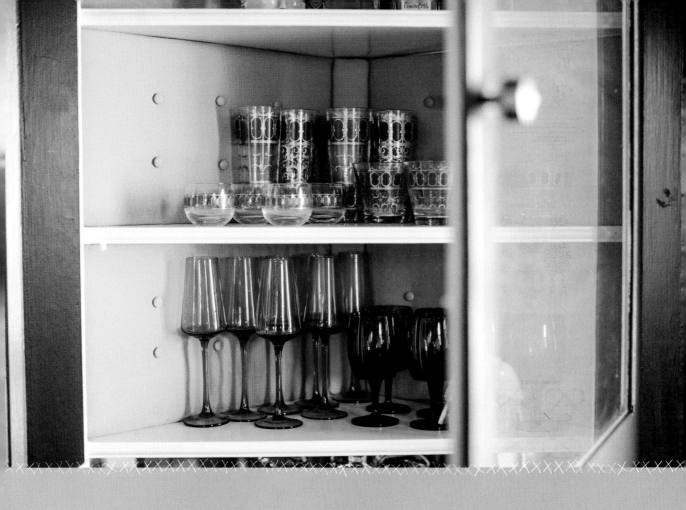

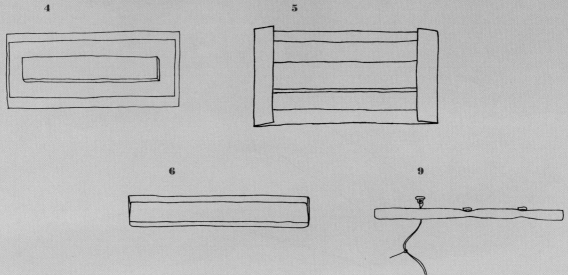

4

5

6

9

Tufted Panels

Custom upholstery on a wall can be luxurious as well as visually striking. With a simple
starter project like this one, you'll find it's also surprisingly easy to execute.
Turn any plain bookshelf into an eye-catching piece with tufted fabric panels.

MATERIALS

Measuring tape

Pencil

$^3/_{16}$"- (5-mm-) thick polystyrene (Styrofoam), a piece
  large enough to cover your desired space

Craft knife

Mid-loft polyester batting (see step 3 for amount)

Scissors

Fabric (we used a linen/rayon blend; see step 3
  for amount)

Hot glue gun and glue sticks

½"- (12-mm-) diameter button cover kit, to make
  fabric-covered buttons

Chalk

Hand sewing needle

Coordinating thread

Removable adhesive putty (optional)

INSTRUCTIONS

1 Measure the space you want to cover with a tufted
   panel. Use a pencil to mark these measurements on the
   foam core.

2 Cut the foam core to size with a sharp craft knife.

3 Cut a piece of batting that is 4" (10 cm) wider and 4"
   (10 cm) longer than the foam core. This will give you
   a piece of batting that is 2" (5 cm) larger on all sides.
   Now cut a piece of fabric that is 6" (15 cm) wider and
   6" (15 cm) longer than the foam core. This will give
   you a piece of fabric that is 3" (7.5 cm) larger on all
   sides.

4 Place the fabric wrong side up. Center the batting on
   top of the fabric and center the foam core on top of the
   batting.

5 Wrap the short sides of the fabric and batting around
   the foam core and hot glue them into place, making
   sure the fabric is taut, but not tight.

6 Wrap the long sides of the fabric and batting around
   the foam core and hot glue them into place.

7 Repeat steps 1 to 6 to make additional panels, if
   desired.

8 On the front side of the panel, measure and mark
   where the fabric-covered buttons will go using the
   chalk. Then prepare as many buttons as needed,
   according to the kit's instructions.

9 Attach each button to the panel by sewing through all
   three layers using a needle and thread. Tie the thread
   off on the backside of the panel.

10 Slide the panels into place on the wall of your bar,
   bookshelf, or nook. If extra staying power is needed,
   use removable adhesive putty.

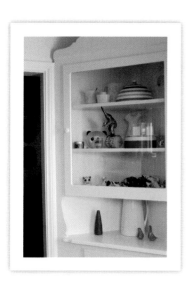

Before

How to Stencil an Outdoor Floor

Plain concrete patios, steps, and entryways are practically begging to be stained, polished, or in this case stenciled. Jaime gave new life to the drab front porch of her bungalow with this bold, tile-inspired pattern that reflects the Spanish and Mexican influences of her sunny southern California city. It's prettier—and more whimsical—than tired old gray concrete.

MATERIALS

Outdoor Floor Stencil template (see page 220)

Craft knife or scissors

Stencil film material (available at any art supply store, we used Mylar brand)

Marker or pen

Cutting mat

Cement sealer (available at any hardware store)

Four paint trays (one for the sealant and three for the paint colors)

Two paint rollers (one for the sealant and one for the background paint color)

Paintbrush (for applying the sealant to corners and tight spaces)

Pencil

Painter's tape

Two stencil brushes, one for each color on the "tile"

Three colors of outdoor cement floor paint (a background color, a "tile" color, and a contrasting color for the center diamond shape)

INSTRUCTIONS

1   Photocopy the Outdoor Floor Stencil template, enlarging it to work with the area you'll be painting. Cut out the center diamond using a craft knife or scissors. Position the template on the stencil film. Trace around the outside edges of the paper template and the diamond shape using the marker. Remove the template. Place the stencil film on the cutting mat and use the craft knife to cut along the drawn lines. This is the first stencil. Set it aside.

2   Using the same paper template from step 1, cut along the stepped lines. Place the template on a second piece of stencil film. Trace around the outside edges of the paper template and the stepped lines with the marker. Remove the template. Place the stencil film on the cutting mat and use the craft knife to cut along the drawn lines. This is your second stencil.

3   Thoroughly wash your outdoor floor. Scrub, scrub, scrub with warm soapy water to remove as much dirt as possible. Let it dry.

4   Following the manufacturer's instructions, apply the cement sealer to the floor to create an even surface for the paint to adhere to. Use both a paint roller and a paintbrush (for those hard to reach places). Let the floor dry completely before proceeding.

5   Paint the entire floor with a single background color using a paint roller. Let the paint dry completely before adding a second coat. Continue adding coats of paint until the background color is uniform and completely dry.

6   Place the second stencil you made in the center of the cement floor. Mark the four corners on the outside edges of the stencil lightly with a pencil. (This will help you identify the exact position the stencil needs to be in as you move it around the floor.)

7   Working out from the center, place your stencil on the floor next to the first marks, and lightly mark the outside corners. Repeat until the entire floor has been covered with a grid.

8   Review your marks and the overall pattern of the grid. Is your pattern even and centered? If so, it's time to paint.

9   Place your stencil again at your center mark, aligning the four corners with your pencil marks. Tape the stencil in place with painter's tape.

10 Use your stencil brush to apply a very light coat of paint. Allow the paint to dry up to a minute between coats, but be sure to lift the stencil while the paint is still wet on the final coat (this will give your work nice, crisp edges).

11 Move the stencil to the next mark and repeat the painting process. When you start the second and third rows, be careful not to tape your stencil to wet paint. And above all, be patient.

12 When the paint is dry, touch up any areas that may need it. Allow the paint to dry completely.

13 Repeat steps 9 to 12 to paint the center diamonds using the first stencil and a fresh stencil brush.

14 Apply another layer of cement sealer to the entire floor to ensure a long lifetime for your design. Let the sealer dry completely.

15 Walk all over your hard work.

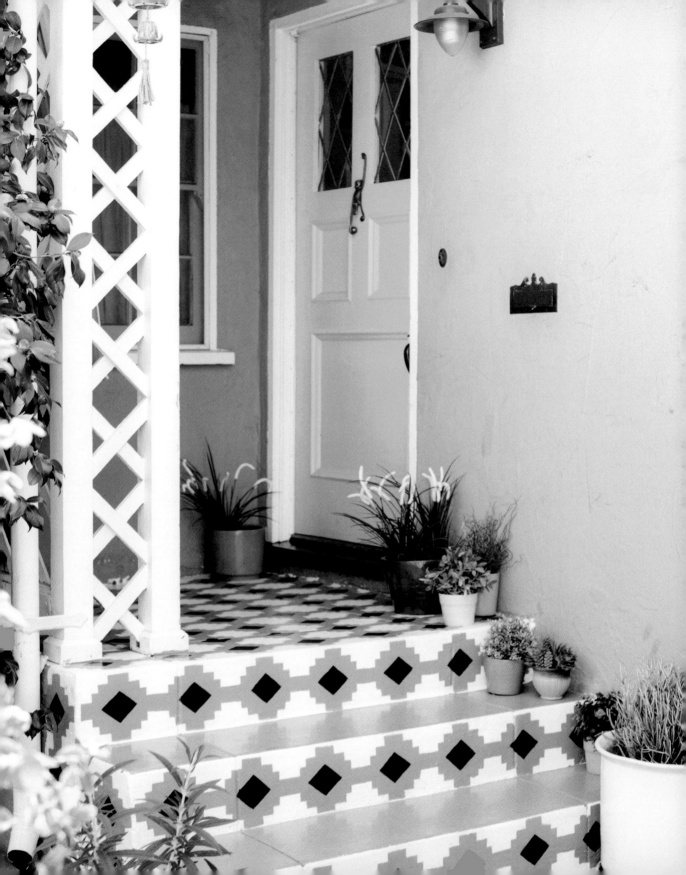

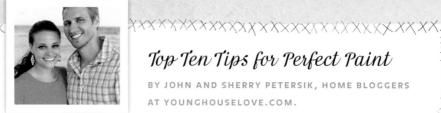

Top Ten Tips for Perfect Paint

BY JOHN AND SHERRY PETERSIK, HOME BLOGGERS AT YOUNGHOUSELOVE.COM.

1   Thin and even coats is our mantra. If you brush or roll paint on too thickly (on walls, a piece of furniture, a cabinet, or you-name-it), you can end up with marks, splatters, drips, and all sorts of other bad news.

2   Our favorite paintbrush for cutting in and painting trim is one of those 2" (5-cm) angled brushes with a short rubber handle. They usually sell them by the register at most home improvement stores. The combination of the short handle and the angled bristles makes controlling the brush a lot easier.

3   We have painted rooms in all different orders—ceiling first, walls first, trim first—but the approach that seems to make the most sense is to tackle the ceilings first. Next go for the trim, then finally, you can paint those walls.

4   We don't always use primer when we paint walls since many wall paints are now of good enough quality to hold up well without it, but it's always best to use a primer in these scenarios: your drywall is new or unprimed/unpainted; you're going from a very light paint color to a very dark one; you're going from a very dark wall color to a lighter one.

5   Whenever we paint wood—be it wood furniture, wood trim, or wood cabinets—we always use a stain blocking primer. This primer will help you avoid one of the most annoying paint issues: wood bleed.

6   When picking paint colors, tape potential swatches to the wall for at least 48 hours before making a decision, so you can compare them all in different kinds of lighting scenarios. The one you like most in the natural light of day might be the one you like least at night when the overhead lights are casting a more yellow tone.

7   If you're still unsure, then spend a few bucks on a test pot of paint (or three). It's one of the easiest ways to avoid having to repaint a whole room because you hate the color.

8   When it comes to washing our brushes after a paint job, regular old water is all that we use for latex-based paint, but we rinse them for a good long time (around five minutes), until the water runs clear. For oil-based paint or primer, we use mineral spirits, but we like to do that outside while wearing a mask, since they can be pretty fumy to work with.

9   When it comes to picking a paint finish, we tend to prefer flat paint for ceilings (it hides imperfections), semi-gloss paint for doors and trim (it's nice and wipe-able) and eggshell paint for the walls of most rooms, except kitchens and bathrooms—a satin finish makes those rooms easier to wipe down.

10 Never paint without good music or on an empty stomach. Seriously, it's a bad idea.

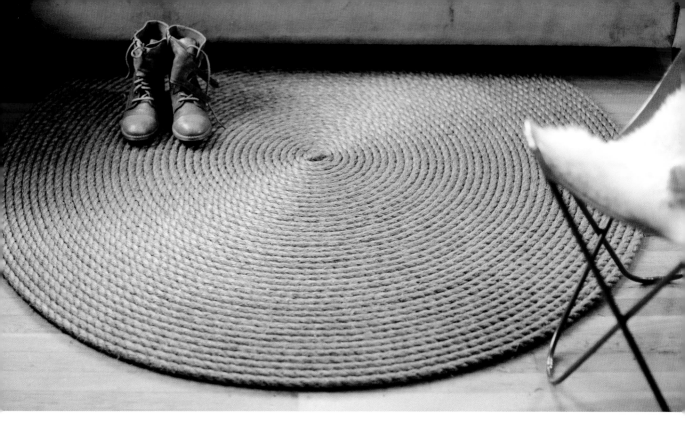

Nautical Rope Rug

Create a decorative and durable rug with a dash of maritime style. Guests
will never suspect that this rug was a hardware store supply DIY project!

MATERIALS

300 yards (274 m) of ¾"- (2-cm-) diameter natural fiber rope
  (we used two 150-yard (137-m) spools)
Hot glue gun and glue sticks

INSTRUCTIONS

1   Coat one end of the rope in hot glue to seal it and to
    prevent it from fraying.
2   Start to coil the rope around the sealed end; secure with
    hot glue. Hold this section tightly until the glue cools
    and it can retain its shape. (Be careful not to burn your
    fingers!) This will be the center of your rug.
3   Place the center coil, wrong side up, on the floor. (This
    should be the side with more visible glue.) Continue to
    wrap the rope around the center, securing it with hot
    glue as you go. Keep the rope flat on the floor as you

work. Work slowly and carefully to prevent the hot glue
from dripping between the coils (if glue drips between
the coils, it will be visible on the right side of the rug).
Hot glue on the bottom of the rug is no problem—it
will act as a non-slip rug mat!

4   When you reach the end of the first spool of rope, seal
    the raw end with hot glue. Then seal the free end of the
    new spool with hot glue too. Line the two ends up and
    glue them together, making sure the glue does not show
    on the right side of the rug. Continue to coil and glue
    the rope until you reach the end of the second spool.
5   Finish the final raw edge of the rope with glue and
    secure it to the rug. Then, check the rug for any gaps
    and secure those areas with glue if necessary. Let the
    glue cool and turn the rug over. Ahoy!

Not-So-Granny Square Crochet Rug

This rug puts a new twist on the traditional granny square and it also takes it someplace unexpected—the floor. If you've ever crocheted a granny square, this project requires no further explanation. Go grab some paracord and an oversized crochet hook and get going.

MATERIALS

550 paracord: 200' (961 m) in charcoal;
  200' (961 m) in safety orange; 400' (122 m) in goldenrod;
  500' (152) in aqua
Crochet hook, size N/15 (10 mm)
Scissors
Fabric glue
Brush
Non-skid rug coating (we used MCG textiles rug backing by Saf-T-Bak)

INSTRUCTIONS

1. To make the foundation chain, start by making a loop.
2. Chain stitch (ch) 6.
3. Slip stitch (sl st) to first ch to form a ring.
4. Round 1: ch 3—counts as first double crochet (dc), 2 dc in ring, [ch 3, 3 dc in ring] 3 times, ch 1, half double crochet (hdc) in top of turning chain (t-ch). Do not turn. Total: 12 dc.
5. Round 2: ch 3—counts as first double crochet (dc), 2 dc in space created by previous row's hdc, *ch 1, [3 dc, ch 3, 3dc] in ch-3 space (sp); repeat from * 2 times, ch 1, 3 dc in ch-1 sp, ch 1, hdc in top of t-ch, do not turn. Total: 24 dc.
6. Round 3: ch 3—counts as first double crochet (dc), 2 dc in space created by previous row hdc, *ch 1, 3 dc in ch-1 sp, ch 1, [3 dc, ch 3, 3 dc] in ch-3 space (sp); repeat from * 2 times, ch 1, 3 dc in ch-1 sp, ch 1, 3 dc in ch-1 sp, ch 1, hdc in top of t-ch, do not turn. Total: 36 dc.
7. Rounds 4–12: work as for round 3, always working 3 dc in each ch-1 sp and [3 dc, ch 3, 3 dc] in the corners and working ch 1 between 3 dc clusters.
8. Dab fabric glue on the ends of each cut cord; let dry.
9. Use the hook to weave the ends of the cord back through the rug toward the backside of the piece.
10. Turn the rug over, wrong side up. Brush on a layer of non-skid rug coating to the entire backside; let the glue dry. (Be careful not to use it in excess, as it dries white.)

note: To change the color of the cord for each new round as we did here, complete the last stitch in the round, a half-double crochet, and pull the loop on the hook out to the side about 5" (12 cm) and cut. Pull the cord still attached to the skein out through the piece and pull tightly on the remaining cord tail. Weave the end through the work to secure and hide it. (You can do this after you complete each round or you can hide all the ends at once when you complete the rug.) Make a loop in the next color and pull it through the same space, on your hook, to begin the next row.

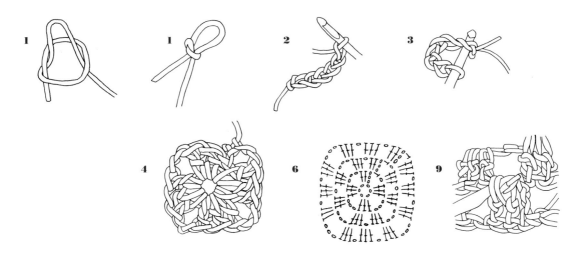

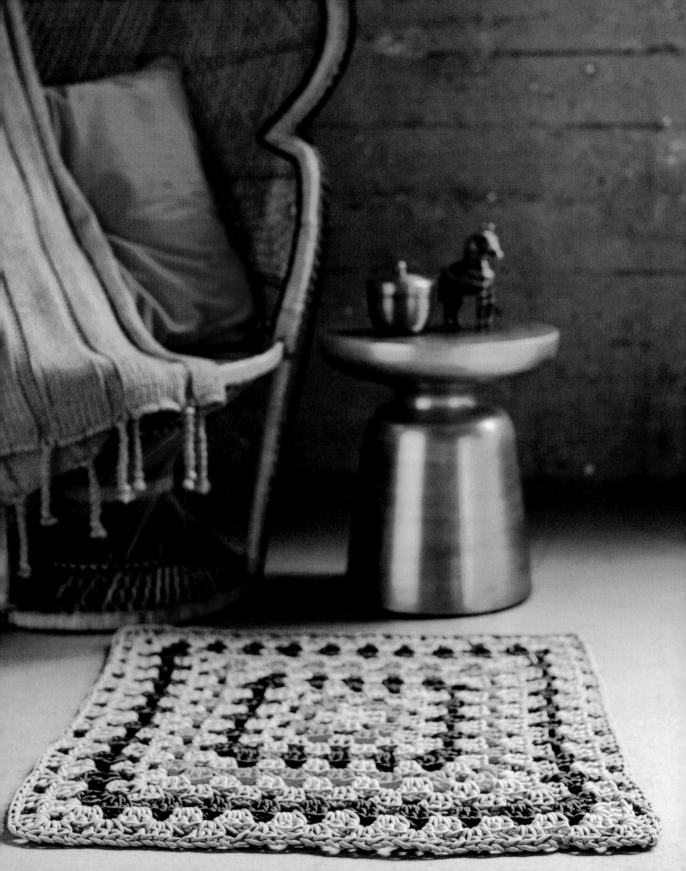

CROCHET KEY

* This indicates the beginning of a stitch pattern that will be repeated. Repeat the directions following a single asterisk as directed.

[ ] Follow the directions within the brackets as many times as directed.

T-CH

turning chain

SP(S)

space(s)

CH

chain stitch—With a loop (slipknot) on the hook, wrap the yarn over the hook and pull it through the loop.

SL ST

slip stitch—Insert the hook into the stitch. Wrap the yarn over the hook and draw the yarn back through the stitch and the loop on the hook.

HDC

half double crochet—Yarn over and insert the hook into the stitch. Yarn over and pull through (3 loops on hook). Yarn over and pull through all loops on hook.

DC

double crochet—Yarn over and insert the hook into the stitch. Yarn over and pull through (3 loops on hook). Yarn over and pull through 2 loops. Yarn over and pull through remaining 2 loops. Typically the first dc in a series will be replaced by 3 ch.

CURTAIN TIEBACKS

Fish need to swim, birds need to fly, and curtains need to hang. Let them drop to the floor and puddle for a classic, romantic look, pull them up to create a more dramatic, even regal appearance, or simply tie them back to let in the light of day. Here are some ideas for inexpensive, easy tiebacks that will complement your room without busting your budget.

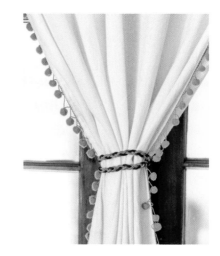

Braid suede cord with a loop at one end and a knot at the other. Pop the knot into the loop to create a simple tieback with a modern yet well-worn look.

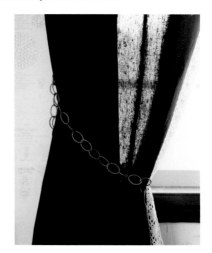

Simple loops of chain can complement a minimalist industrial look or add a bit of shine and polish to any room. Just use pliers to open a link of chain, drape the length of chain around the curtains, then hang the open link on a hook.

For instructions on how to sew a pair of traditional tiebacks (opposite), visit prettyprudent.com.

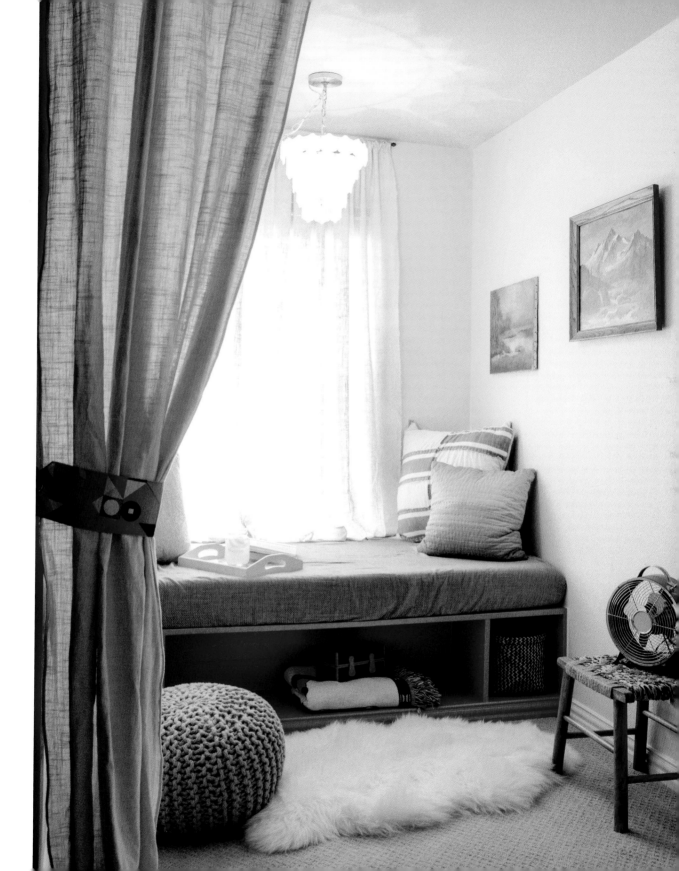

Tie-Top Curtains

This easy, DIY curtain project uses ribbon to create a charming row of ties along the top of a basic curtain panel.

MATERIALS

Two 40" x 25" (100 x 63.5 cm) pieces of fabric in coordinating prints
(We made this reversible café curtain for a 17"- [43-cm-] wide window.)
Eight 16" (41-cm) lengths of 1½"- (4-cm-) wide grosgrain ribbon
Measuring tape
Scissors
Air-erasable fabric marker
Straight pins
Sewing machine
Coordinating thread
Point turner
Iron and ironing board
Trim (optional)

INSTRUCTIONS

1 To customize these curtains to your particular window dimensions, you first need to determine the width and length you'd like them. Start by measuring the width of your window. A good rule of thumb is that a curtain should be two to three times this amount. Once you have your width, add 2" (5 cm) to this measurement for the seam allowances.

2 Now determine how long you want the curtains to be. This really depends on the height of the window and the style you prefer. The ones pictured here are 24" (61 cm) long. Once you've determined the length, add 1" (2.5 cm) to this measurement for the seam allowances.

3 Next calculate the number of ribbon ties you'll need. You want an even number of ribbon ties evenly spaced across the top of the curtain every 5"–10" (12–25 cm). (Adjust your measurements, if necessary, to get an even number of ties.) Each pair of ribbon ties should be cut to a length that's equal to one-third the length of your top panel of fabric.

4 Place the fabric for the back side of the curtain right side up on your work surface.

5 Measure and make a mark 1" (2.5 cm) from the left edge. (This is your seam allowance.) Pin a pair of ties at this 1" (2.5-cm) mark. The ends of the ribbons should be even with the top, unfinished edge of the panel. Continue to pin evenly spaced pairs of ties every 5"–10" (12–25 cm), leaving another 1" (2.5 cm) seam allowance on the opposite end of the panel. Optional: To add trim, pin it along the bottom edge of the panel with the raw edges even.

6 Place the remaining piece of fabric (the front side) on top of the back panel with right sides together and raw edges even. (The ties and trim should be sandwiched between the two layers of fabric.) Pin together. Sew around all four sides of the panel with a ½" (12-mm) seam. Leave a 5" (12-cm) opening on one side of the panel for turning the curtain right side out in the next step. Clip the corners.

7 Turn the panel right side out through the opening and use a point turner to push out the corners. Tuck the seam allowances into the opening so they don't show, and iron flat.

8 Top stitch all the way around the panel with a ¼" (6-mm) seam.

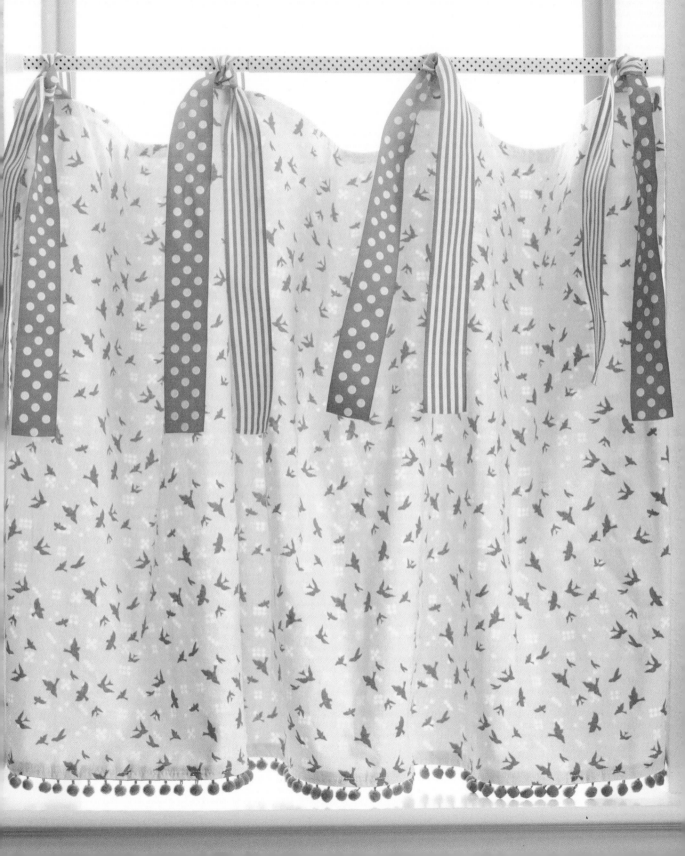

Dip-Dye Curtains

Turn this DIY project upside down by dip-dying the tops of your curtains.
These window dressings make a bold statement with an easy-breezy vibe.

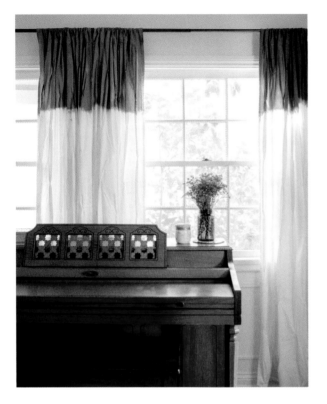

INSTRUCTIONS

1 Decide how much of the curtain you want dyed, and mark each side with a clothespin. Neatly fold up the remaining length of the curtain, (the portion you want to remain un-dyed), and secure it with clothespins.

2 Place the plastic tub in a bathtub and put your gloves on. Following the manufacturer's instructions, mix together the dye, water, and salt in the plastic tub (we used two parts denim blue dye, one part teal dye).

3 Dip the top of your curtain into the dye up to your clothespin markers. Use the spoon to ensure this portion is completely submerged. Let it soak for a minimum of ten minutes.

4 Remove the curtain from the dye bath and rinse the dyed portion only with warm water, then cold, until the water runs clear. Hang the curtain to dry (hang it upside down so drips don't fall onto the un-dyed part).

5 Repeat these steps to dye additional curtains. Then hang and enjoy!

MATERIALS

Curtains made from a natural fabric like cotton or linen (synthetic fabrics, even a poly blend, won't take the dye)

Clothespins

Plastic tub

Disposable gloves

Fabric dye (we used Rit Liquid Dye in denim blue and teal)

Water

Salt

Large metal spoon (for stirring)

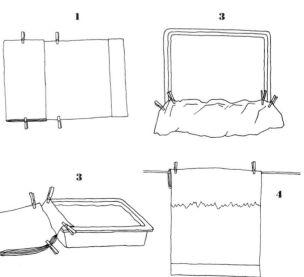

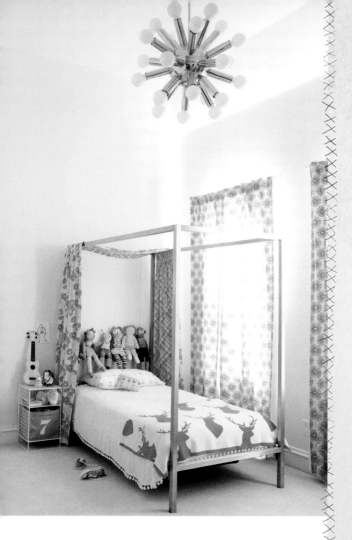

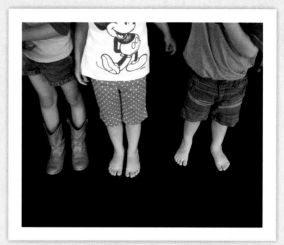

Five Floor Tips
for Living with Kids

1   Dark wood shows every footprint and every speck
    of dust.

2   Consider skipping a rug under the kitchen table;
    this makes for easy food cleanup.

3   Bamboo floors are very delicate. They will bear
    the scars of every dropped toy, high heel, or roller
    skate. Also, do not roller-skate in the house.

4   Use an area rug to define a play space, even
    on top of carpet.

5   Splurging on carpet and padding will pay off
    in luxurious softness under your feet. Higher-
    quality carpet typically is also more durable and
    stain resistant.

Five Window Treatment Tips
for Living with Kids

1   Consider cordless blinds, or follow the
    manufacturer's instructions for cutting cord length.

2   Plantation blinds block light well and can be
    custom-made to fit irregularly shaped windows.

3   Curtains lined with black-out fabric help to control
    light in baby's room during the day.

4   Kids will play in floor-length curtains. They just
    will. Pick fabric types and colors that can tolerate
    being kid-handled.

5   Curtains can be altered to any length—no sewing
    involved!—using iron-on adhesive strips.

pillows & linens

Anyone can personalize a prudent home with fabrics regardless of skill level—we promise. These basic home-sewing lessons help you outfit your home in custom coziness at a deep cost cut, even if you've never sewn before. So get ready to start stitching your own ammunition for the next big pillow fight, and the linens you'll snuggle up in after.

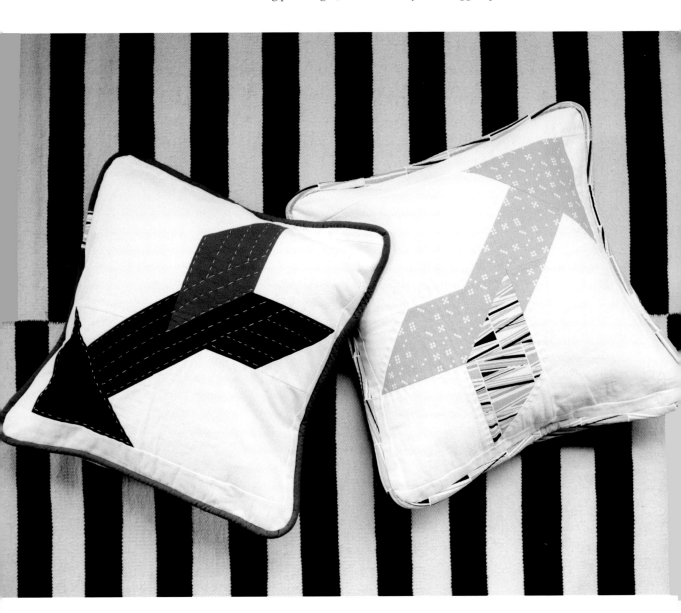

These geometric arrow pillows take quilting from cozy and cute to bold and sophisticated. Find instructions for making them on prettyprudent.com.

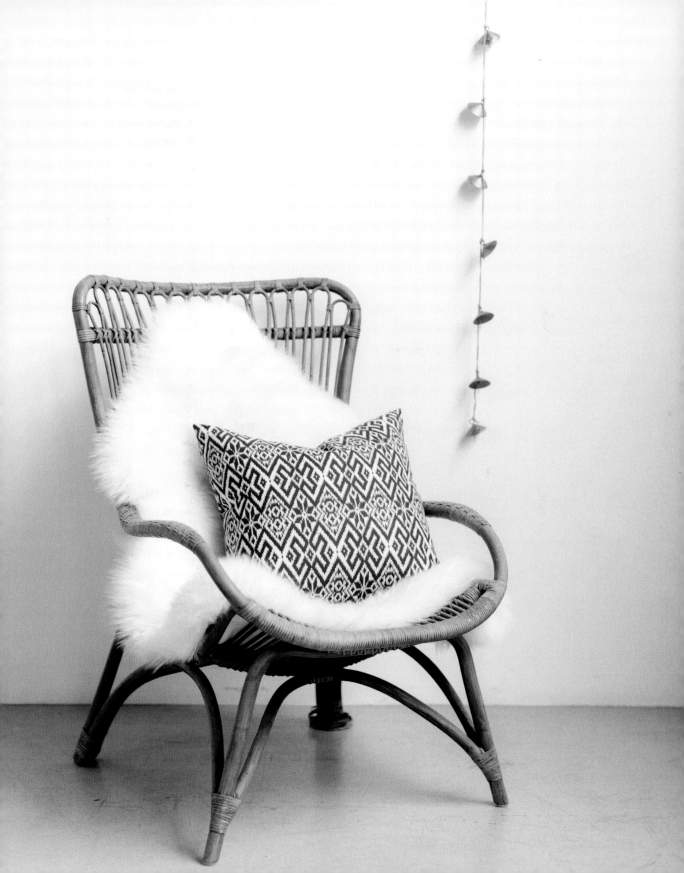

Basic Zipper Pillow

Don't fear the zipper! Once you make one zipper pillow, it will quickly become
your new favorite sewing project (trust us!). Your spouse will love it too—apart
from complaints about twenty pillows taking up all the space on the bed!
But jokes aside, *do* make a zipper pillow because they're fun and easy to make,
and we promise you won't be disappointed with the results.

MATERIALS

Pillow insert

Measuring tape

Cotton fabric (see step 1 for amount)

Scissors

Pinking shears or serger (optional)

Straight pins

One all-purpose zipper, 2" (5 cm) shorter
in length than your pillow insert

Air-erasable fabric marker (or chalk)

Sewing machine

Coordinating thread

Iron and ironing board

Zipper foot

Seam ripper

INSTRUCTIONS

1 To determine the amount of fabric you'll need, measure
the length and width of your pillow insert; then add 1"
(2.5 cm) to the width and 1" (2.5 cm) to the length. Cut
two pieces of your fabric to this size.

2 Finish the left-hand edge of each piece of fabric by
sewing it with a zigzag stitch, or by trimming it with
pinking shears or using a serger. Pay attention to the
direction of the pattern on your fabric to ensure that
you'll like the way it will line up on both the front and
the back of the pillow when the fabric pieces are sewn
together. Adjust the fabric's orientation, if necessary.

3 Align and pin your two fabric pieces together, with right
sides facing; place the finished edges on the left-hand side.
Center the zipper along the left edge on the top piece of
fabric. Mark the fabric at the top and bottom zipper stops
using the air-erasable fabric marker. Remove the zipper.

4 Using a straight stitch, sew from the bottom edge of
the fabric up until the line that marked the bottom of
the zipper, backstitching at the beginning and end to
secure the stitches. The stitches should be parallel to and
½" (12 mm) away from the left finished edge. (Use the
illustration as a guide.) Repeat this procedure to sew from
the top edge of the fabric down to the line marking the
top of the zipper.

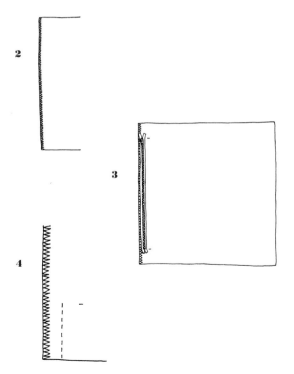

5 Use a basting stitch (basting can be done by setting your machine to its longest stitch length, usually a 5) to sew between the stitches you made in step 4.

6 Open up the fabric, with the wrong sides facing up, and press the seam allowances open.

7 Center the zipper, face down, on the seam. Pin it in place.

8 Using a straight stitch and the zipper foot, sew the zipper in place down each side and across the bottom. (When you reach the zipper slider, drop your needle down in the fabric, lift the presser foot, and zip, or unzip, the zipper to move the slider out of the way so you can continue stitching the rest of the zipper.) Be careful not to stitch through the metal stopper at the end of your zipper or it will break your needle.

9 Open your fabric and place it right side up on your work surface. Use a seam ripper to remove the previous basting stitches and reveal the zipper. Unzip the zipper halfway so you'll be able to turn the pillow cover right side out later.

10 Align the raw edges of the two fabric pieces with right sides facing; pin the three unsewn edges.

11 Sew with a ½" (12-mm) seam, backstitching at the beginning and end of the seam to secure your stitches.

12 Clip the corners and finish the raw edges by sewing them with a zigzag stitch, or by trimming them with pinking shears or using a serger.

13 Turn the pillow right side out through the open zipper and place the pillow insert inside.

14 Lay your head down and rest.

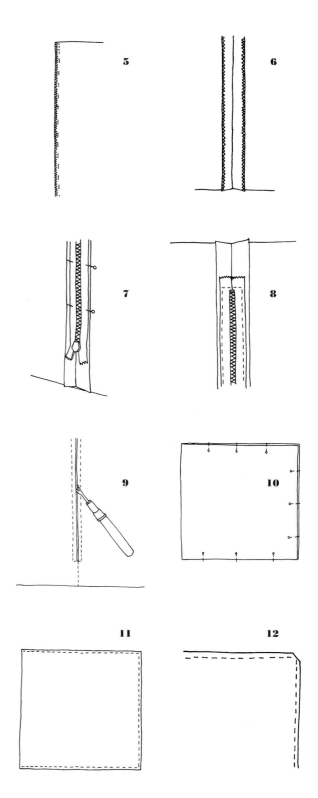

Metallic Painted Pillow

Bold metallic stripes add a touch of sophistication to basic canvas pillow covers, and they add shimmery accents to your home.

MATERIALS

Pillow with removable cover made from heavy-duty canvas (to sew your own, see Basic Zipper Pillow on page 98)

Iron and ironing board

One roll of 2" (5-cm) painter's tape

Foam brush

Gold paint, fabric or all-purpose craft

Gesso or gel medium (optional)

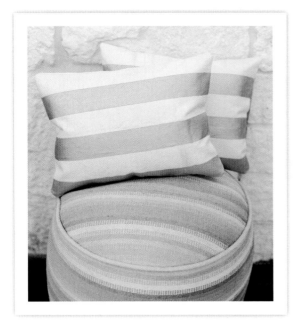

INSTRUCTIONS

1   Remove the insert from your pillow and iron the cover flat. (Even if you make your own pillow cover, paint it after you've sewn it together. We find that machine stitching over painted fabric gums up the sewing machine.)

2   Run strips of tape across both sides of the pillow cover 2" (5 cm) apart. You're taping off the negative spaces to create 2"- (5-cm-) wide stripes that will alternate between the canvas color and a single paint color—metallic gold.

3   Use the foam brush and metallic paint to paint the spaces between the strips of tape. Apply additional coats of paint if necessary, building the color until you are satisfied with the result. Let the paint dry completely between coats. (Note: If your pillow cover is made from cotton or home-décor weight fabric, seal the fabric first with a layer of gesso or gel medium before you paint it.)

4   When the pillow cover is completely dry, remove the tape and insert your pillow form.

5   Get cozy!

2

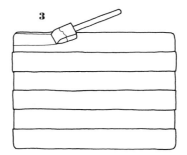

3   **4**

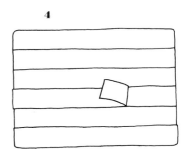

Pear-Shaped Pillow

There's nothing wrong with being shaped like a pear, just ask this cute pear-shaped pillow.
Go green for a dash of fruity color or just keep it neutral like the one we made.
This is an extremely simple project that even a kiddo can try.

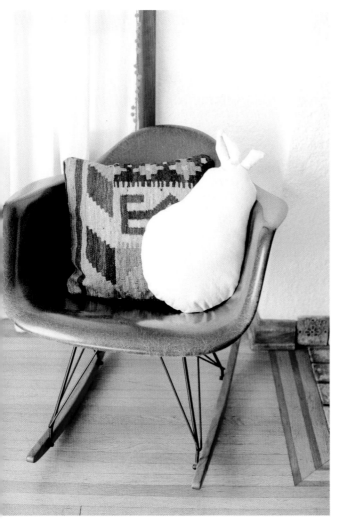

MATERIALS

1 yard (91 cm) of cotton fabric
Pear Pillow template (see page 220); enlarged
  so it will fit twice on the fabric and cut out
Air-erasable fabric marker
Scissors
Straight pins
Sewing machine
Two spools of all-purpose thread (one that matches
  your fabric and one spool of green)
Point turner or chopstick
Pillow stuffing
Hand sewing needle (optional)

INSTRUCTIONS

1 Place your fabric on your work surface wrong side up.
   Position the Pear Pillow template on top of the fabric
   and trace around the outside edge with the air-erasable
   fabric marker. Turn the template over, reposition it on
   the fabric, and trace around its outside edge. Cut out
   both pear shapes. When you're done, they should be
   mirror images of each other.

2 Pin the two pear shapes together with right sides facing
   and raw edges even. Sew around the edges of the pear
   with a ⅜" (1-cm) seam, leaving a 4" (10-cm) opening at
   the bottom of the pear.

3 Turn the pear right side out through the opening.
   Use the point turner or chopstick to gently push out
   the stem and leaf parts, then fill the pillow with stuffing
   until it's firm.

4 Tuck in the seam at the bottom of the pillow and sew
   it closed by machine or by hand.

5 Using green thread and the zigzag stitch on the sewing
   machine, sew a decorative line of stitching down the
   center of the leaf.

6 You're done! Cuddle up and enjoy the fruits of your
   labor.

Pocket Pillow

This cozy and convenient pocket pillow was made for Jaime's daughter, Scarlet, to keep her books, craft supplies, and treasures close by in her reading nook. Everyone who's seen it has fallen in love with it and wants a grownup version for themselves. Just think—with pockets for your cell phone, a small notebook, magazines, and maybe even a little snack, you'd never have to leave your hiding place! This fun and easy project makes great use of fabric without posing the challenge of making a whole quilt.

MATERIALS

Ruler

Scissors

1 yard (91 cm) linen blend or home-décor weight cotton fabric (for the front and back of the pillow)

1 yard (91 cm) printed cotton fabric (for the pockets and pocket lining)

One 12" × 36" (30.5 cm × 91 cm) pillow insert (see the note in step 1)

Straight pins

Sewing machine

Coordinating thread

Point turner or chopstick

Iron and ironing board

1 spool metallic thread (optional)

1 all-purpose 28" (71-cm) zipper

INSTRUCTIONS

1 Measure and cut two 37" × 13" (94 cm × 33 cm) pieces of fabric for the front and back of your pillow. Set them aside. (Note: If you're using a pillow insert that's a different size than ours, simply measure the pillow then add 1" [2.5 cm] to both the width and length to get your fabric measurements.)

2 Cut six pockets in the following sizes from the printed fabric: one 10.5" × 10.5" (26.5 cm × 26.5 cm); one 4.5" × 7.5" (11 cm × 19 cm); one 9.5" × 4.5" (24 cm × 11 cm); and two 5" × 4.5" (12 cm × 11 cm). You'll want to "fussy cut" your fabric. (This means you want to cut your pocket pieces so they feature the cutest bits and pieces of your printed design.) Set these pieces aside. Now cut a second set of pocket pieces for the pocket lining in the same sizes using the remaining fabric. (Note: To customize your pocket design, add ½" [12 mm] to both the width and length of your final desired pocket's dimensions to determine your measurements.)

3 Prepare the pockets. Align and pin one cut pocket piece to its matching lining piece with right sides facing. Stitch around the edges with a ¼" (6-mm) seam, leaving a 1½" (4-cm) opening for turning the pocket right side out. Trim the seam allowances, except for those at the opening, to ¼" (6 mm) and clip the corners. Repeat these steps to sew the remaining pockets.

4 Turn one pocket right side out and gently push out its corners using a point turner or chopstick; iron flat. Repeat with the remaining pockets.

5 To finish a pocket, tuck in the seam allowances at the opening; then press. Next sew around the entire edge of the pocket with a ⅛" (3-mm) seam allowance to close the opening and to finish the pocket. For added interest, use metallic thread, decorative stitches, or concentric rows of straight stitching. Finish the remaining pockets in the same way.

6 Place the piece of fabric that will be the front of the pillow right side up on your work surface. Position all the pockets right side up on the fabric. When you're satisfied with the arrangement, pin them in place.

7 Sew one pocket to the front side of your pillow by stitching along the left side of the pocket, across the bottom, and then up the right side with a ¼" (6-mm) seam. Carefully backstitch at the beginning and end of the seam to secure your pocket. (Do not sew the top of your pocket closed!) Use decorative thread, if desired, knowing that these stitches will show on the front of your pillow. Repeat these steps to attach the remaining pockets.

8 Complete your pillow by following steps 2 to 13 of the instructions for the Basic Zipper Pillow on page 98.

9 Stuff the pockets with goodies!

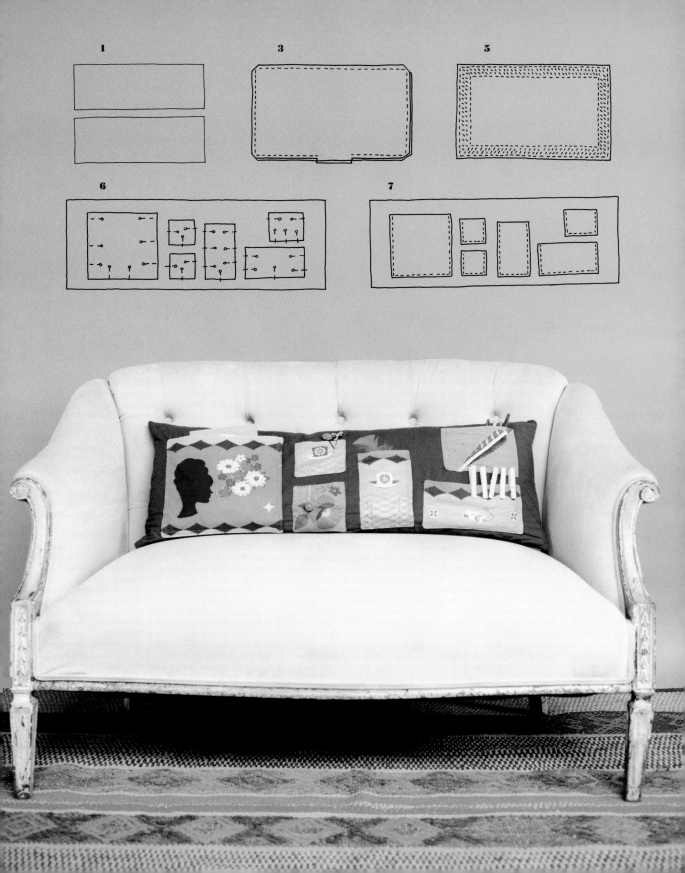

Striped Crochet Blanket

Chunky yarn and a jumbo-sized hook make for speedy crochet work. This luxurious and warm blanket comes together so quickly that it makes it hard to resist loved ones' requests for a warm stripy blanket of their own. Be prepared—they will ask. Black and white is a beautiful accent for the home, but consider a version in school or team colors for the always elusive man-friendly handmade gift.

MATERIALS

5 to 10 skeins of super chunky yarn (we used black and white)
Crochet hook, size S/35 (19 mm)
Scissors

INSTRUCTIONS

1 To make the foundation chain, start by making a slip knot.

2 Chain stitch (ch) until you reach your desired width of the blanket. (The final width measurement will increase by about fifty percent due to stretching, so adjust accordingly.)

3 To make the first single crochet (sc), insert the hook into the second stitch from the hook under the top loop.

4 Bring the yarn over the hook and draw the loop back through the stitch. Now there will be two loops on the hook. Bring the yarn over your hook again and draw the loop back through both loops on your hook. You've finished your first single crochet (sc) and should have only one loop remaining on the hook.

5 Repeat step 4 in every stitch of the foundation chain.

6 Holding the hook stationary, turn the work away from you so that the back becomes the front. (This is so you always work in one direction.)

7 At the beginning of the row "chain up" by adding one chain stitch (ch).

8 To begin the next row, work one single crochet stitch (sc) into the first stitch of the previous row. Now work a single crochet stitch (sc) in each of the remaining stitches across the previous row.

9 Repeat steps 6 to 8 until you reach the desired stripe width. At the end of the row, change the yarn color by leaving the last single crochet stitch (sc) unfinished. (When there are two loops still on the hook.)

10 Pick up the new color of yarn with the hook. Pull the loop through using the second color while holding the tail of the first color to avoid loosening the work. This will finish the previous single crochet stitch (sc).

11 Turn the project, "chain up," and begin a new row.

12 Cut the end of the first color so it's a few inches long. Given the looseness of this type of yarn, tie the end to the body of the blanket before weaving the end into the work.

13 Continue adding rows and alternating yarn colors until the desired size is reached, remembering that the finished blanket will stretch.

14 Be prepared to make more—this one is a family favorite!

See the Crochet Key on page 90 for more information on crochet terminology, including detailed illustrations.

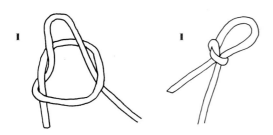

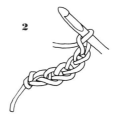

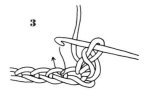

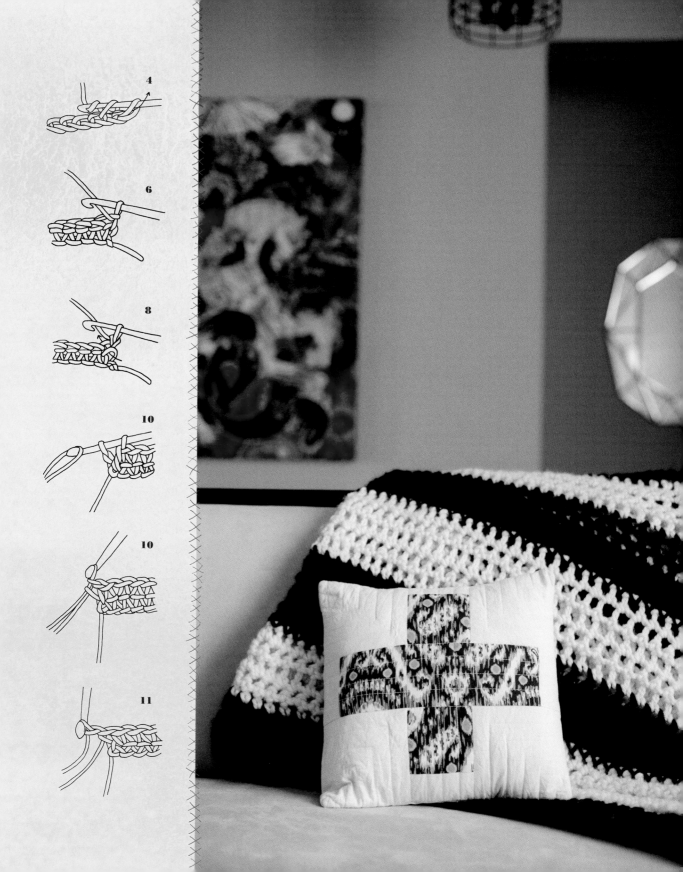

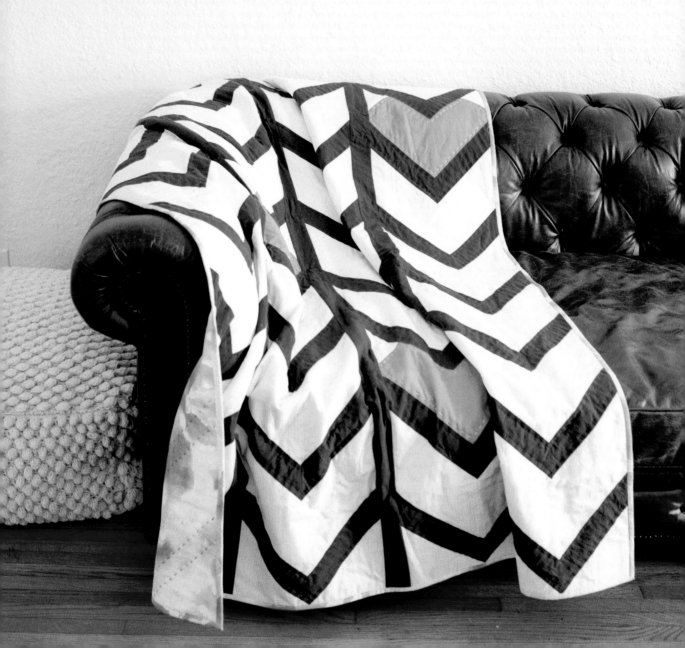

Herringbone & Heart Quilt

Just like my three tiny Texans, this quilt design is 80 percent bold and 20 percent sweet. Erin Schlosser took my vision for this quilt and designed a beautiful and easy-to-execute pattern using my own Texas Modern fabric collection combined with some gorgeous solids.

Finished Size: 54" x 68" (137 cm x 173 cm)

MATERIALS

Ruler

Rotary cutter

Cutting mat

2⅔ yards (2.4 m) of 44"- (112-cm-) wide white quilting cotton fabric for the background

2 yards (1.8 m) of 44"- (112-cm-) wide dark gray quilting cotton fabric for the chevron strips

½ yard (46 cm) of 44"- (112-cm-) wide coral quilting cotton fabric for the accent hearts

3½ yards (3.2 m) of 44"- (112-cm-) wide coordinating print quilting cotton fabric for the backing

½ yard (46 cm) of 44"- (112-cm-) wide coordinating print quilting cotton fabric for the binding

Straight pins

Sewing machine

Coordinating thread

78" x 92" (198 cm x 234 cm) mid-loft polyester batting

Iron and ironing board

Air-erasable fabric marker

Walking foot (recommended for quilting and binding)

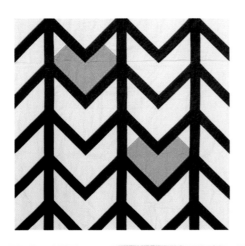

Quilting by Erin Schlosser, who shares her craft on schlosserdesigns.com.

INSTRUCTIONS

1   Using a ruler, rotary cutter, and cutting mat, remove the selvage then prepare the following pieces:

FROM THE WHITE BACKGROUND FABRIC, CUT:

12 strips each 7" × width of fabric (WOF) [17 cm × WOF]; from these strips cut 58 squares each 7" (17 cm)

1 strip 5½" × WOF (14 cm × WOF); from this strip cut 3 squares each 5½" (14 cm)

FROM THE DARK GRAY CHEVRON STRIP FABRIC, CUT:

22 strips each 2½" × WOF (6 cm × WOF); from these strips cut 64 strips each 13" × 2½" (33 cm × 6 cm)

6 strips each 2½" × WOF (6 cm × WOF); sew 2 of the strips together along the short ends to make 1 long 88" (2.25-m) strip; repeat this process to make a total of 3 long strips

FROM THE CORAL ACCENT HEART FABRIC, CUT:

1 strip 7" x WOF (17 cm x WOF); from this strip cut 6 squares each 7" (17 cm)

FROM THE BACKING FABRIC, CUT:

2 rectangles each 1¾ yard × WOF (1.6 m × WOF); sew the two rectangles together along the 1¾-yard (1.6-m) sides

FROM THE BINDING FABRIC, CUT:

8 strips each 2¼" × WOF (5.7 cm × WOF); sew the strips together along the short ends to make one long strip

1   You'll need a total of 52 white standard background blocks with a diagonal dark gray stripe: 26 blocks with the stripe oriented one way, and 26 blocks with the stripe oriented the opposite way (the mirror image).

2   If you're using directional fabric like we did (our white cotton had a faint pattern), you'll need to cut 26 of the 7" (17-cm) background fabric squares in half on the diagonal. For the remaining 26 mirror-image blocks, cut in half on the diagonal in the opposite direction. (If you're using non-directional fabric, go ahead and cut all 52 of the 7" (17-cm) background fabric squares in half on the diagonal without worrying about the orientation.)

3   Place one "top" triangle piece right side up on your work surface. Position one dark gray chevron fabric strip right side down on top of it, as shown. (Start the chevron strip on the upper right. Its short end should only extend past the corner of the triangle by approximately ¼" (6 mm). Pin, then stitch in place using a ¼" (6-mm) seam allowance; unfold and press the seam to the dark side.

4   Place the sewn piece from step 3 right side up. Position the remaining triangle right side down, and with raw edges even, as shown. Make sure the bottom edges of the triangles are aligned. Pin, then stitch in place using a ¼" (6-mm) seam allowance; unfold and press the seam to the dark side. Trim away the extra strip fabric.

5   Repeat steps 3–4 to make the remaining 25 standard background blocks in this orientation. Then make 26 standard background blocks with the stripe oriented in the opposite direction in the same manner.

CREATE THE HEART BLOCKS

6   Each heart is made up of four blocks. The top two blocks form one "V" block and the bottom two blocks form a second "V" block. To make the top half of one heart, place one of the coral 7" (17-cm) heart fabric squares right side up on your work surface. Position a white 5½" (14-cm) square right side down on top of it, aligning the top left corners and two edges. Mark a diagonal line on the white square starting at its top right corner and ending at its bottom left corner. Stitch on

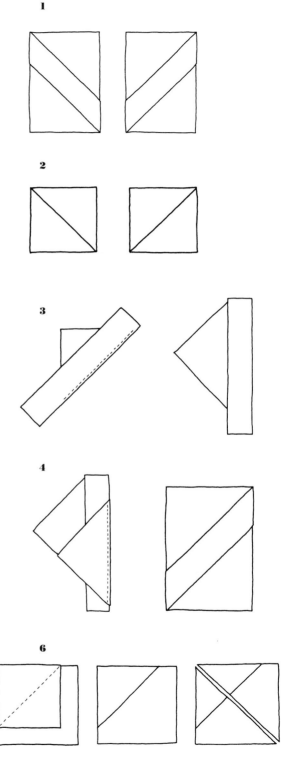

the line. Trim away both layers of the top half of the triangle, leaving a ¼" (6-mm) seam allowance, unfold the fabric, and press the seam to the dark side. Cut this square in half on the diagonal from the top left corner and ending at the bottom right corner.

7   Cut 2 white 7" (17-cm) background squares in half on the diagonal. Set them aside. Place 1 sewn triangle piece from step 6 right side up on your work surface, positioning it so the coral corner is on the bottom left and the white portion is on the top left. Position 1 dark gray chevron fabric strip right side down on top of it, just as you did in step 4 to make a standard block. Pin, then stitch in place using a ¼" (6-mm) seam allowance; unfold and press the seam to the dark side. Place the sewn piece right side up. Position 1 white background triangle, right side down and with raw edges even, as you did in step 4 to make a standard block. Make sure the bottom edges of the triangles are aligned. Pin, then stitch in place using a ¼" (6-mm) seam allowance; unfold and press the seam to the dark side. Trim away the extra strip fabric.

8   Use the remaining sewn triangle from step 1 and 1 dark gray chevron fabric strip along with the remaining white triangle from step 2 to make the mirror image of the piece you completed in step 2. These two blocks make up one "V" block and the top half of one heart.

9   To make the bottom half of the heart, cut 1 white 7" (17-cm) background square and 1 coral 7" (17-cm) heart fabric square in half on the diagonal. Sew together 1 white triangle, 1 dark gray chevron fabric strip, and 1 coral triangle, following the directions to make a standard block. One finished block should have the coral triangle on the top right side and the white triangle on the bottom left side, while the second block should be the mirror image.

10 Lay out the 4 heart blocks as shown. Sew the blocks together using a ¼" (6-mm) seam allowance to make one heart; press flat.

11 Repeat steps 6–10 to make 2 additional hearts so you have 3 total.

10

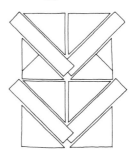
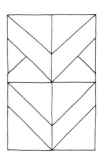

12

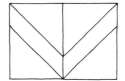

COMPLETE THE QUILT

12 Lay one standard background block right side up with the dark gray strip oriented diagonally from the upper left to the lower right on your work surface. Lay a mirror-image standard background block right side down on top. Pin, then stitch along the right-hand long side using a ¼" (6-mm) seam allowance. Unfold and press the seam open to make a "V" block.

13 Continue sewing together the remaining 50 standard blocks until you have 26 "V" blocks.

14 Sew together 4 columns of 8 "V" blocks each, adding in the heart blocks as shown or as desired. Sew your 88" (2.25-m) dark gray strips between the columns to complete the quilt top. Trim excess strips so the edges are even.

15 Layer the backing, batting, and quilt top. Use your sewing machine and walking foot to quilt and bind as desired or send it off to your local sewing shop to be made into a beloved family heirloom.

Beginner's Guide to Machine Appliqué

My daughter and I started this quilt when she was only four years old; we were just hanging out in my studio, picking out pretty scraps of fabric, and playing with my embroidery machine together. An embroidery machine is a great place to start sewing with young ones because, unlike regular sewing machines, there are no opportunities for little fingers to get close to the needle while at the same time, magnificent images made of thread take shape in front of your eyes. Yes, once you know how to machine appliqué, it's so easy even a kid can do it. Give it a try and in a few years' time, you will have enough blocks to stitch together a quilt top and send it off to your local sewing shop, to be quilted into a beloved family heirloom.

MATERIALS

note: The finished size of the quilt we made is 80" × 100" (203 cm × 279 cm) and the fabric requirements listed here will make a quilt top in that size. But it's easy to change the size: simply adjust the number of squares you use, or their size!

Ruler

Rotary cutter

Cutting mat

9 yards (8.25 m) of a solid color cotton, linen, or linen blend fabric, solid, for the base

6 yards (5.5 m) of light- or medium-weight tear-away stabilizer

Machine-embroidery hoop

Embroidery machine

Coordinating thread

2 yards (2 m) total of patterned cottons, linens, or linen blend fabrics, for the hearts

Spray adhesive

Embroidery scissors

INSTRUCTIONS

1   Using the ruler, rotary cutter, and cutting mat, cut the base fabric and stabilizer into fifty-six 11" (28-cm) squares. (If you'd like to make squares of a different size, simply add an additional ½" [12 mm] to each side for seam allowances.)

2   Place one fabric square on top of one stabilizer square and insert them into the embroidery hoop. Tighten the hoop and adjust the fabric until it is taut with no wrinkles.

3   Create a pattern for a heart (or whatever shape you choose or is available from your embroidery machine) using a straight stitch.

4   Insert the hoop into the embroidery machine. Stitch the heart shape in the center of your fabric. (The fabric should still be in the embroidery hoop.)

5   Cut out a heart, slightly larger than the stitched one, from a 6" (15-cm) square of the patterned fabric. Spray the wrong side with spray adhesive, and then adhere it over the stitched heart in the embroidery hoop.

6   Repeat the stitch of the same pattern through all three layers (patterned fabric, base fabric, and stabilizer).

7   Remove the hoop from the embroidery machine but don't remove the fabric from the hoop. Carefully trim around the patterned heart, just outside the stitch line using sharp embroidery scissors.

8   Re-insert the hoop into your embroidery machine and select the same pattern at the same size, but this time use a satin stitch. Sew using the satin stitch to finish the edges of your heart.

9   If any remaining fabric pokes out from your stitch lines, trim it with your embroidery scissors.

10 Remove your fabric from the hoop, tear off the stabilizer, and trim any loose threads.

11 To copy our quilt design, make fifty-five more heart-embroidered quilt squares. Arrange your blocks so you have eight rows, with seven squares in each row. Sew together with a ½" (12-mm) seam.

12 Send your quilt top off to your local quilt shop to be finished.

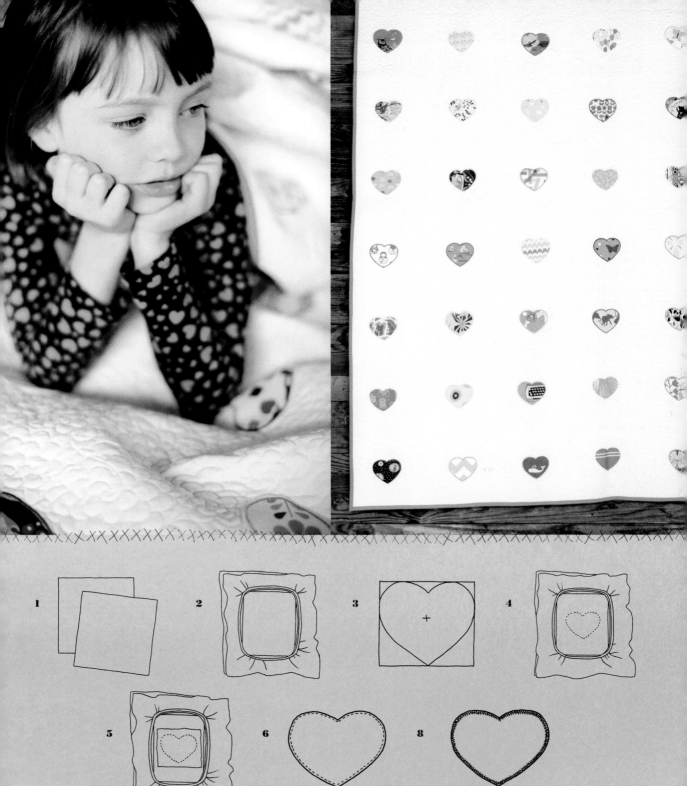

PRETTY PRUDENT DÉCOR

the details

Discover the flourishes and final touches that make a house feel like home, and then
add your own twist using your crafty talents and our easy DIY instructions.
There's so much fun to be had establishing and refreshing the tone of your home with
inventive ideas for the little details. Bring life to your walls with art and
vitality to your surfaces with vines, shrubs, flowers, and plants.
We make fun, lively projects easy to imagine and even easier to execute.

WALL DÉCOR

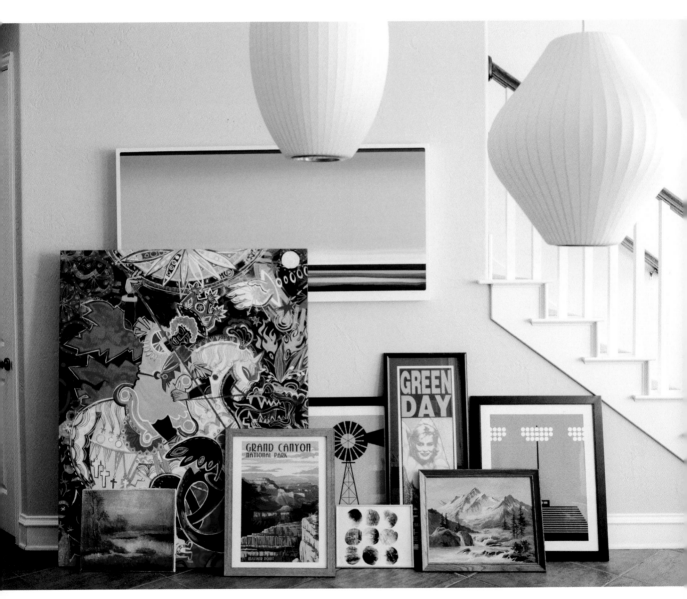

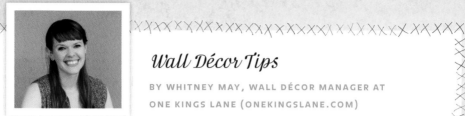

Wall Décor Tips

BY WHITNEY MAY, WALL DÉCOR MANAGER AT
ONE KINGS LANE (ONEKINGSLANE.COM)

1   Try framing vintage flash cards or game cards and arranging them salon-style with smaller prints or paintings for a dynamic wall display. Never be afraid to mix high- and low-end pieces.

2   Always be on the lookout for great vintage posters to add color to a hallway, kitchen, or living room. If there's a bit of wear or damage to the poster you love, take a risk and purchase by bargaining. You can always take your find to a great framer who can repair or disguise any minor tears or fraying.

3   Start a collection of ephemera with items like colorful vintage post cards, vintage ribbons, or wallpaper samples, and frame them. These items are some of the cheapest and most beautiful flea market finds, but most buyers aren't sure how to use them.

4   Always be on the lookout for the perfect marquee or pub letters for your loved ones. When the holidays or their birthdays come around, you'll have a unique gift that will add vintage flair, as well as their initials, to their walls.

5   If you spot a lackluster mirror with great carved details when you're at a thrift store or flea market, consider refinishing it yourself in a bright color that will pop while also complementing your walls.

6   Keep an eye out for vintage game boards with great colors and hand-lettering. If you add some hanging hardware, you can incorporate one into your family room or kids' room. And, if someone wants to play, just unhook it and grab the dice.

7   Buy up as many vintage pennants as you can when you're at thrift stores or flea markets. Most people don't purchase these if they fail to advertise a college or school that they attended. As a result, they're often offered at bargain prices, and they look great in every family room.

8   Smaller framed maps make for the most thoughtful gifts. Everyone loves receiving a beautiful print of his or her hometown or current abode. Even a map of a favorite destination spot always does in a pinch.

9   Jere-style metal wall sculptures from the 1960s and 1970s are back. Try hanging one of these abstract sculptures above your bed instead of a headboard for *Mad Men*–like appeal and some serious glamour.

10 Keep your wall displays fresh and in regular rotation. While people rearrange their furniture from time to time, they often forget to change out the walls, don't be afraid to buy and hang what you adore now and switch it out later.

Decoupage Backsplash

Despite the best intentions and sincere New Year's resolutions, many family photos remain solely in digital form. We suggest moving them off-line and onto your walls. Gather a few of your favorite life moments in pictures and create an elegant, conversation-starting backsplash for your kids and your friends to enjoy.

MATERIALS

Measuring tape

Lightweight acrylic glass (we used Plexiglas, which is available at most hardware stores), as large as the backsplash area you want to cover

Permanent marker

Two C-clamps

Heavy-duty plastic cutter (this is a type of utility knife designed to cut Plexiglas, acrylic, and Lucite)

Ruler or straight-edge

Printed photos, enough to cover your backsplash area

Clear acrylic (or polyurethane) spray sealant

16 oz. (473 ml) decoupage medium, gloss or matte finish

Two brushes, soft bristle or foam

Clean rags or soft cloths

Screwdriver (optional)

Industrial-strength ¾"- (2-cm-) wide hook and loop tape with adhesive backing (we used Velcro)

INSTRUCTIONS

1   Measure the dimensions of the space where you want to add a backsplash. Trace the shape of the space you measured onto the acrylic glass using the permanent marker.

2   Secure the acrylic glass to your work surface using the C-clamps. Use strong, steady pressure and make several passes with the heavy-duty plastic cutter (held firmly against the edge of the ruler) to cut the acrylic glass to size. Once you've cut halfway through the plastic, align the cut line with the edge of a table and press on the plastic edge until the excess snaps off.

3   If the backsplash area has an electrical outlet, fit the acrylic glass over the space. Then mark a rectangle slightly smaller than the outlet cover using the permanent marker.

4   Return the acrylic glass to your work surface, secure it with the C-clamps, and cut along the marked lines until you can slowly push out the cut piece. Set the prepared piece of acrylic glass aside.

5   Place all your photos, face up, on a work surface in a well-ventilated (but low wind) area. Spray them with a light coat of acrylic sealant. Be sure to coat the edges of the photos too. Let the sealant dry. Apply a second and then a third coat of sealant, letting the pictures completely dry between coats. When the photos are completely dry, position them on the front side of the acrylic glass until you have the desired composition.

6   Lift up just one photo at a time and apply a layer of decoupage medium (as thick as the photo paper) to its entire backside using the brush. (Be careful not to get any decoupage medium on the front of photo.) Adhere the photo to the acrylic glass in the same place you removed it, and smooth it with a clean, dry cloth. Continue gluing in this manner until all photos are applied; let dry for at least twenty minutes or overnight.

7   Using a new, dry brush, apply a thin layer of decoupage medium to the entire front of the backsplash. Let dry at least 20 minutes. Repeat these steps two more times.

8   Spray the front of the backsplash with the acrylic sealant.

9   If necessary, remove the electrical outlet plate from wall with a screwdriver.

10   Cut the industrial-strength hook and loop tape into 6" (15-cm) strips. On the back side of the acrylic glass, adhere the strips on all four corners and every 8" (20 cm) around all four sides of the acrylic glass.

11   Remove the backing paper on the hook and loop tape and press the backsplash against the clean, dry wall.

12   Replace the electrical plate (if necessary) and admire your new backsplash.

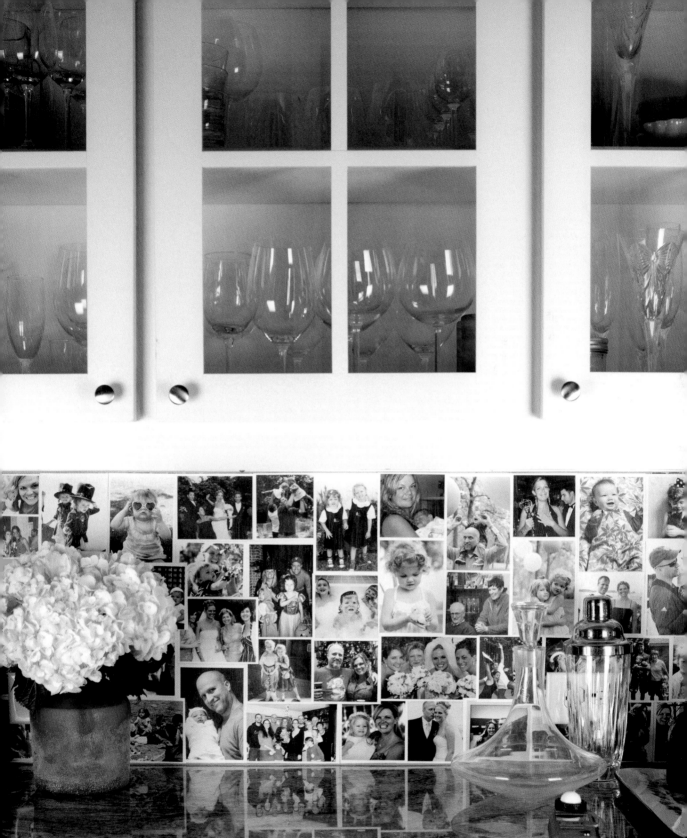

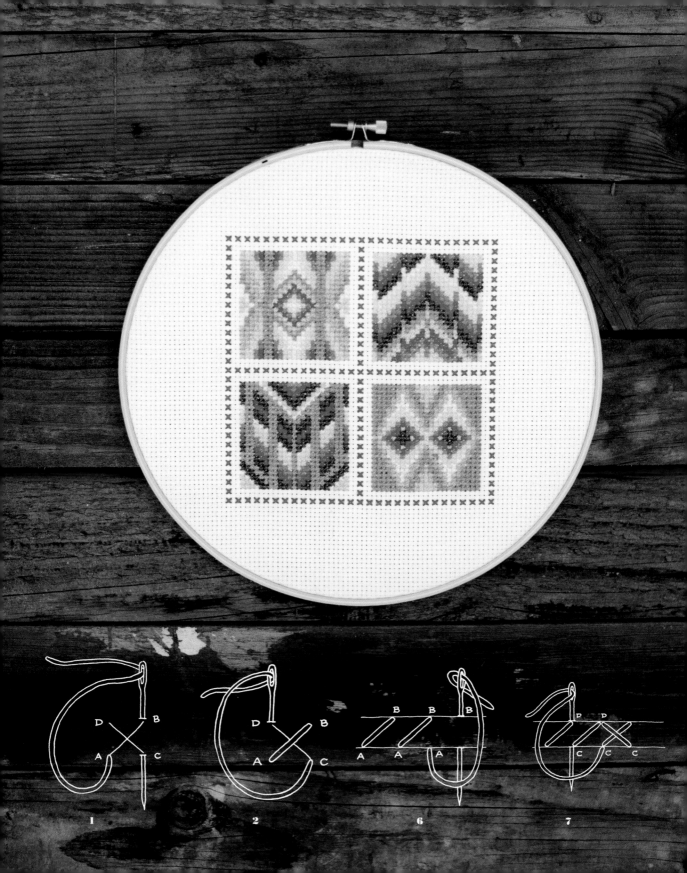

Hot Cross-Stitch

This western-inspired sampler pulls together elements of Texas wildlife, cowboy culture, and Native American–influenced designs to create a piece of artwork perfect for a baby's nursery or the bedroom of a kid obsessed with the Wild West. Use the lettering patterns to personalize the sampler shown on page 5 or stick to the smaller hooped design for a simple project with the feel of a Comanche weaving.

MATERIALS

MATERIALS FOR PATTERN 1 (SEE PAGE 5)

Finished size of artwork: 9" × 12" (23 cm × 30.5 cm);
  Frame size: 11" × 14" (28 cm × 35.5 cm)
One 16" × 20" (40.5 cm × 50 cm) piece of 14-count Aida cloth
Scroll frame
Embroidery floss (see note)
Hot Cross-Stitch 1 pattern (see page 220);
  enlarged for easier reading if necessary
Embroidery needle, size 1/5
Scissors

note: We used DMC Pearl Cotton, size 5, in the following amounts and colors: Two skeins each of red #999, turquoise #597, black #310, and light gray #415. One skein each of light turquoise #598, dark gray #413, bright yellow #726, orange #946, peach #353, white (blanc), auburn #400, brown #938, gold #676, green #988, light green #3348, and cream #712.

MATERIALS FOR PATTERN 2 (OPPOSITE)

Finished size of artwork: 5½" × 5½" (14 cm × 14 cm);
  Hoop size: 9" (23 cm) diameter
One 12" (30.5-cm) square of 14-count Aida cloth
Embroidery floss (see note)
9" (23 cm) wooden embroidery hoop
Hot Cross-Stitch 2 pattern (see page 221);
  enlarged for easier reading if necessary
Embroidery needle, size 1/5
Scissors

note: We used one skein each of DMC Pearl Cotton, size 5, in the following colors: red #999, turquoise #597, light turquoise #598, light gray #415, dark gray #413, bright yellow #726, orange #946, peach #353, white (blanc), and cream #712.

Cross-stitch by Gina Seaman.

INSTRUCTIONS

1 Depending on which project you've chosen, place the Aida cloth in the embroidery hoop or in the scroll frame and tighten the closure. Pull the fabric taut on all sides.

2 Thread your needle with a 12" (30.5-cm) length of pearl cotton and if you prefer, knot the long end.

3 Follow your desired pattern, using the stitch instructions below.

HOW TO CROSS-STITCH

Cross-stitch is one of the easiest stitches to learn. Master these basics, and there will be no stopping the possibilities!

CREATE A SINGLE CROSS-STITCH

1 Insert the needle from underneath the hoop or frame up through point A; pull the needle through. Insert the needle down into point B and back up through point C; pull the needle through.

2 Insert the needle down into point D; pull the needle through.

CREATE A ROW OF CROSS-STITCH

4 Insert the needle from underneath the hoop or frame up through point A. Insert the needle down into point B.

5 Repeat by inserting the needle up through the next point A and down into the next point B across the row.

6 At the end of the row, insert the needle down into the last point B, then back up through point C; pull the needle through.

7 Insert the needle down into point D. Repeat to complete the row.

Tattoo-Inspired Hand Embroidery

These days hand embroidery is hot. It gives a touch of handmade charm to any décor, but requires a certain sense of nostalgia to pull off. Everyone loves an embroidery hoop with a semi-ironic quote lovingly detailed within. We found a kinship between tattoo art and the newly revived art of hand embroidery, so we asked world-renowned artist Lewis Hess (who designed and executed Jaime's famous Scarlet and pomegranate tattoos) to imagine our crafty saying as an embroidered wall hanging. Here's the template he came up with. Use these steps to create a custom wall hanging; even if you are beginner and want to say something else, these steps will get you on your way to the embroidery + irony hall of fame. But watch out, crafters are a harsh crowd: It's no joke; we will cut you.

MATERIALS

I Will Cut You embroidery template on page 221
Iron and ironing board
14" (35.5 cm) square of white cotton or linen fabric
14" (35.5 cm) square of graphite transfer paper
Pencil or stylus
Air-erasable fabric marker
12"- (30.5-cm-) diameter embroidery hoop
Embroidery floss, one skein each in black, gray, white, and red
Embroidery needle, size 3
Scissors
Craft glue

INSTRUCTIONS

1   Photocopy the I Will Cut You embroidery template, enlarging it to fit your fabric. To transfer the template design onto the center of your ironed fabric, place the fabric, right side up, on your work surface. Position the graphite transfer paper on the fabric and place the template on top of the transfer paper. Use the pencil to trace over the design on the template. Remove the template and the transfer paper to reveal the image. If desired, redraw the design directly onto the fabric using the fabric marker.

2   Center the fabric in the embroidery hoop and tighten the closure. Pull the fabric taut on all sides.

3   Thread your needle with black embroidery floss. Bring the needle to the midpoint and tie the two cut ends into a knot.

4   Start with the outline of the banner using stem stitch (see Embroidery Stitches on page 120). We did ours partially in black and partially in gray to create depth. Continue adding stem stitches, changing colors if you wish, until the banner is complete.

5   Next, you'll create the handles of the scissors and the screw using black embroidery floss and blanket stitch (see Embroidery Stitches on page 120). Keeping your stitches very close together, continue to add blanket stitches until you have filled in the handles of the scissors.

6   Now embroider the blades of the scissors using satin stitch that increases in width along with the pattern (see Embroidery Stitches on page 121). Use the gray embroidery floss. Continue adding satin stitches until each blade is complete.

7   Finish by embroidering the phrase in the banner with split stitch (see Embroidery Stitches on page 121). Use black and red embroidery floss. Continue adding split stitches, changing colors if you wish, until each word is complete.

8   When you've finished embroidering, neatly trim away the excess fabric around the embroidery hoop, leaving ½" (12 mm). Apply a thin line of craft glue all the way around the backside of the embroidery hoop. Press the fabric onto the hoop to adhere it and let dry.

9   Hang that baby!

Embroidery by Julia Perry. Julia writes about family, faith, food and all of the things that make her life as a modern Southern momma. Find her at her blog, Bless Her Hearth (blessherhearth.com). Illustration by Lewis Hess of Atlas Tattoo.

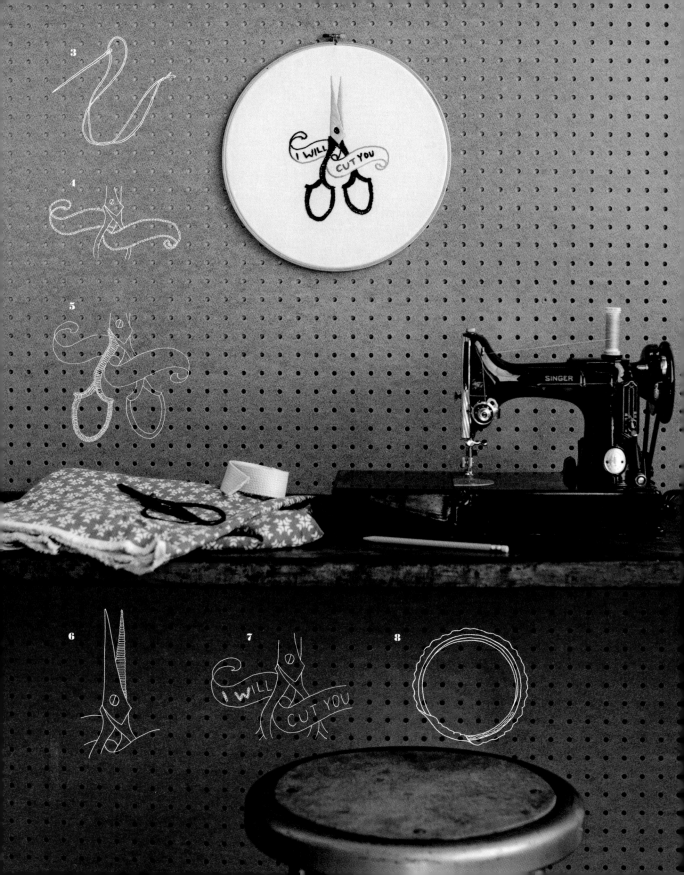

EMBROIDERY STITCHES

With just these four stitches you can create a wall-worthy work of art!

STEM STITCH

1 Insert the needle from underneath the hoop up through point A; pull through.

2 Insert the needle down into point B and back up through point C, which should be halfway between points A and B. Before you pull the needle through, hold the floss that exits point A below the stitch line. Then pull the needle through above point A (above the stitch line).

3 To make the next stitch, insert the needle down into point D and back up through point E. (Point E should be directly in front of the last stitch.) Hold the floss below the stitch line and pull the needle through above the stitch line.

BLANKET STITCH

1 Insert the needle from underneath the hoop up through point A; pull the needle through.

2 Insert the needle down into point B and back up through point C. Loop the floss under the needle, as shown.

3 Pull the needle through (over the looped thread), which should bring the looped thread into a taut (though not overly tight) line. Insert the needle down into point D and up through point E, pulling the needle through (over the looped thread).

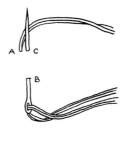

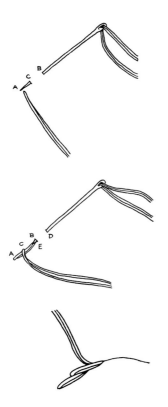

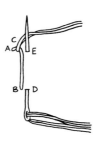

SATIN STITCH

1   Insert the needle from underneath the hoop up through point A. (In this tattoo-inspired project, it should be a point on the edge of one scissor blade.) Pull the needle through. Insert the needle down into point B. (Choose a second point directly opposite the first on the opposite edge of the same blade.) Pull the floss through so the stitch is tight, but not so tight that the fabric bunches. The key to a neat satin stitch is ensuring uniform tension with each stitch.

2   Insert the needle from underneath the hoop up through point C, which should be next to point A; pull through. Insert the needle down into point D, which should be next to point B.

SPLIT STITCH

1   Insert the needle from underneath the hoop up through point A; pull the needle through. Insert the needle down into point B and back up through point C, which should be halfway between points A and B.

2   Pull the needle through the center of the two threads that exit point A. (This is like a stem stitch, but instead of pulling your needle above point A, you're going through the center of the floss at point A.) We've been using a double-threaded needle. If you do this stitch with a single strand of embroidery floss, simply separate it into two halves. (Most embroidery floss has six threads that make up one strand, so separate it into two sections with three threads each.)

3   Repeat the above steps to create the next stitch, as shown.

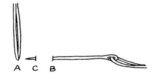

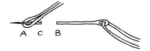

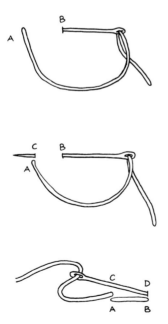

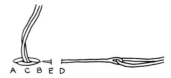

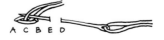

Wood-Burnished Wall Art

One of my favorite pieces of advice in Jaime's first book, *Prudent Advice*, is "You Have a Garden." To summarize her heartfelt explanation, it means that if you don't have a yard or even a planter on a balcony, you still have all of the beautiful gardens of the world. You don't need to own a garden to have one. Amen to that.

When we asked Jackie Miller to design these lovely wood-burning projects, we knew this beautiful line was the perfect place to start. Then to balance out the earnest poetry of "you have a garden," we went to a great quote from the movie *Jaws*. "We're gonna need a bigger boat" basically sums up family life, with a bit of ominous humor.

MATERIALS

One 7" × 9" (17 cm × 23 cm) or larger unfinished wooden plaque (you can also use any other unfinished wood surface)

180- or 220-grit sandpaper or soft sanding block

Bigger Boat Wood Burning Template or You Have a Garden Wood Burning Template (see page 221), enlarged to fit the plaque

Masking tape

Tracing paper

Pencil and soft eraser

Wood burning tool, fitted with a small cone-shaped tip (it's the one that looks most like a pencil)

Pliers

Heat-resistant surface (a dinner plate will do)

Watercolor, craft, or acrylic paint (see note)

Paintbrush

Ruler

Heavy-duty staple gun and staples (or a hanging bracket)

Hammer

note: If you're using craft paint or acrylics instead of watercolors, use a palette where you can thin the paint with water.

INSTRUCTIONS

1 To prep your wooden plaque, smooth the surface and edges using the sandpaper. Wipe the dust off, and set it aside.

2 Photocopy the template you want to use. Tape a sheet of tracing paper over the template. Using a pencil, trace the design. Lift the tracing paper off the template and place it wrong side up on your work surface. Use the pencil to draw the traced lines onto the wrong side of the paper. Now, tape the same sheet of tracing paper, right side up, onto the plaque. Trace over the image once again to transfer the graphite lines from the wrong side of the tracing paper onto the wood. (You have now drawn the design three times total.)

3 Remove the tracing paper. Use the pencil directly on the wood to touch up any faint lines, if necessary.

4 Prep your wood burning tool using the Safety Suggestions on page 125. Wait 5 to 10 minutes for the tool to heat.

5 Holding your tool at a 45-degree angle like a pencil, trace over your lines with light to medium pressure. (Start with the part of the design that is closest to your hand.) Check the tip periodically and use the pliers to tighten it, if necessary.

6 When you are satisfied with your design, unplug the wood burning tool. Place it on the heat-resistant surface and make sure it's secure as it cools.

7 Erase any pencil marks from your wooden plaque.

Wood burning by Jackie Miller. Through her craft, Jackie aims to express innocence, humor, and whimsy inspired by stories and objects of childhood.

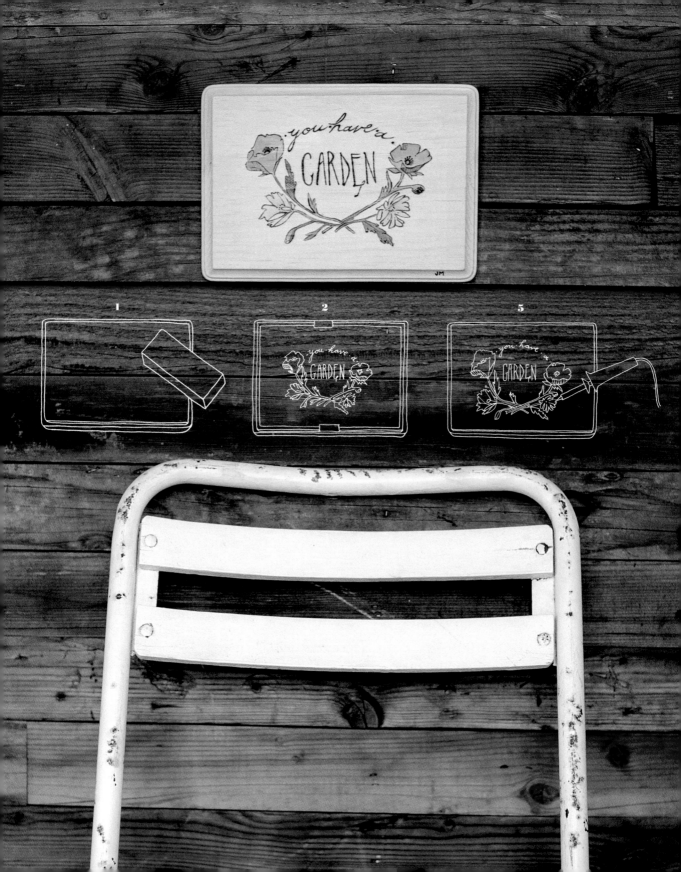

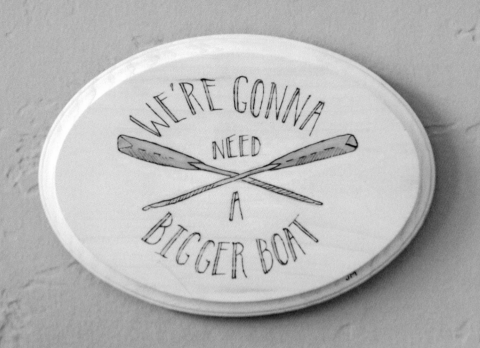

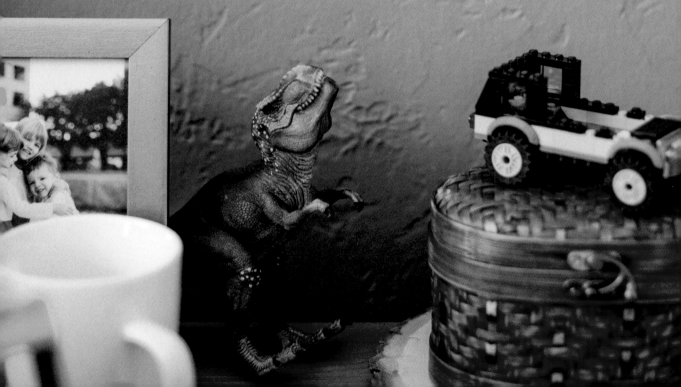

8   To paint the "You Have a Garden" plaque, begin by painting the center of the flowers, then move to the petals, and end with the stems. There is no suggested starting point for painting the "We're Gonna Need a Bigger Boat" plaque.

9   When the paint is dry, place the plaque wrong side up on your work surface. Measure and mark the center of the plaque 3" (7.5 cm) from the top edge. Add a heavy-duty staple at this point for hanging. Hold the stapler slightly above the wood so the staple won't go in all the way. Be careful though, the staple sometimes bounces off the wood! If it goes in all the way, use the claw of the hammer to remove it slightly, or pull it out completely and try again.

10 You're done! No need to seal it—just don't get it wet.

9

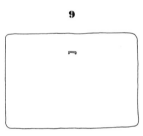

Try the following color ideas
for each plaque:

YOU HAVE A GARDEN
poppy petals = coral
poppy center = gray-blue
poppy stem = yellow-green
daisy center = yellow
daisy petal = pale yellow and white
daisy stem = grass green or blue-green

WE'RE GONNA NEED A BIGGER BOAT
oars = orange-red, teal, orange-brown
lettering = red
center = blue-tinted white

Safety Suggestions

Because the wood burning tool can reach up to 900 degrees F, take these precautions:

1   Make sure your tool rests on a heat-resistant surface, like a dinner plate.

2   The tool should not be stretched far from the outlet—if needed, use an extension cord.

3   For extra peace of mind, use masking tape to hold the cord in place, reducing the chance of the tool rolling off your work surface. If it rolls, your first instinct is to catch it, which will burn you!

4   Never leave the tool unattended.

5   Keep the tool away from curious children and pets.

6   Don't hold the tool directly under your hand—heat rises, and it's very hot!

7   Don't be alarmed. There is a small amount of smoke produced.

Four Tips for Wood Burnishing

1   Practice on a scrap of unfinished wood to get a feel for the tool.

2   When using the tool, move it away from you, not toward you.

3   Rotate your wood as needed to get the best angle.

4   Vary the pressure to get a thinner or thicker line, just like calligraphy.

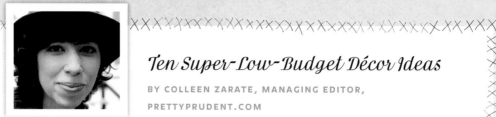

Ten Super-Low-Budget Décor Ideas

BY COLLEEN ZARATE, MANAGING EDITOR,
PRETTYPRUDENT.COM

1   **TURN PRODUCTS INTO ART** For my birthday my boyfriend gave me a giant-size photo of the couch he bought me that hadn't yet arrived. We hung the photo on the wall and quickly realized it had turned into a piece of art. Bring a pop of color and art into your home by finding a high-res photo and have it printed out extra-large to hang directly on the wall.

2   **INDOOR GETAWAY** Use blankets and pillows to create a fort that can be easily propped up and put away. We use ours for movie nights and as a reading nook.

3   **HANG IT UP** Decorate a blank wall in the kitchen by hanging antique kitchen utensils from nails. Decorate a blank wall in your bedroom or living area by doing the same thing with hats. This is a great solution that you can continue to add to as time goes by.

4   **LANTERNS AND LIGHTS** Make your bedroom extra cozy by hanging paper lanterns or stringing globe lights over your bed.

5   **DECORATING WITH JEWELS** Frame a piece of corkboard in a frame without glass. Push thumbtacks into the corkboard and use them as hooks for your necklaces. This also helps to keep your jewelry from getting tangled.

6   **DREAMING OF ADVENTURE** Collect small knickknacks from your travels (shells, twigs, trinkets, etc). When you get home make a dream catcher and hang your findings on the end. Hang your dream catchers on one wall, or scatter them around the house.

7   **LOVE LETTERS** This is a great way to add a little rustic charm to your room. Take a piece of wood and paint it with watered-down acrylic paint. Write a message to your sweetheart on it like "kiss me quick" and hang it from a piece of twine or rope over the bed.

8   **DIVIDE YOUR SPACE** Make a macramé-inspired room divider by hanging several pieces of rayon cord or rope from a piece of wood. Dye the ends of the rope to add a pop of color and add beads or weave section together if you'd like. When you're done, hang it from the ceiling to divide your two spaces.

9   **INSPIRED BY NATURE** One of the easiest ways to bring a bit of nature into your home is by hanging dried herbs and flowers from the wall or ceiling. Dried lavender is one of my favorites, because it makes the whole house smell wonderful. When you take them down you can use them to make potpourri.

10 **BUY A BLANKET** For those days when you feel like you want to sell everything you own and completely redecorate, start by buying a blanket. You will find that a blanket can go a long way toward changing the mood of a room.

Simple & Stunning Living Succulent Wreath

Succulents are going strong in today's gardens and planters, and that makes these Texas and California girls pleased as champagne punch. After all, what's easier to care for than succulents? (Find directions for making the wreath at prettyprudent.com.)

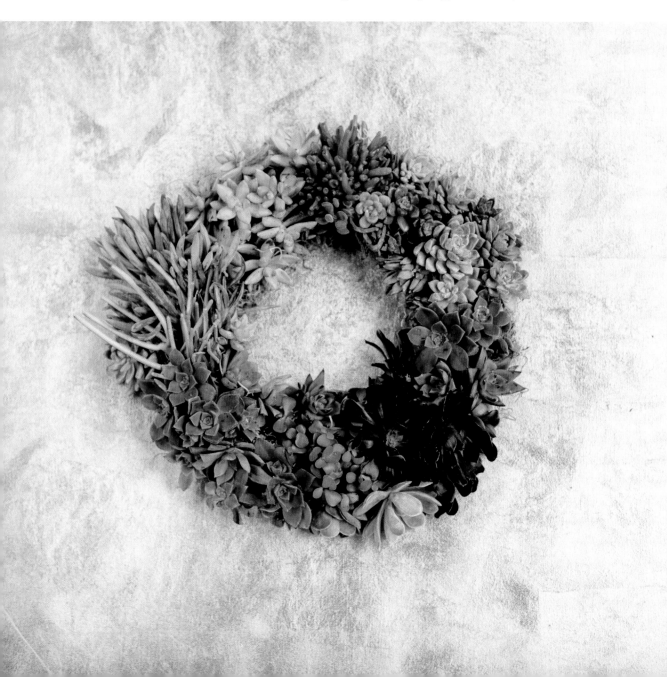

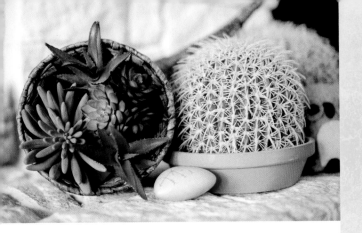

SUCCULENT CORNUCOPIA

There's only one thing easier than caring for succulents, and that's caring for fake succulents. The succulent trend is going strong, and this has resulted in beautiful artificial succulents being widely available everywhere from high-end home stores to bins at the craft shop. Grab a seasonal basket like this woven cornucopia for fall and fill it generously with fake succulents. Use a piece of floral foam if you need to secure the stems.

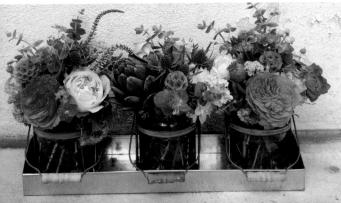

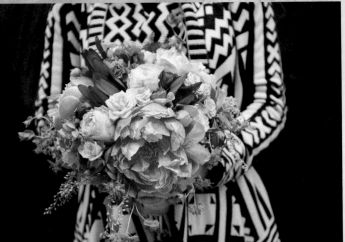

Tips for Decorating with Succulents

BY GRETA PECHTER, FLORAL DESIGNER AND OWNER OF GLASSWING FLORAL, LOS ANGELES

1   Succulents thrive both indoors and outdoors. They require plenty of natural light, but too much direct sun may be damaging. Placing your succulents near a south-facing window is ideal.

2   Water your succulents about every two weeks. Choose a planter with good drainage, and let the soil dry completely between waterings. Do not overwater your succulents, as this can cause irreversible root damage.

3   Pay attention to the leaves. Soft, plump leaves are a sign of over-watering, while leaves with brown spots are a sign of under-watering. Crispy, dry leaves are a sign of too much sun.

4   Sansevieria is a great choice for homes with low light. Its leaves also act as an air purifier.

5   Incorporate succulents into a bouquet or floral arrangement for added visual interest. Replant the succulents after you are finished with the flowers.

CONTAINER GARDENS FOR EVERY SEASON

Container gardens look gorgeous overflowing with bountiful spring and summer blooms,
but don't forget that fall and winter might need a splash of outdoor color or even just a bit of greenery too.
And, if you throw in a few herb plants that thrive in the weather du jour, you'll have fresh
ingredients at your fingertips all year round! Of course, if you live on snowy tundra,
you may want to pull the hardiest of plants indoors for the coldest months.

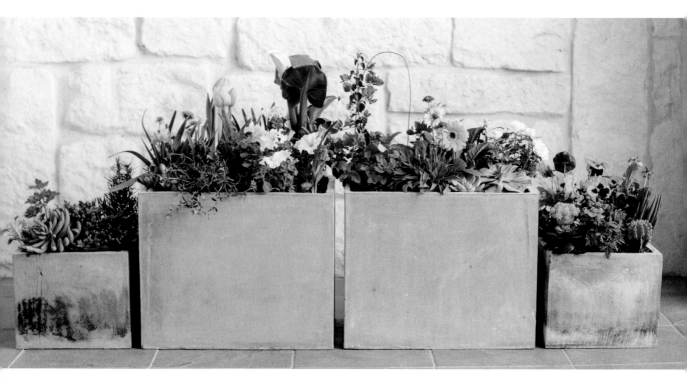

1 WINTER CONTAINER

Winter is tricky, of course, but hearty evergreens, strong herbs like rosemary and parsley, and perennial ground cover like Dusty Miller make an elegant and aromatic arrangement in shades of green. Sneak in a fake succulent to add a modern twist or a holly for a bit of color.

2 SPRING CONTAINER

There's no shortage of options to add to a beautiful spring planter. Calla lily, tulips, daffodils, hyacinth, and pansies make a stunning combination in shades of white, yellow, and indigo. A succulent and a fresh herb or two, like oregano, that enjoys mild temperatures, and some beautiful flowering ground cover combine for a stunning display.

3 SUMMER CONTAINER

In most of the United States, summer means gorgeous, easy gardening. In Texas we worry about everything drying up to a crisp, but we still persist with trying to keep the prettiest summer blooms alive. Bougainvillea is perfect for a big planter, as it needs to move inside during winter. Add roses, Gerber daisies, Morning Star, and succulents all in shades of pink and green.

4 FALL CONTAINER

Fall planters start to get challenging. Hearty cactus and herbs, like chives, complement pansies, decorative kale, and marigolds all in shades of red, purple, and yellow. There are even a few fake succulents in there for when the temps start to dip below freezing.

The Tape Trick

Transform a supermarket bouquet and inexpensive drugstore vase into a little floral work of art with our favorite trick for making any skimpy bouquet look full and vibrant.

MATERIALS

Bouquet of flowers
Empty vase
Transparent adhesive tape (we used Scotch tape)
Garden shears or scissors

INSTRUCTIONS

1 Fill the vase with water.

2 Use the tape to form a grid over the mouth of your vase as shown.

3 Add a ring of tape around the edge of the vase to hold your grid in place.

4 The key to making this cheapo bouquet look gorgeous is to take it apart and reassemble it. First, remove all the leaves from the stems. (It'll look cleaner and last longer. Leaves rot under the water, making your water dirty and grimy-looking.) Next, trim the stems so that the flowers sit right above the top of the vase. (You don't want to see a lot of empty stems above the rim.) Now, start reassembling the bouquet by evenly distributing the most colorful flowers throughout the grid.

5 Keep adding flowers and greens into your grid until your arrangement looks nice! A dome shape is usually a good one to go for. Position filler flowers around the rim of the vase to cover your tape (or artfully arrange your flowers to cover it).

6 There you have it—a beautiful arrangement on a budget.

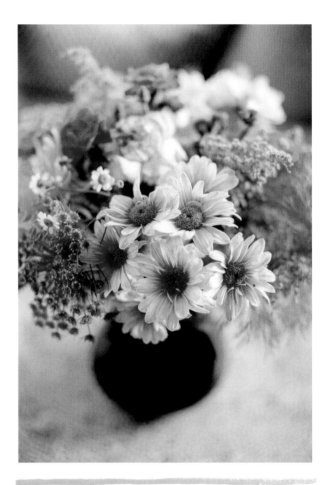

You won't need to use all of your filler because now the grid holds your flowers up. If your bouquet has a lot of baby's breath, pull it all out, gather it together, and put it in its own vase. It looks so nice on its own. And you get two bouquets for the price of one!

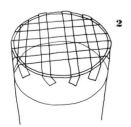 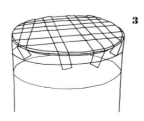 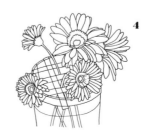

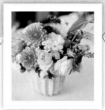

Top Ten Tips for Flower Arranging

BY HEATHER WILLIAMS OF TWIG & TWINE (TWIGANDTWINEDESIGN.COM)

1 Keep it simple, both stylistically and in the mechanics. As with all design, less can be more. If you're a beginner, take on a project that is doable for you; then as you start to feel more comfortable working with flowers, take on more a more challenging approach or design.

2 Use a monochromatic range of colors. You can't go wrong with this. An arrangement with too many colors may take on that dreaded "grocery store bouquet" look. Keep it simple and in a single palette and you'll make it easy on yourself. Fuchsia flowers mixed with touches of blush and medium pink still has depth and an array of colors without feeling gaudy.

3 Use your garden and surrounding area for greenery and other accents. Don't forget about the beauties that might be in your own backyard. Forage for a few pieces to add a specialized touch that you may not be able to get from your local flower shop or market.

4 Invest in a good vase—one that not only goes well with your existing décor but is also practical to build your arrangements in. It will be worth it. A wide mouth vase may take a lot of product or require tape to make your arrangement look nice, so keep that in mind when searching out suitable vases for your home.

5 Mono-floral arrangements: These are a very easy and elegant solution. Choose a single type of flower and make sure you buy enough bunches of them to fill your vase completely. "Chop and drop," as we like to call it in the floral world.

6 Keep the existing décor of your house in mind when buying flowers. Flowers are meant to accent and complement what is already in place so build around the color scheme and style of your home décor. If the room is elaborate you may opt to tone down the flowers in color, design style, etc. If the room is simple you can have more fun with the flowers as they won't clash with an already busy room.

7 Use unexpected vases or items you have around the house as vessels. Be sure they are watertight or else slip another simple clear glass vase in as a liner. You can turn a somewhat mundane object into a lovely vessel for a centerpiece.

8 Don't be afraid to decorate with something other than flowers. A tablescape made from fruit and vegetables or even living plants can be a great alternative to a traditional floral centerpiece. You can use bowls to gather items or even place them directly on the table. Build out from the middle and pay attention to your color scheme and textures.

9 Always cut your flowers after they have been out of water—even if it's only been just a few minutes. Just give them a little snip so they will be able to drink water and reach their maximum livelihood.

10 Use a few large-faced flowers strategically placed in your arrangements as a resting place for the eye. Often times they look best bunched together, most often in odd numbers (three or five). This will make the arrangement feel balanced and well-composed.

3

prudent entertaining

Life can feel like a string of obligations—meals that need preparing, events that need attending, gifts that need giving. We try to cast these duties in a different light: Rather than tasks to be checked off endless to-do lists, we see a series of milestones to celebrate in a neverending cycle of meaningful commitments, reciprocal appreciation, and collective joy. Whether setting a beautiful table, icing a pretty cake, wrapping a lovely package, or sending a hand-written card, what we are really doing is honoring each other and the community we share.

Even when executed in the simplest way, the act of cooking a meal, hosting a gathering, or giving a gift is a gesture that represents our essential connection to one another. These obligations are actually opportunities—chances to care for our family and friends, in the spaces we share, with food, drink, and thoughtfulness. Seizing these opportunities not only rewards the ones we love, but also allows us to nurture the most creative, attentive, and giving parts of ourselves. Learning to be a good host doesn't come down to memorizing the rules of proper table settings; at its heart, it's about setting the scene for a single beautiful day and the endless beautiful memories that follow. We invite you to make a meal, throw a party, give a gift, and feel grateful.

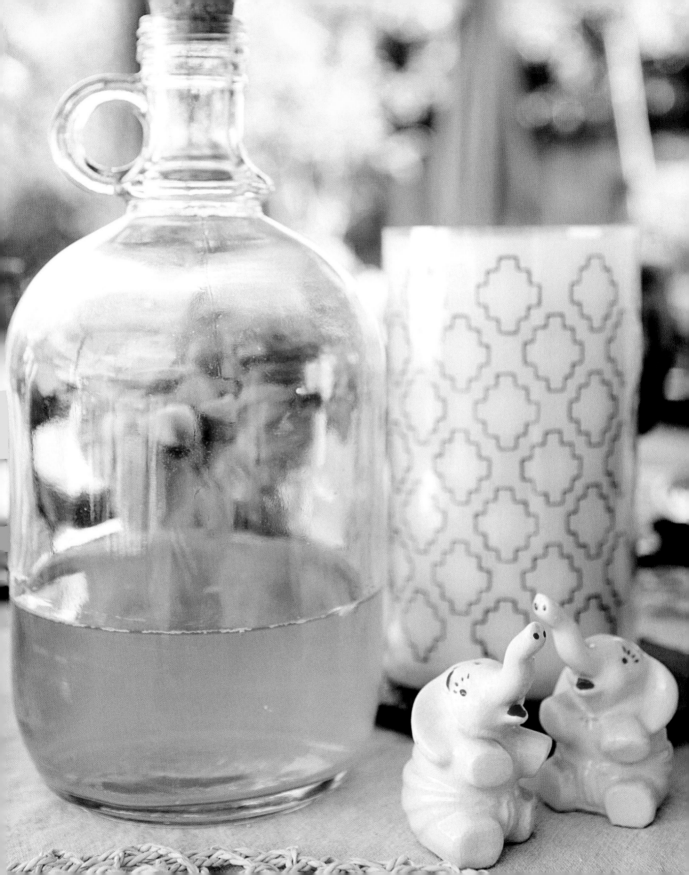

party planning

It's easy to get caught up in the stress of planning a perfectly decorated party, with just the right food served at just the right moment with just the right decoration topping your table. But truly, your guests are just happy to be with you: a well-rested hostess who didn't go to all that much trouble, is the single best addition to any party. We have a few ideas, tips, and tricks for low-stress celebrations everyone will enjoy—even the host.

TEN PARTY BASICS TO HAVE ON HAND

We love to throw parties and having these basic supplies on hand makes it simple to pull together a classy little gathering.

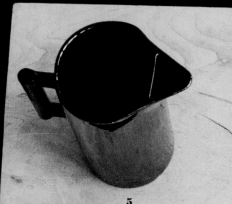

3
Party straws don't take up much storage space and give your events a special touch. Red and white stripes work for Christmas, Valentine's Day, Independence Day, and beyond.

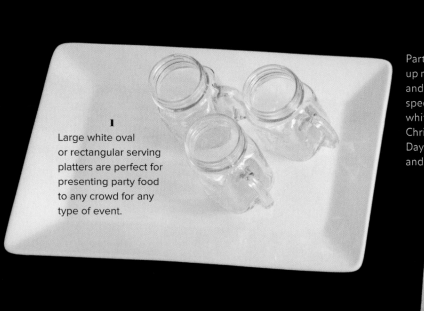

1
Large white oval or rectangular serving platters are perfect for presenting party food to any crowd for any type of event.

4
A classic pitcher in black or white can work as a beverage server or a vase.

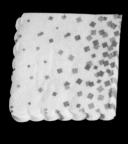

2
Festive paper napkins make a party feel special. Pick up a pretty pack when you see them on sale. These metallic confetti napkins are perfectly neutral for any event.

5
Woodblock cutting boards serve you (and your guests) well both for food prep and for serving.

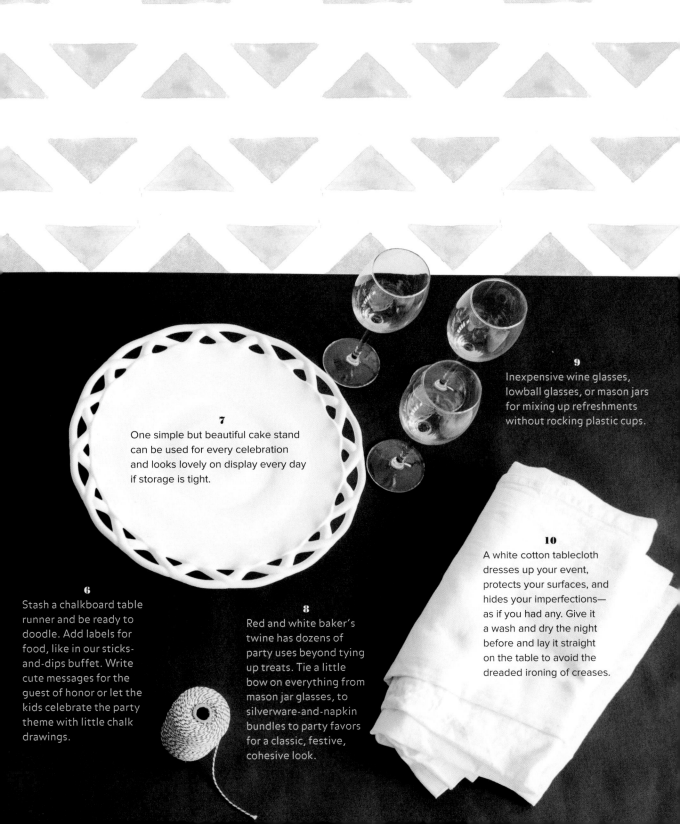

7

One simple but beautiful cake stand can be used for every celebration and looks lovely on display every day if storage is tight.

9

Inexpensive wine glasses, lowball glasses, or mason jars for mixing up refreshments without rocking plastic cups.

10

A white cotton tablecloth dresses up your event, protects your surfaces, and hides your imperfections— as if you had any. Give it a wash and dry the night before and lay it straight on the table to avoid the dreaded ironing of creases.

6

Stash a chalkboard table runner and be ready to doodle. Add labels for food, like in our sticks-and-dips buffet. Write cute messages for the guest of honor or let the kids celebrate the party theme with little chalk drawings.

8

Red and white baker's twine has dozens of party uses beyond tying up treats. Tie a little bow on everything from mason jar glasses, to silverware-and-napkin bundles to party favors for a classic, festive, cohesive look.

PANTRY SPREADS THAT ALWAYS WORK

Throwing impromptu gatherings may feel like something from your childless past. Pulling together a last-minute party can easily turn into a stressful and expensive affair that just isn't possible at the end of the day. Here's the thing: Your friends, like you, just want to visit, laugh, and share a bit of food and wine.

Stock up on the items in these four delicious spreads, and you'll be ready to pull together a last-minute fête straight from the cupboard.

Keeping the Kids Entertained

Even if you're not throwing a "kid" party, there are bound to be a few (or a few dozen) pint-size tagalongs. Here are a few low-maintenance ideas for keeping kids of any age entertained at a boring grown-up party.

AGES 0–2
Bubble machine, a cozy corner with blankets and pillows

AGES 2–4
Balloons, a sandbox, parachute, cardboard playhouse

AGES 4–6
Simple craft kits, sidewalk chalk, scavenger hunt

AGES 6–10
Beanbag toss game, watercolor supplies, karaoke machine

AGES 10–14
Bocce ball set, water guns, beading kits

AGES 14–18
Movies and projector, badminton set

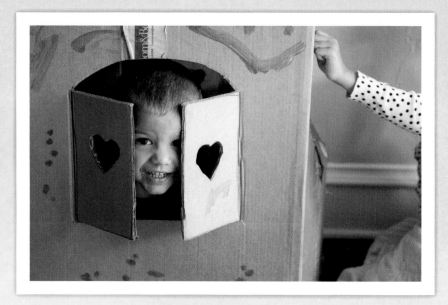

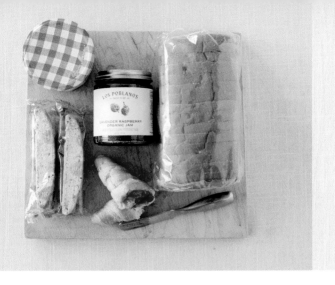

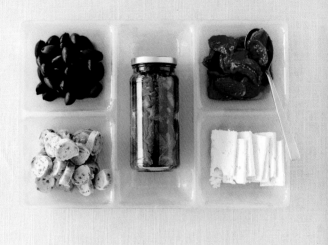

MORNING DROP-IN BRUNCH

Set out lovely jams, lemon curd, and cream cheese to spread on cinnamon bread and English muffins. Add a few berries from the fridge for a fresh touch. Serve with Mimosas and coffee.

GREEK PLATE

Sun-dried tomatoes, Kalamata olives, herb-seasoned crackers, and feta cheese, plus grape leaves from the pantry, combine for a satisfying luncheon hors d'oeuvre.

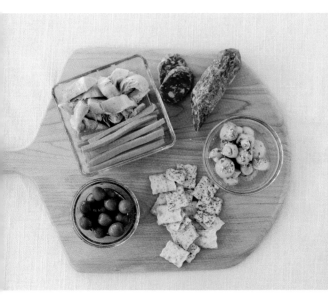

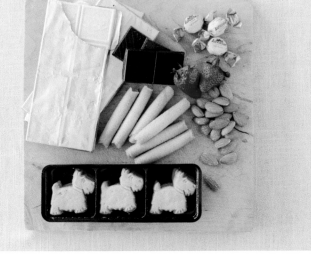

PANTRY ANTIPASTI

The jarred options are virtually endless when it comes to this Italian staple. Marinated artichokes and mushrooms plus pickled veggies pair deliciously with dry salami and crackers or a loaf of fresh bread.

DESSERT IN A PINCH

Adorable shortbread Scotty dogs, plus biscotti and rolled wafer cookies accompany an assortment of chocolate and fine caramel candies.

tabletop design

While table basics in white will always work, sometimes your table needs a special touch for a big day, or just for every day. These projects use everything from luxurious leather and gold leaf to rustic wooden beads and garden flora to give your presentation a pop of fabulous.

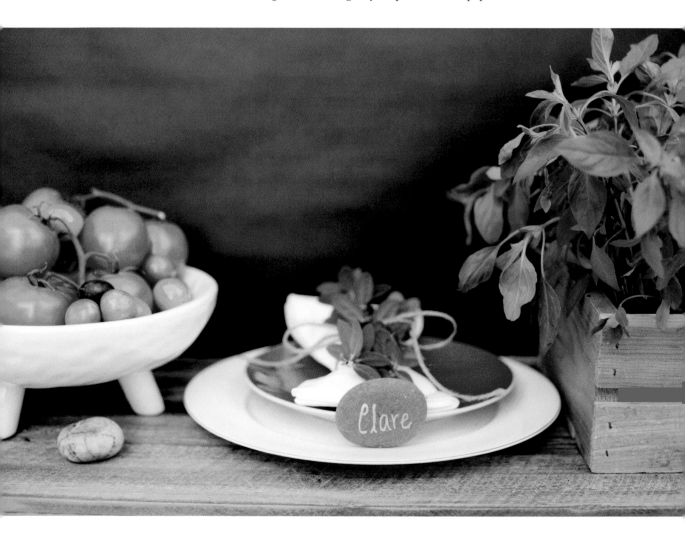

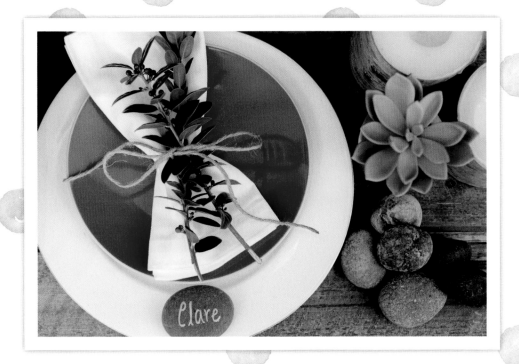

GARDEN TO TABLE PLACE SETTINGS

No need to spend mad dollars on florals. The most beautiful table décor might come right from the woods, your garden, or even a swamp. Use twigs and branches of leaves to make a statement.
Write on river stones or a small succulent for a creative place card. Wrap candles or vases in birch bark.
Create a beautiful, fragrant centerpiece from a bowl of bright tomatoes or a carafe of fresh herbs.

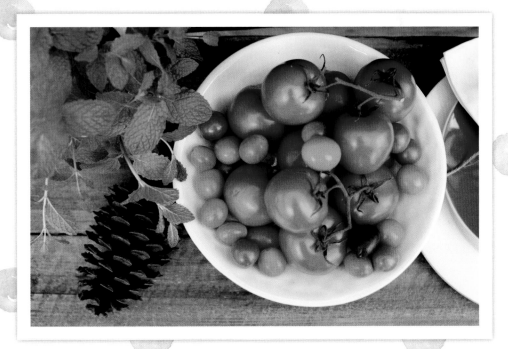

Neon Wood Bead Trivet

Brighten up your backyard cookouts while protecting your table from hot food right off the grill. All you need are some wooden beads, bright paint, and a little patience, which is always easiest to come by on a sunny day.

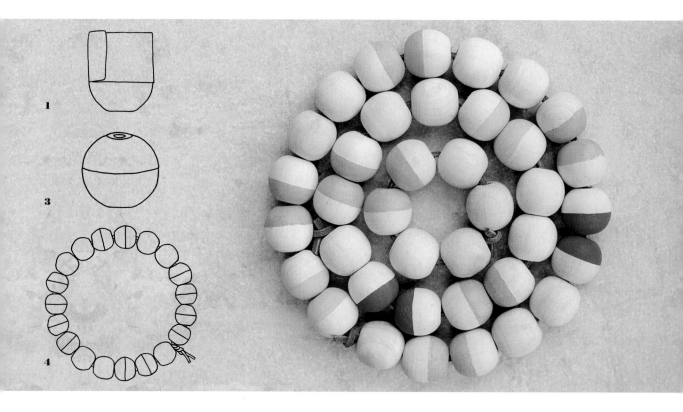

MATERIALS

38 wooden beads, 1" (2.5 cm) diameter
Painter's tape
Craft paint in 4 to 5 different bright colors (we used
   light blue, dark blue, orange, yellow, and pink)
Paintbrush
1½ yard (1.4 m) suede cord
Scissors

INSTRUCTIONS

1   Set aside 16 wooden beads. With the remaining 22, wrap a piece of painter's tape around half of each bead.

2   Paint the exposed half of the beads. (We painted 6 light blue, 4 dark blue, 4 orange, 4 yellow, and 4 pink.) Let them dry. Add a second coat of paint, if necessary.

3   Peel off the painter's tape.

4   String 19 beads onto the suede cord. (We combined 7 plain beads with 6 pairs of painted ones with the painted sides facing.) Bring both cord ends together and tie them with a tight double knot; trim the excess cord. This is the trivet's outer ring.

5   To make the middle ring, string 13 beads onto a second piece of cord. (We combined 5 plain beads with 4 pairs of painted ones.) Tie the cord ends together and trim.

6   To make the innermost ring, string 6 beads onto a third piece of cord. (We combined 4 plain beads and a pair of painted ones.) Tie the cord ends together and trim.

7   Place the rings one inside the other to create your trivet.

Scratch-Off Labeled Party Cups

You know that thing where you throw a party and everyone uses four cups because they don't know which one is theirs and which one is covered in kid-germs? We've solved that problem with our scratch-off party cup labels. Make the labels, stick them to your adorable cups, and let each guest scratch their name into their cup before filling it. When the party is over you'll have a lot less trash headed to the landfill and also a lot less cleaning up to do. Meanwhile, guests will be impressed with your DIY conservation methods. Also, you know everyone thinks it's fun to scratch their initials into things; better to give them a paper cup than a tree.

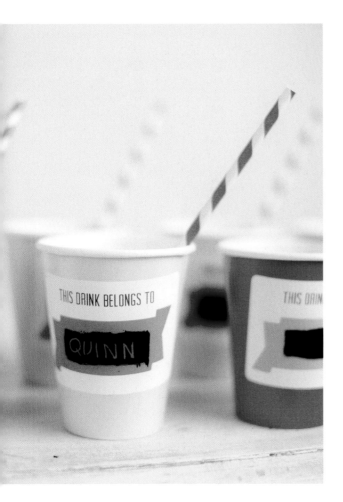

MATERIALS

2 oz. (56 g) black acrylic paint
Dish soap
Clear packing tape
Sticker paper or labels
Foam brush
Paper cups
Toothpick or key (for scratching the names)

INSTRUCTIONS

1   To make the scratch-off paint, mix 2 parts paint with 1 part dish soap.
2   Adhere a piece of packing tape to each sticker label where you want the scratch-off name.
3   Paint a loose rectangle on top of the tape with the foam brush; let dry.
4   Adhere a sticker to each cup.
5   Scratch names into cups using a toothpick, key, or your pinky nail to claim them as your own.

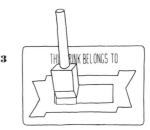

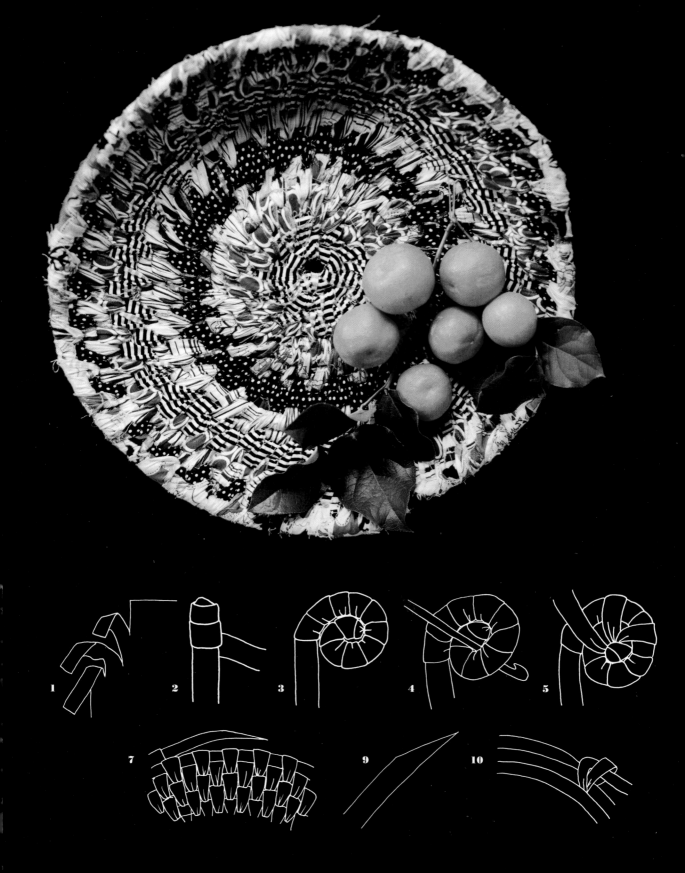

Fabric Wrapped Bowl

A while back, my extremely crafty and creative mother, Nancy, sent me a fabric-wrapped bowl
that she had made many years before. I copied the project, and it quickly became one of my favorites.
It's a great use of fabric scraps, a fun exercise in pattern making, a mindless project you can make
in front of the TV, and has stunning finished results. We use them for storage but also just as pretty
décor that doesn't break when a kid or a kitten knocks it off the counter.

MATERIALS

3 yards (2.7 m) total quilting cotton fabric
(we used ¼ yard (23 cm) each of 12 different fabrics)
12 yards (11 m) piping cord, ½" (13 mm) diameter
(to make an 18"- [46-cm-] diameter bowl)
Scissors
Small crochet hook

INSTRUCTIONS

1 Tear your fabric into 1"- (2.5-cm-) wide strips along
the full length of the fabric. (Our strips were 1" × 44"
[2.5 cm × 112 cm].) Pull off any loose threads. (No need
to go crazy though; there will be more to trim later.)

2 Wrap 1 strip around the end of the cord until it's
completely covered, including the tip.

3 Continue wrapping the same strip of fabric around the
cord, keeping the fabric flat and completely covering the
cord as you work. As you wrap, begin to curl the end
of the fabric-covered cord into a tight spiral, holding it
in place with your fingers until you secure it in step 5.
(This is the beginning of the base of your bowl.)

4 When you've wrapped enough cord and have enough
coils to enclose the end of the cord, as shown here,
use the crochet hook to pull the end of fabric strip up
through the center of the spiral.

5 Using the same fabric strip, continue wrapping the
bare cord where you left off. To secure each portion of
newly wrapped cord to the main coil, alternate between
single wraps (pulling the fabric strip from underneath
and wrapping it around the outer coil of cord) and
double wraps (pulling the fabric strip from underneath
and wrapping it around the two outer coils of cord).
Periodically place your coils on your work surface to
ensure that they lay flat.

6 If your fabric strips are fairly short, you can sew a few
together, end-to-end, but don't make them longer than

about 1 yard (1 m). (They become too difficult to work
with.) To change to a new fabric strip without sewing
two together, wrap the end of the first fabric strip
around the outer cord. Cover it with the end of the new
fabric strip and wrap it tightly, at least once around, to
secure it. Proceed with a double wrap, and continue as
before.

7 Once you have the base of your bowl (our base was
about eight coils, but how big you make it is completely
up to you and your supply of fabric strips and cord),
you can begin to build up the sides. As you make each
new coil, angle the cord about 45 degrees, then continue
wrapping with alternating single and double wraps.

8 Continue adding each new coil at a 45-degree angle to
make a shallow bowl like we did here, or change to a
steeper angle for a deeper bowl.

9 To finish, cut the cord at an angle to help even out the
lower side of the bowl.

10 Continue wrapping the cut cord with the fabric strip
until it's completely covered. Then pull the fabric strip
through the previous coil to secure it to the bowl. Pull
the fabric strip through once again, but this time leave
the loop loose. Insert the end of the fabric through the
loop and pull tight to secure it.

11 Trim the end of the fabric strip, and you are done! If
you have lots of loose threads, just snip them off. No
need to get all of them; it's part of the charm.

Leather Bow Place Mats

If you think you can't sew leather, you're wrong. All you need is a heavy-duty needle in your sewing machine and a good local source for cheap hides. Once you have those two items, sewing leather is a breeze and costs a fraction of buying the real deal at a home store. This tutorial adds a fun twist by including a napkin ring in the form of a bow to stylishly corral your flatware. Whip this table setting together and impress all of your guests.

MATERIALS

1 piece leather, at least 19" × 14" (48 cm × 35 cm)
(to make one place mat)
1 piece leather in a contrasting color, at least 6" (15 cm)
square (to make one bow napkin ring)
Ruler
Rotary cutter
Cutting mat
Quilting clips or binder clips
Sewing machine with heavy-duty needle
Coordinating heavy-duty thread
Scissors
Hand-sewing needle
¼ yd (23 cm) vinyl (to back one place mat)

INSTRUCTIONS

1   From your main piece of leather, cut four leather strips, each 4¾" × 14" (12 cm × 35 cm), using a rotary cutter and cutting mat. (You'll need four strips for each place mat.)

2   Place 2 strips, right sides together, edges even. Secure them with clips. (Don't use straight pins, to avoid poking holes in your leather.) Straight stitch along the long side using a ¼" (6-mm) seam allowance.

3   Repeat step 2 to add the remaining 2 strips of leather, until all 4 pieces are sewn together.

4   Finger-press the seams to one side and secure them with a clip at top and bottom. Top stitch ⅛" (3 mm) from each seam, as shown, to ensure that the leather lays flat. Set this aside.

5   To make one bow, cut a 4" (10-cm) square and 1" × 2" (2.5 cm × 5 cm) rectangle from the contrasting leather.

6   Fold the square in half, right sides together, edges even. Sew along the long side using a ⅛" (3-mm) seam allowance.

7   Turn it right side out. You should have a tube.

8   Wrap the rectangle of leather around the center of the tube and hand-sew it closed.

9   Turn the bow over to the right side (stitches are on the wrong side) and set it in the center of the last panel of the place mat. The left side of the bow should be ⅛" (3 mm) from the inside seam, and the right side of the bow should be ¼" (6 mm) from the outside edge of the place mat. Clip the bow in place, then sew each raw edge to the place mat with a straight stitch using a ⅛" (3-mm) seam allowance.

10   To add a backing to your place mat, use the scissors to cut the vinyl to the exact size of your sewn leather piece.

11   Place the leather and vinyl pieces right sides together, edges even, and clip together to hold in place. Sew along all four outside edges using a ¼" (6-mm) seam allowance and leaving a 3" (7.5-cm) opening for turning along one side; backstitch at the beginning and the end.

12   Turn the place mat right side out. Tuck in the raw edges at the opening and clip in place. Top stitch around all four outside edges of the place mat using a ⅛" (3-mm) seam allowance and closing the hole as you go.

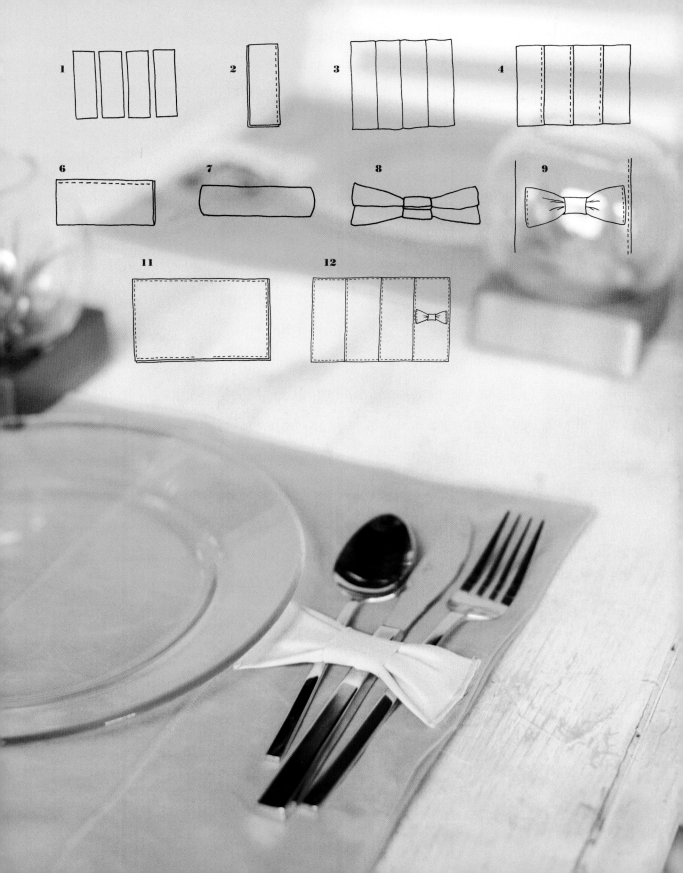

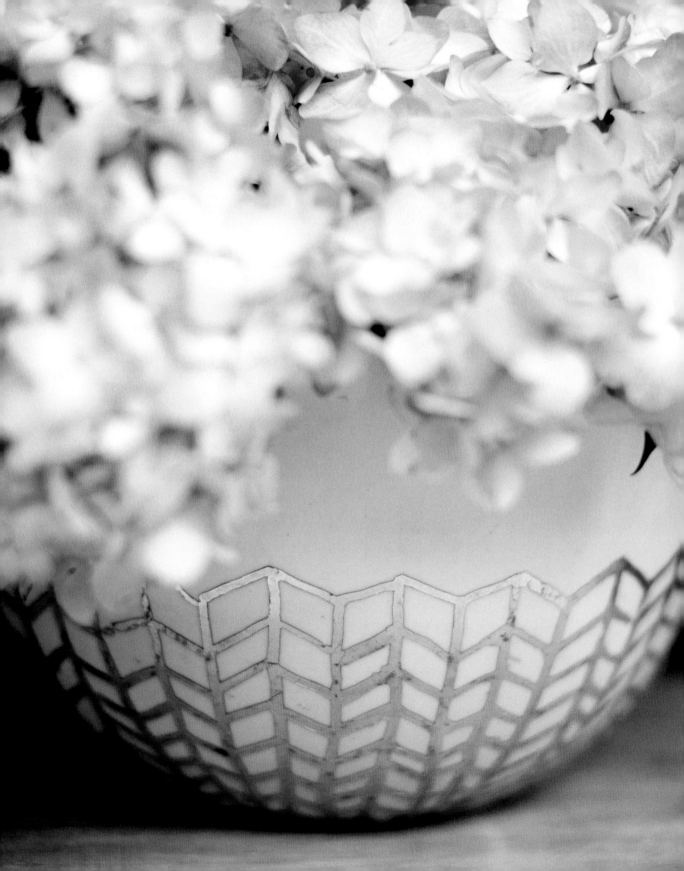

Gold Leaf Vase

★

Use this
technique to gold
leaf anything!

★

Create a hand-drawn herringbone pattern around the base of an inexpensive ceramic bowl and turn it into beautiful showpiece for the holidays. By using a bowl as a vase, you double its usefulness in a cozy home.

MATERIALS

Bowl or vase (we used a ceramic bowl)

Adhesive pen for use with metal leaf

Imitation gold leaf sold on sheets of waxed transfer film, see note, or real gold leaf, if you are a millionaire

Cotton gloves

Cheesecloth

Paintbrush

Acrylic clear-coat sealant

note: Metal leaf affixed to sheets of waxed transfer film is easier to apply and creates less waste than the traditional metal leaf booklet.

INSTRUCTIONS

1   Prepare your surface. If you're using a sealed ceramic or porcelain bowl like we did, you don't have to do a thing. If you want to apply gold leaf to a porous surface like wood, sand and seal it first.

2   Draw your design, as shown or as desired, with the adhesive pen, filling in the design completely with adhesive.

3   Let the design dry for 15 to 30 minutes. It's ready when you touch it with your knuckle and the adhesive is tacky but doesn't come off on your finger.

4   Put on the cotton gloves (to avoid fingerprints) and carefully apply a sheet of gold leaf to the bowl, pressing it flat with a piece of cheesecloth for about 30 seconds. Repeat this step to cover the entire design with additional sheets of gold leaf. Let it sit for at least 30 minutes.

5   Remove the sheets of gold leaf, leaving the gilded design. (Only those parts of the gold leaf not adhered will peel away.) Save any sheets that still have gold leaf on them for touch-ups or future projects. Keep in mind that with multiple applications of the sheets, your gilding will look more worn and rustic.

6   Burnish the gold leaf with a piece of cheesecloth that's been folded in half. Gently rub the cheesecloth back and forth over the gilded areas to remove any excess flakes.

7   If necessary, apply more adhesive and gold leaf to fix any spotty areas.

8   Use the paintbrush and acrylic clear coat to seal only your gilded design. This will add a slight shine to the metal and ensure that it lasts.

9   To care for your gilded items, never put them in the microwave! Microwaves and metal don't mix. We also suggest you hand wash your gilded accessories, just to be on the safe side.

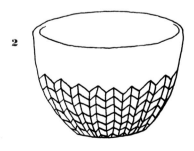

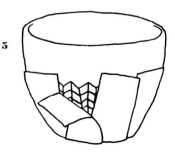

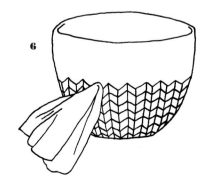

Dowel Table Runner

Create a bold wooden dowel table runner woven with only supplies from the craft store.
This black and white version has a pop of bright green that is eye catching but still neutral
enough to use all year long. Top it with a pretty succulent arrangement.

MATERIALS

32 straight wooden dowels, 36" (91 cm) long
  and ⅜" (1 cm) in diameter

Small handsaw

Fine sandpaper

1 can black spray paint

1 can white spray paint

2 oz. (56 g) green all-purpose craft paint

Small paintbrush

Clear acrylic (or polyurethane) spray sealant

Scissors

8 yd (7.3 m) leather or suede lacing

Clothespins

INSTRUCTIONS

1   Using the handsaw, cut each of the dowels so you now have 64 dowels, each 18" (46 cm) long. (The best way to cut dowels without them splintering or splitting them is to stop sawing halfway through, rotate the dowel 90 degrees, and then start sawing again.)

2   Set 2 dowels aside. With the remaining 62 dowels, sand the ends and any rough spots. Wipe away any dust or debris.

3   Place the 2 dowels you set aside on your work surface 12" (30.5 cm) apart. (These will elevate the sanded dowels while you paint them.) Place a handful of sanded dowels across the first two. Spray paint the dowels black; let dry. Turn them to the opposite side and finish painting them. Continue until you have 32 black dowels.

4   Paint the remaining 30 dowels white.

5   Using a paintbrush, paint the ends of all 62 dowels green; let dry.

6   Spray all the dowels with acrylic sealant; let dry.

7   Cut four pieces of leather lacing, each 2 yd (1.8 m) long. Gather 2 lengths together and tie the ends into a knot. Repeat with the remaining 2 lengths.

8   Place 1 black dowel on your work surface vertically. Slide 1 pair of knotted lacing onto the dowel, 2" (5 cm) from the end, as shown. (One lace should be on top of the dowel, the other underneath.) Cross the laces, then secure them with a clothespin. Repeat this step on the opposite side of the same dowel with the other pair of knotted lacing.

9   Repeat step 8 to add another black dowel, followed by 2 white dowels. Continue adding 2 dowels at a time and alternating colors. Since you began with 2 black dowels, end the runner with 2 black dowels as well.

10 To finish, knot each pair of lacing as you did when you started. Trim the ends to about 1" (2.5 cm) long.

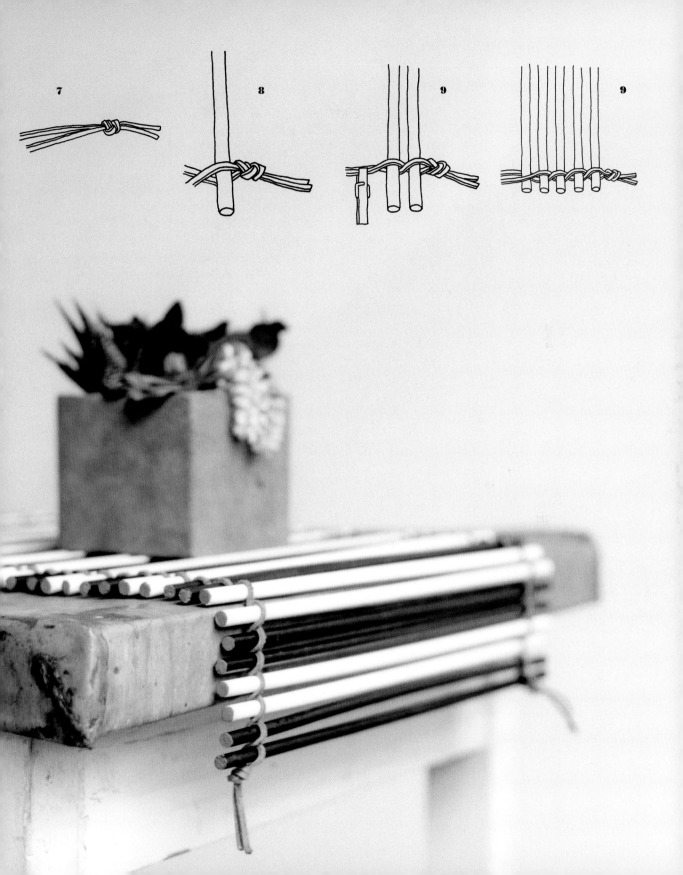

7   8   9   9

Polymer Clay Cake Toppers

Use just a few supplies to create a stunning cake topper
that you can use year after year for all of your celebrations.

MATERIALS

Two 2-oz. (56-g) packages polymer clay
  (such as Sculpey or Fimo)
Rolling pin
Ruler
Craft knife
Parchment paper
Cookie sheet
2 metal skewers
Clay embossing set (such as Walnut Hollow)
Aluminum foil
Oven
8 fl. oz. (236 ml) Martha Stewart Crafts®
  Decoupage Multi-Surface Durable Matte Finish
1"- (2.5-cm-) wide soft-bristle brush
Paper towels
Toothpicks

INSTRUCTIONS

1   Knead a package of polymer clay for several minutes
    until it's soft and pliable.
2   With clean hands, roll the clay into a long, log shape
    and place it on a clean surface. Using the rolling pin,
    roll out the clay ¼" (6 mm) thick, then using a ruler
    and craft knife, cut a strip approximately 1" x 10"
    (2.5 cm x 25 cm). (Store the unused clay in a plastic
    bag so it doesn't dry out.)
3   Lift up the piece of clay and transfer it to a parchment
    paper–lined cookie sheet.
4   Set the type for your message in reverse on the tool
    handle. Center it on the clay and with a steady, firm
    hand, press the letters into the clay. If your message
    is longer than the tool, or if you are using individual
    letters, use a piece of parchment paper to create a

baseline for the type. Don't worry if you make a
mistake; polymer clay is very forgiving. Most marks
will rub smooth with a clean fingertip.

5   Carefully lift up the left end, fold it under itself and
    back out again, curving the clay into a backward "S"
    so it resembles a folded ribbon. Slide the top of one
    skewer between the last two layers of the clay ribbon.
    (Press firmly enough for the layers to mold to the
    skewer, but not so hard that you make a mark.) Repeat
    these steps to add a skewer to the right side.
6   At both ribbon ends, use the craft blade to cut away
    a "V" shape.
7   Place scraps of aluminum foil under the folds of the
    ribbon and skewers so that they hold their shape
    during baking.
8   Bake at 275 degrees F for 15 minutes. (If your ribbon
    is thicker, or thinner, adjust the baking time by a minute
    or so.) The clay may still feel slightly soft when it comes
    out of the oven, but it will harden completely once cool.
9   Apply a few thin layers of food-safe sealant to the
    clay ribbon using the brush. (You can also add glitter
    between the layers for added shine.) To remove any
    sealant from inside the letters, wrap a bit of paper
    towel around a toothpick and dab each letter to absorb
    any excess.
10 Now you're prepared to congratulate everyone you
    know with a celebratory confection when they do
    something awesome!

You can use cookie cutters to create smaller toppers
for cupcakes. Place thinner layers of clay (in two
colors) back to back to make reversible toppers. We
used metal food picks and Milestone® Stone Stamps:
Letters and Numbers to make ours.

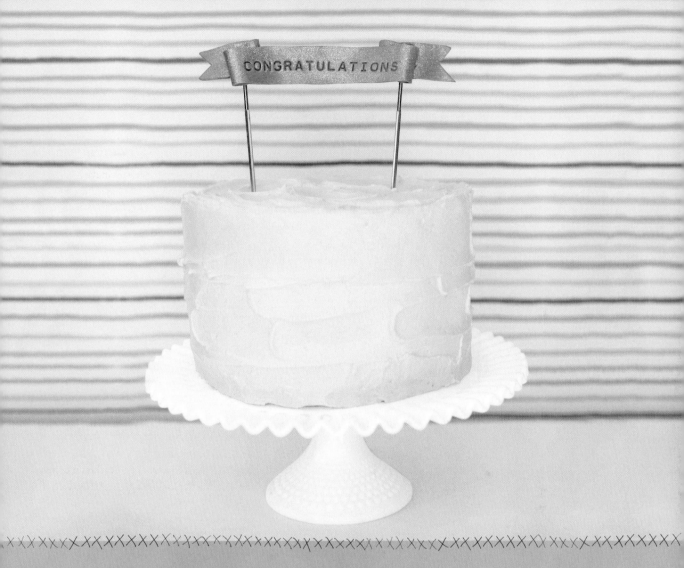

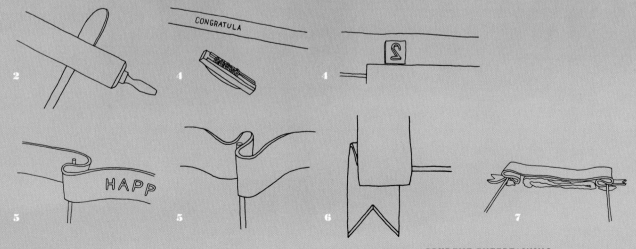

2

4 CONGRATULA

4

5 HAPP

5

6

7

wall décor

Creating inexpensive, festive décor is a fun way to bring a lighthearted, cheery touch to any bash. These deceptively simple adornments can be made in a jiff, then pulled out to display on special days, or left up year round as you see fit. Bonus: Most of these projects are simple enough to do as a family.

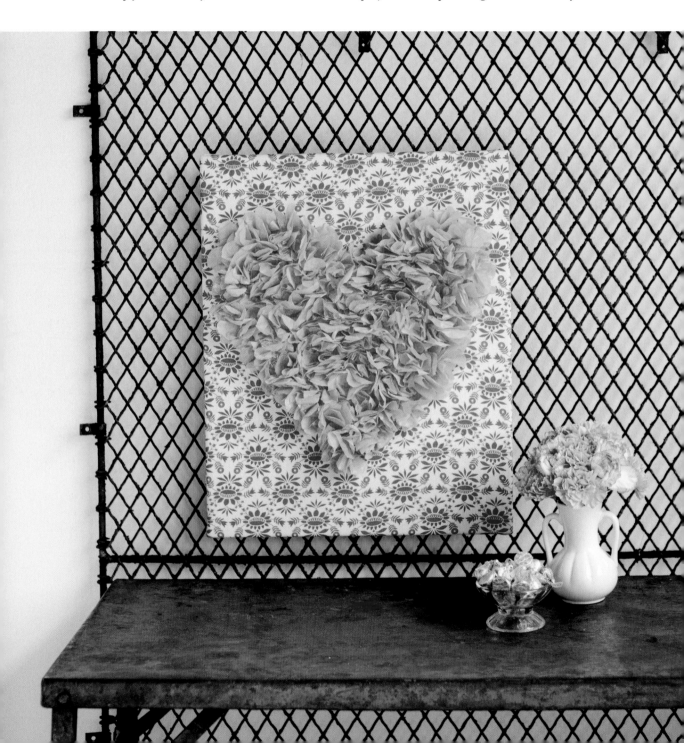

Tissue Paper Party Signs

While we love decorating for Christmas and Halloween, the thought of decorating for Valentine's Day, Easter, St. Patrick's Day, the winter solstice, Independence Day, etc. etc. etc. gets us a bit stressed out. But we have these little humans who are delighted by any excuse to fill our home with decorations, so we are easily swayed into decking out the place for every celebration. This embellished canvas is a decoration that goes a long way toward satisfying their merry tendencies without exhausting our creative energy. We've made a cat for Halloween, a dreidel for Hanukkah, a heart for Valentine's Day, and a star for Independence Day, but with a simple outline of a holiday image you can create a canvas for any celebration—try a numeral for a birthday. Pop it up on the mantle with a few other decorations, and it goes a long way in making the home feel festive.

MATERIALS

Artist's canvas
Fabric 2" (5 cm) wider on all sides than your canvas
Staple gun and staples
Chalk
Tissue paper
Scissors
Hot glue gun with glue sticks

INSTRUCTIONS

1   Place the fabric on your work surface wrong side up. Center the canvas, right side down, on top.

2   Wrap one long side of the fabric to the backside of the canvas and staple it in place at the center point along the wooden frame. Repeat on the remaining long side and both short sides, making sure to pull the fabric taut to avoid wrinkles. At the corners, neatly fold fabric before stapling it in place.

3   Turn the fabric-covered canvas right side up. Use chalk to draw a freehand outline of a holiday image onto the fabric. Set aside.

4   Cut the tissue paper into 3" (7.5-cm) squares.

5   Stack 6 squares of tissue paper. Fold them in half. Now fold each corner as shown to form a triangle. Use scissors to round the top edge as shown.

6   Unfold the stack of tissue paper squares to reveal their flower shape.

7   Take a tissue paper flower, pinch the center, then twist it to form a short stem for gluing.

8   Use hot glue to attach each flower inside the outline you drew on your fabric. Repeat steps 5–7 to make more flowers as needed, gluing them to the fabric until the entire shape is filled in.

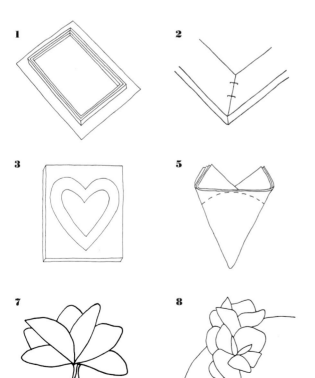

Fan Bunting

This classic decoration typically found in Independence Day parades and car dealerships gets a pretty makeover when the mini-fans are made from designer fabric. This garland can be used for any event, depending on your fabric choice, and once you are done, it makes a gorgeous decoration for above the bed.

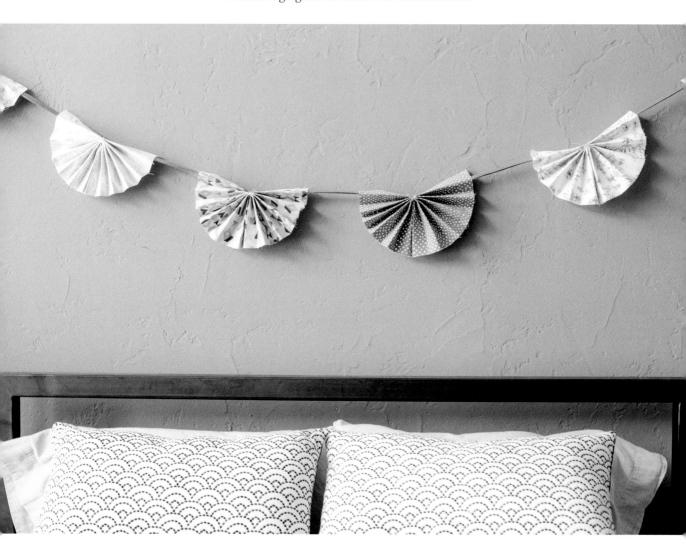

INSTRUCTIONS

1 Place the fabric on your work surface wrong side up. Follow the manufacturer's instructions to iron the interfacing to the backside of the fabric.

2 Cut the fabric into 10" × 15" (25 cm × 38 cm) rectangles (one for each fan you want to make) using the ruler, cutting mat, and rotary cutter.

3 Place 1 fabric rectangle on your work surface wrong side up, oriented vertically. Leaving a 12" (30.5-cm) tail of ribbon for hanging, position the ribbon wrong side up across the top of the fabric, ¾" (2 cm) from the edge. Secure in place with paper clips. Machine stitch the ribbon to the fabric with a ¼" (6-mm) seam allowance. Repeat these steps to add more fabric rectangles to the ribbon, spacing them as desired.

4 Place the ribbon and all the fabric rectangles wrong side up. Begin with 1 fabric rectangle and, starting at the top, fold the edge down 1½" (4 cm). Turn this rectangle to the right side and fold down another 1½" (4 cm), using the first fold as a guide. Turn it back to the wrong side and fold again. Continue turning and folding the fabric, accordion-style, until you reach the bottom. Secure the folds with the clips. Repeat these steps to accordion-fold the remaining fabric rectangles.

5 For each fan, hand-sew the folds together by piercing the needle through the center and pulling the thread through all the layers. Knot the thread at the bottom to secure it.

6 For each fan, bring the bottom fold on both the right and left together. Machine-stitch the folds together on the wrong side, as shown.

7 Trim away any loose threads or uneven edges, and hang!

MATERIALS

Fabric, see note
Medium-weight iron-on interfacing, see note
Iron and ironing board
Ruler
Rotary cutter
Cutting mat
Ribbon or trim, ½" (12 mm) wide, for hanging
Scissors
Paper clips or quilting clips
Sewing machine
Thread
Hand-sewing needle

note: Use a variety of matching fabrics! Each fan requires a piece of fabric and interfacing that is 10" × 15" (25 cm × 38 cm), but it's easiest to work with larger pieces of fabric that you affix the interfacing to and later cut to size.

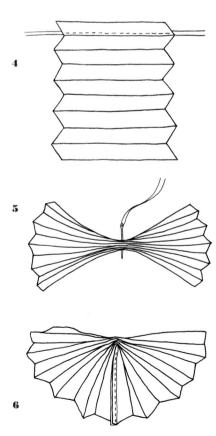

Spring Wreath

Cameroonian juju hats are beautiful swaths of feathers on a raffia base,
splayed out in a disk shape. They make beautiful wall art, with a hefty price tag.
We made our own version inspired by the headdresses to celebrate spring.

MATERIALS

Two 12"- (30.5-cm-) pieces of twine, ribbon, or string
12" (30.5-cm) diameter polystyrene (Styrofoam) disk
Pencil
Lots and lots and lots of feathers, various colors
Nail
Hammer

INSTRUCTIONS

1   Cross 2 pieces of twine and place them on the disk to identify the center point. Mark the center using a pencil and remove the twine.

2   Insert a few feathers perpendicularly into the center of the disk.

3   Working toward the outside edge, continue adding feathers in various colors in concentric circles.

4   Create a gentle transition between the colors or make very defined spaces by planning each feather's placement.

5   Add feathers until the top of the disk is completely covered. Now cover the edges with feathers too. (This will give it a three-dimensional appearance and hide the polystyrene base.)

6   Hammer the nail into your wall where you want to hang the piece; push the foam onto the nail to secure it.

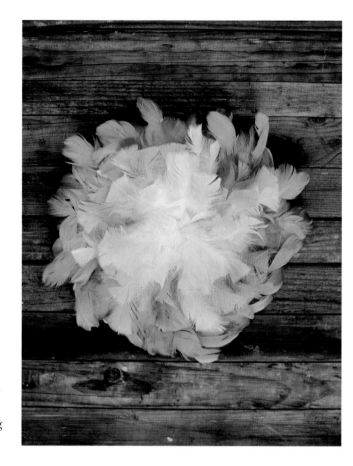

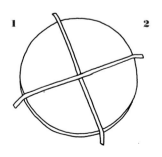 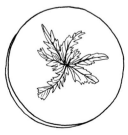 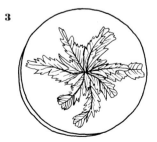 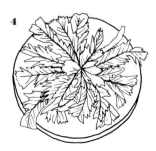

Winter Wreath

Winter is the traditional season of wreaths, and while we love a ring of pine or juniper as much as the next girl, we find it fresh to take a sleek approach to the season of shine. Modern metallic studs lend a crisp edge to this seasonal favorite without evoking the winter blahs.

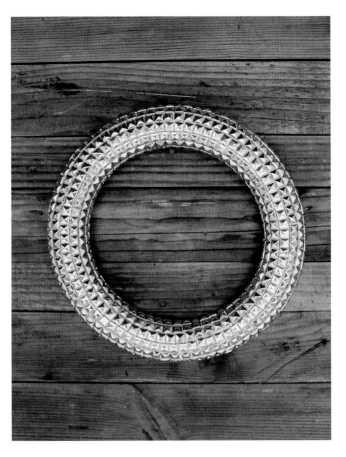

MATERIALS

12"- (30.5-cm-) diameter full-round
polystyrene (Styrofoam) wreath form
Pencil
Approximately 800 silver-finish square pyramid
prong studs, ⅜" (1 cm) wide
Polystyrene-safe glue
(we suggest E6000® industrial strength adhesive)

INSTRUCTIONS

1 On the inner circumference of the wreath form, mark the center, all the way around, using a pencil.

2 Insert the studs, one at a time, into the polystyrene along the marked pencil line to complete one full ring.

3 Working outward, add a second ring next to the first. You'll need to offset this second ring to account for the curvature of the wreath form.

4 Continue adding rings of studs until the wreath form is completely covered. If necessary, secure any loose studs with glue.

5 Hang the wreath on a nail, or loop a ribbon or chain around the top to hang it. Studly.

1
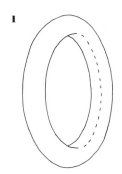

2
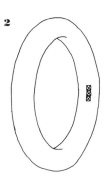

3
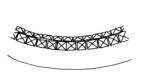

4
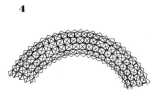

PRUDENT ENTERTAINING

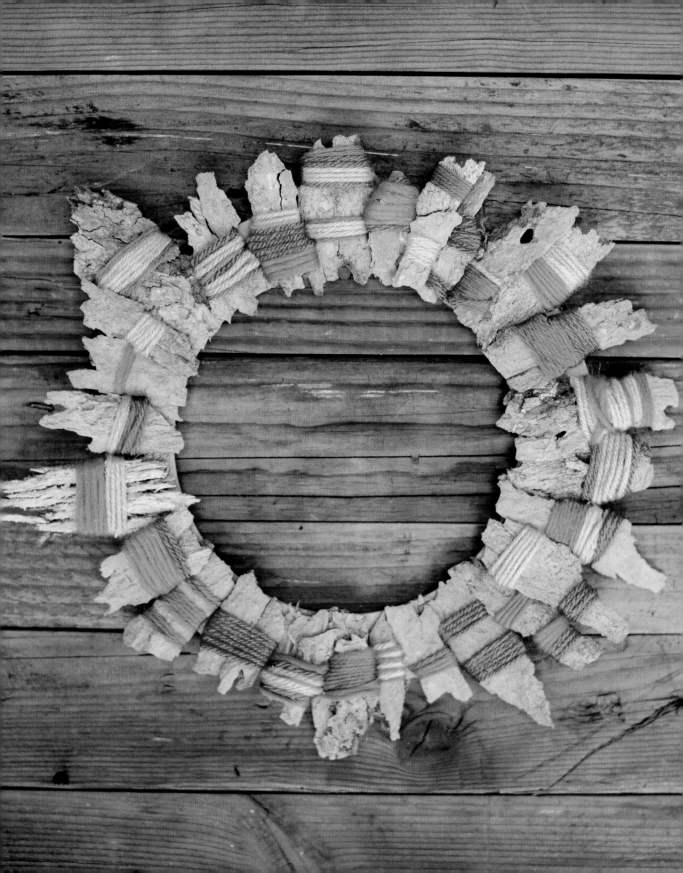

Fall Wreath

Gather up scraps of bark from your fall trees and cozy them up in their own fuzzy scarves.
When you yarn bomb your own front door, you feel welcome every time you come home.

MATERIALS

Approximately 35 pieces bark, each approximately
  2" (5 cm) wide and 2"–8" (5–20 cm) long
Yarn, 4 colors (we used pink, orange, yellow, and
  blue)
10"- (25-cm-) diameter cardboard wreath form
Hot glue gun and glue sticks

INSTRUCTIONS

1 Wrap each piece of bark with single or multiple colors
   of yarn, as shown. Change the placement of the yarn on
   each piece by leaving different areas exposed. To finish,
   tie the yarn ends on the back side.

2 Position the pieces of wrapped bark on the wreath
   form, evenly distributing the longer pieces throughout.

3 When your layout feels complete, adhere the bark to the
   form using the hot glue gun.

4 Hang and enjoy!

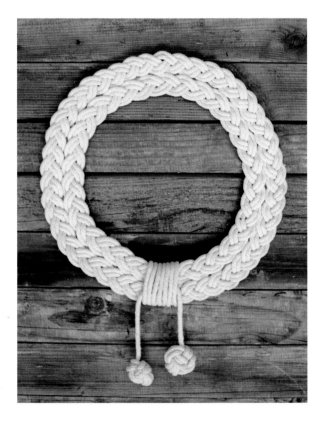

Summer Wreath

Rope elements conjure lazy days with toes in the
sand. We love the industrial edge rope gives to a
traditional wreath form while evoking a seaside
escape. Simply braid two strands of cotton rope,
secure them to a cardboard wreath form with glue,
and wrap the cut edges to finish.

around-the-clock entertaining

Gathering your friends for a celebration doesn't need to be limited to brunch or a dinner party. Why not invite your pals over for breakfast? Spice things up with a Bloody Mary bar! Or how about a kid-friendly buffet? Not that it ever went anywhere, but why don't we bring back the afternoon tea? Here are our favorite super-simple recipes and meal ideas for each time of day. When the event is over, celebrate your success with our signature late-night party for one.

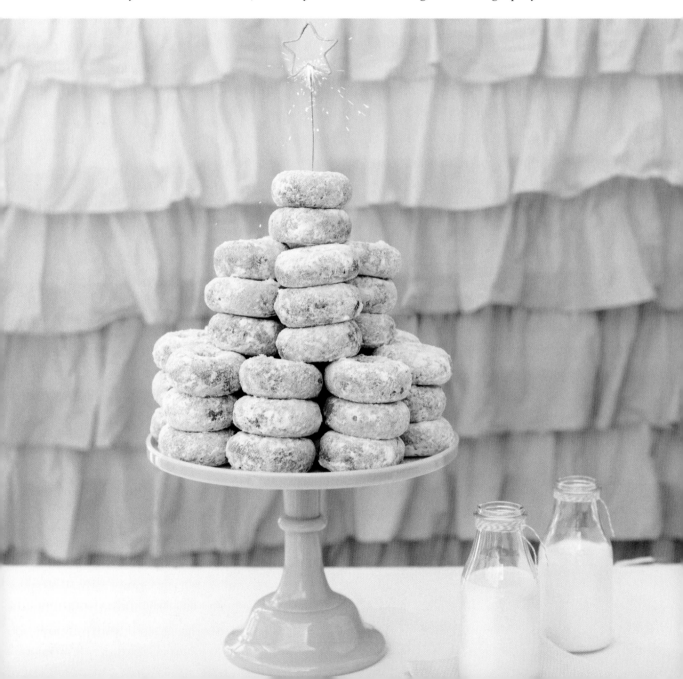

Donut Layer Cake

Ahh, the iconic donut: world's unhealthiest yet most adorable food. These deep-fried, sugarcoated bread rolls are the go-to goodies for early office conferences, last-minute school bake sales, and morning treats on special days. We turn the unassuming, all-American donut into a delightful layer cake worthy of your best birthday parties or maybe even a wedding between two fried-dough lovers.

INGREDIENTS

Lots of donuts (approximately 4 dozen)
Cake stand

DIRECTIONS

For a layer-cake appearance like our powdered donut cake, create a ring of donuts, evenly spaced, around the perimeter of your cake stand. Then place one donut directly in the center. Add two more donuts to each original donut, creating stacks of donuts three high. If the space between your center donut stack and your outside donut stacks is too big to support the next tier, break some additional donuts into pieces and insert them between the stacks. Once your first tier is fully in place, add a second tier of donuts, evenly spaced and three high, positioned above the donuts in the first tier, offset like bricks. Once again, if necessary, fill in the space in the center with broken donut pieces. Add a final stack of donuts; we liked the look of just two donuts for this third tier. If your fingerprints have left any donuts looking a little sparse or spotty, dust with powdered sugar. Add a sparkler, and you are good to go! Your five-minute creation is sure to be the icing on the cake, or hrmm . . . the donut.

Ten Ways to Make Store-Bought Breakfast Special without Firing Up the Stove

1 Create a milk bar with gourmet syrups, boba, fancy straws, and garnishes.

2 Top muffins from your favorite bakery with pretty dessert picks.

3 Display sausage and fried chicken biscuits in rustic baskets.

4 Dye hardboiled eggs in seasonal colors any time of year.

5 Go monotone with all foods and décor in a single color.

6 Create a breakfast punch by combining your favorite fruit juices.

7 Serve unexpected coffee toppings like chili chocolate powder and sweeteners like rock candy.

8 Transfer nostalgic cereals to elegant clear containers as a treat.

9 Everything is cuter when it's tiny. Select all miniature baked goods and line them up neatly on trays.

10 Exotic fruits, served with labels, turn this no-bake breakfast into a culinary experience.

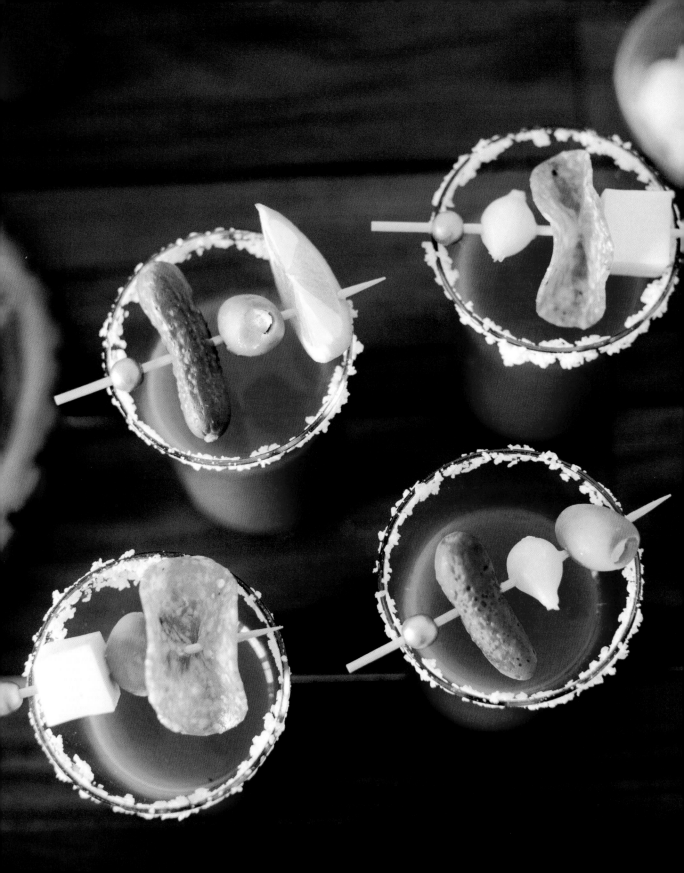

Bloody Mary Bar

For as long as people have had hangovers, there has been the Bloody Mary, a rich, savory, well-garnished elixir, to save the weekend. This morning cocktail was invented by a French bartender working in Paris who brought the drink with him when he began working at New York's St. Regis hotel in the 1930s. It's also one of two drinks that is socially acceptable before 11 A.M., which can come in handy when entertaining parents with children in tow. See the Champagne Cocktail Menu (page 170) for the other. While Jacinda's husband, Rick, and Jaime will both pass on this tomato juice–based delight, Jaime's husband, Carleton, and Jacinda celebrate the Bloody Mary in all its delicious variations as one of their favorites. Here's how to set up a killer Bloody Mary bar for your next brunch.

SUGGESTED GARNISHES

Celery
Lemon
Green olives
Pickled peppers
Cheese and prosciutto–stuffed cherry peppers
Chunks of Parmesan or sharp cheddar cheese
Pepperoni or salami
Jumbo shrimp
Pickled green beans
Pickled onions
Bacon
Blue cheese–stuffed olives
Fresh herbs like Italian basil, cilantro, and dill
Cornichons
Beef jerky

Folks tend to get passionately opinionated about their perfect Bloody Mary. Show your guests how to do it up right with an array of ingredients you have beautifully set out. Let guests create their own custom skewers.

MIX-INS

Salt
Pepper
Worcestershire sauce
Hot sauce
Seafood seasoning
Celery salt
Olive brine
Horseradish

MIXERS

Tomato juice
Tomato and clam juice
Pre-mixed Bloody Mary mix
Vodka, gin, tequila, citrus-flavored vodka (or other flavored vodkas), sriracha, bacon beer, red wine, or port

ICE

Plain water ice
Ice cubes made from fresh juice— like cucumber-basil or tomato-dill

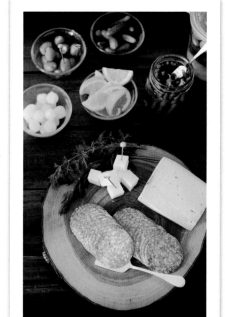

VARIATIONS

BLOODY MARIA
Tequila instead of vodka

RED SNAPPER
Gin instead of vodka

BLOODY CESAR
Add clam juice and rim with celery salt

MICHELADAS
Beer instead of vodka (plus hot sauce!)

RED WINE BLOODY MARY
Last night's leftover Cabernet instead of vodka

VIRGIN MARY
Everything but the booze

PRUDENT ENTERTAINING

Sticks & Dips Buffet

Some kids are picky eaters and some are more adventurous, but one thing that most can agree on is that food on a stick is awesome. Have a kid on the fence about a type of cheese or an exotic fruit? Put a stick in it, and suddenly it's too fun to resist. We love the idea of laying out a buffet of proteins, fruit, and even salad on a stick. It presents a beautiful display of healthy goodies and puts some of the decision-making in the little one's hands.

PROTEINS

Grill or broil steak, marinated chicken breast, seasoned tofu, or our kids' favorite, shrimp. Cut the proteins into bite-sized chunks and skewer them up. Serve with sweet-and-sour sauce, peanut sauce, soy sauce, ketchup, BBQ sauce, and even gravy.

VEGGIES

Stack a variety of veggies, depending on your kids' preferences, on bamboo skewers. We like zucchini, squash, tomatoes, mushrooms, onions, and peppers. Roast or grill and serve with ranch dressing and veggie dip.

SALAD ON A STICK

Skewer items like tomatoes, cucumbers, and mozzarella, or tomatoes, feta cheese, and olives alongside salad dressings.

FRUIT

Create beautiful wands of melon, berries, and pineapple. Cut some into shapes like stars and hearts using cookie cutters. Lay out bowls of seasoning like Tajin Fruit Seasoning, cream cheese dip, and fruit glaze. For a sweeter touch, add bowls of melted chocolate and caramel and plenty of whipped cream.

Lay it all out on a kids' buffet table with chalkboard paper for labeling.

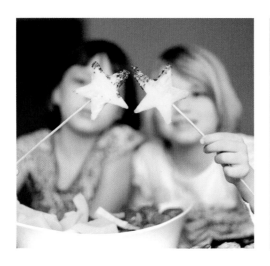
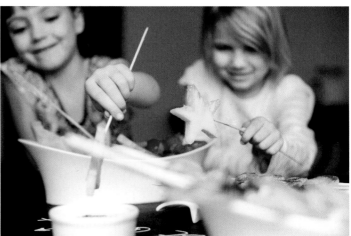

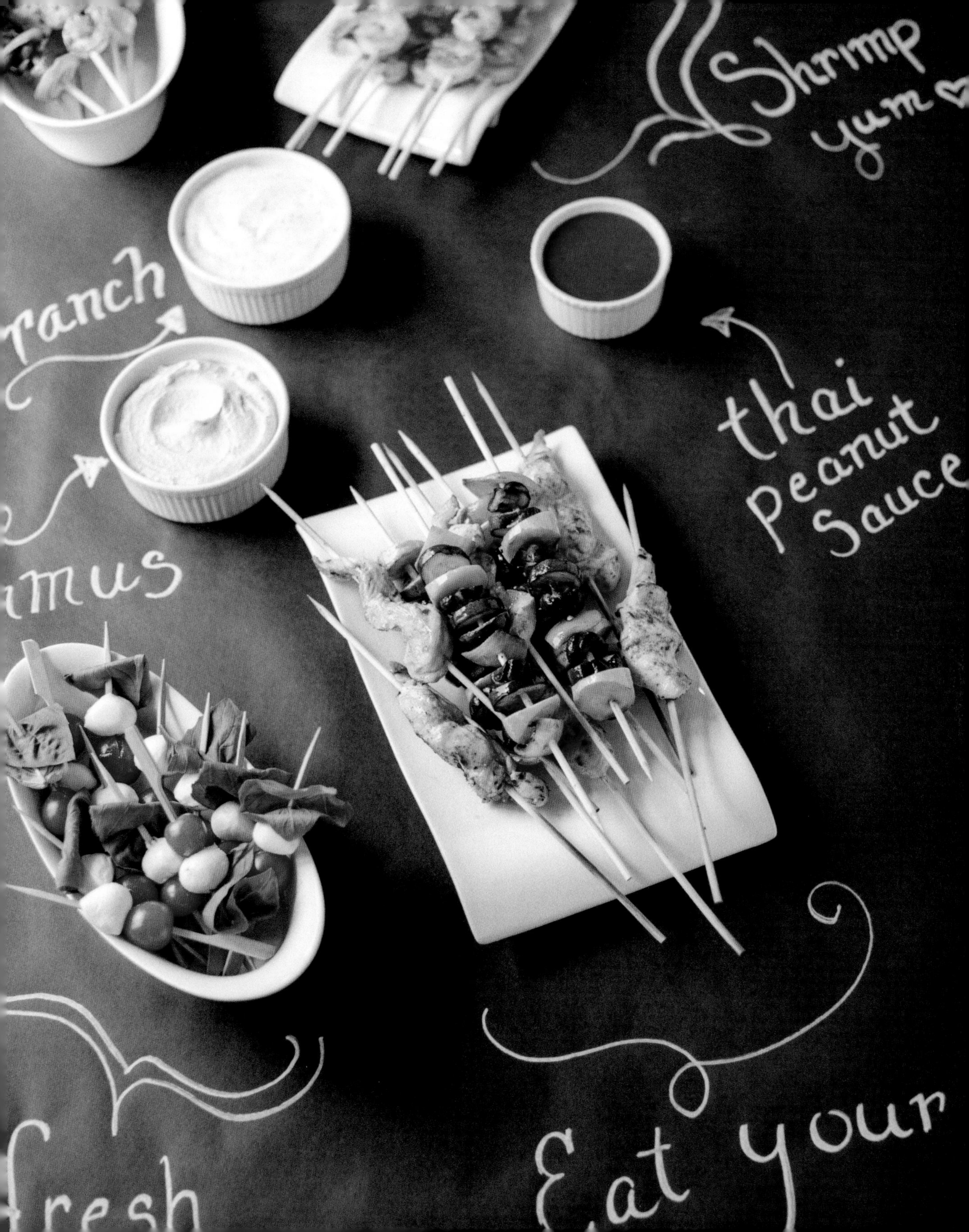

Shrimp
yum ♥

ranch

thai
peanut
Sauce

mus

Eat your

resh

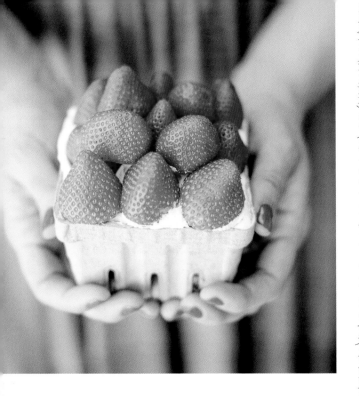

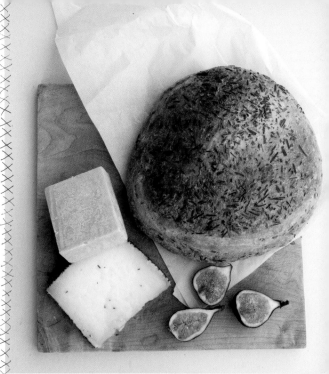

AFTERNOON TEA

Simple Strawberry Shortcake Baskets

Serve a sweet treat that looks like a basket of berries fresh from the farm in no time at all. This recipe is a simple assembly project: Layer three delicious ingredients for a major hit of farm-style charm.

INGREDIENTS

Ladyfingers
Whipped cream
Strawberries, sliced and whole

DIRECTIONS

In a strawberry basket, place a layer of ladyfingers. Cover them with a layer of whipped cream, followed by a layer of sliced strawberries. Continue adding layers until the basket is almost full. Finish with a top layer of whole strawberries: Slice the tops off and place them cut-side down on top of the whipped cream. Arrange on a wooden crate to serve.

Farmer's Market Feasting

The no-bake strawberry shortcake basket at left is also the perfect centerpiece for a party inspired by your neighborhood farmer's market. After a leisurely morning trip through the vendors, pull together an easy afternoon event with fresh local food and natural décor.

Mason jars and pitchers of seasonal blooms

Artisanal cheese and crackers with homemade jam

Rustic sandwiches with ripe heirloom tomatoes and fresh bread

Roasted or grilled seasonal veggies

Herb- and fruit-infused water

Fruit crates for storage and décor

Casual soft fabric napkins

Chalkboard signage

Hand-cut rosemary-scented bathroom soap

Small pots of herbs as parting gifts

Ten Reasons to Host an Afternoon Tea

1. Even the most reluctant entertainer can pull off this simple event.

2. Tea can be a formal and elegant affair or a casual last-minute cup with friends.

3. Requiring only tea, coffee, and a few nibbles, afternoon tea is an affordable party option.

4. You can typically host a last-minute tea with items you already have on hand.

5. Tea parties are intimate events, allowing all of the guests to connect.

6. You can easily add a touch of whimsy by suggesting that your guests wear a hat or fascinator.

7. Afternoon is an easy time of day, ripe for a little break before family dinner.

8. It's easy to wow your guests by presenting each with a small gift, like a simple ribbon corsage.

9. Small touches like a pretty dessert or a handful of garden flowers make a big impact at such an intimate event.

10. An afternoon tea is the perfect gathering to turn into a tradition among a small group of friends.

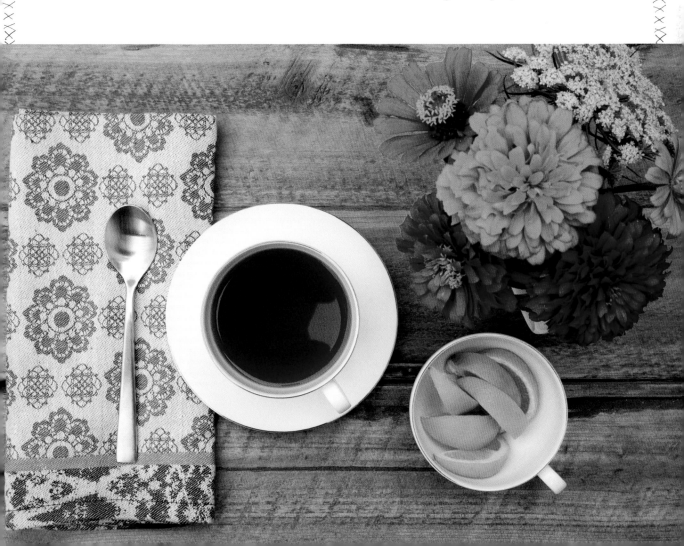

Vietnamese Meatloaf

Back in college at Notre Dame, Jacinda's husband's roommate Drew introduced him to Vietnamese cuisine, and it has been his favorite ever since. Whenever we get together with Drew and his wife, Brookes, we love to cook a big feast that includes fresh rolls made at the table with veggies and rice paper wraps. For years this involved grilling marinated pork to perfection, but a few years ago they introduced us to a new creation they had invented, Vietnamese meatloaf. This turns Vietnamese food into an easy weeknight meal and the meatloaf only requires five ingredients.

INGREDIENTS

SERVES 6 TO 8

FOR THE MEATLOAF

2 pounds (1 kg) ground pork
5 tablespoons (70 ml) fish sauce
¼ cup (60 ml) soy sauce
¼ cup (50 g) sugar
2 tablespoons minced garlic (jarred is fine)

FOR THE FRESH ROLLS

Dry round rice paper wraps, with bowls of hot water
Thin rice noodles, cooked per instructions
Thinly sliced cucumbers
Lettuce leaves with the stalk removed
Julienned carrots
Fresh mint, Thai basil, and cilantro leaves
Chopped green onions
Chopped roasted peanuts
Spicy peanut sauce

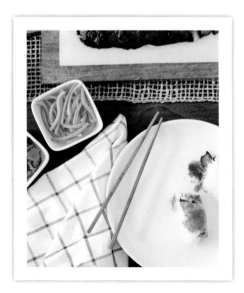

DIRECTIONS

FOR THE MEATLOAF

1 Set a rack one-third from the top of the oven and preheat the oven to 375 degrees F (190 degrees C).
2 Combine all meatloaf ingredients in a bowl until just mixed. The mixture will be wetter than typical meatloaf.
3 Cover a baking sheet with foil, including the sides.
4 Pour meatloaf mixture onto covered baking sheet and form into a rectangle 1–1½" (2.5–4 cm) thick.
5 Bake for 45 minutes to 1 hour. If the surface does not look nicely browned after 1 hour, broil for 3–5 minutes. The sugar escaping the meat may blacken and smoke a little; watch carefully and turn on the kitchen fan.
6 Remove from the oven and let sit for 5 minutes. Transfer to a cutting board and slice thinly.

FOR THE FRESH ROLLS

1 Wet a round rice wrap in hot water for 10–20 seconds, until just pliable.
2 Lay wrap on a plate and top with desired ingredients down the center, with room at the top and bottom. Don't overstuff, or your wrap will split.
3 Fold the top and bottom of the wrap over the edge of the ingredients.
4 Starting from one side, roll up. Eat. Repeat.

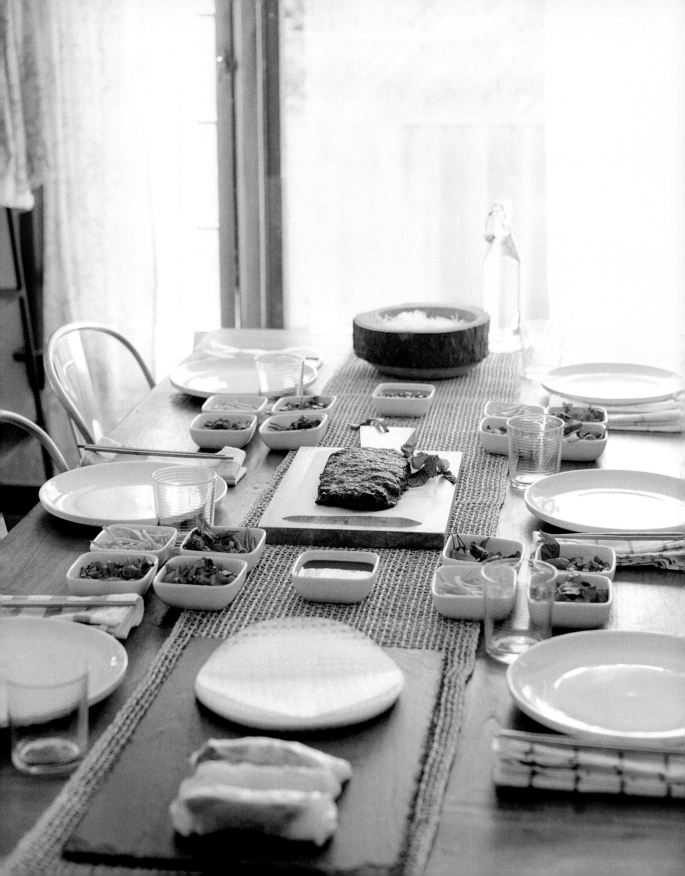

HAPPY HOUR
Champagne Cocktail Menu

Pretty Prudent readers know that when it comes to the bubbly, our cups runneth over. Over years of friendship we've sipped many a magnum, honing our taste for Cava, Prosecco, and of course, Champagne. We've perfected the art of mixing sparkling wine and liquor with fragrant juices, berries, and blooms to create distinctive cocktails sure to make your party pop.

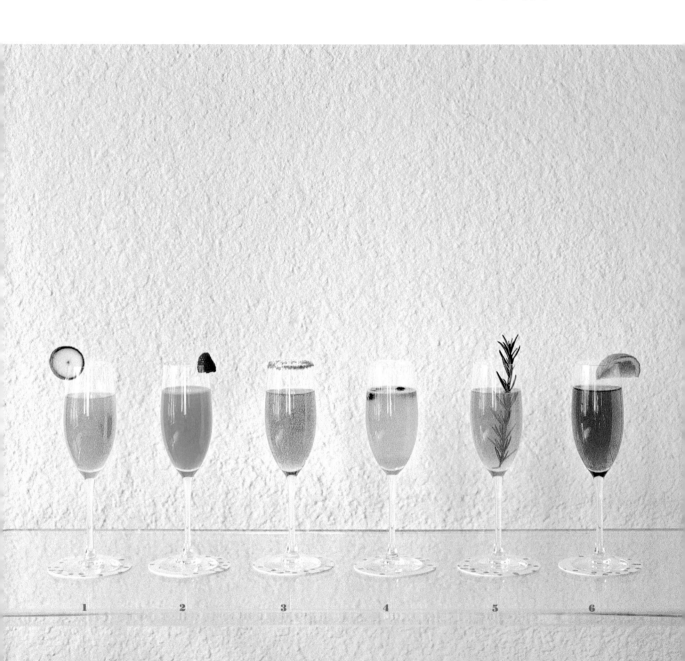

1 SAINT FLORA

1 SERVING

INGREDIENTS

1 jigger elderflower liqueur
¼ cup (60 ml) pear juice
Pear slices, for garnish
Champagne

DIRECTIONS

Add the elderflower liqueur and pear juice to your Champagne glass. Top with Champagne and garnish with a slice of pear.

FIVE PAIRINGS FOR SAINT FLORA

1 A dainty platter of pastel macarons

2 Vintage monogrammed hankies as napkins—any initials will do

3 Baked brie with toast

4 A handful of tiny white flowers in a colored glass bottle

5 Teacups filled with berries

2 CALIFORNIA GIRL

1 SERVING

INGREDIENTS

10–12 raspberries
2 teaspoons sugar
Juice of 4 tangerines
1 jigger brandy
Ice
Champagne

DIRECTIONS

Set 1 raspberry aside. In a small bowl, mash remaining raspberries with a fork into a fine pulp. Add the sugar and mix. Let sit 2 minutes. In a cocktail shaker, combine the tangerine juice, brandy, and ice. Shake to chill, then strain into a Champagne glass. Fill glass with Champagne almost to top. Add raspberry-sugar mixture then garnish with a raspberry on the rim.

FIVE PAIRINGS FOR CALIFORNIA GIRL

1 An array of fresh salsas, guacamole, and chips

2 Bright *papel picado* strung from trees

3 Succulents and palm fronds

4 Raw-edge napkins cut from Mexican cotton

5 Fresh melon, cucumber, and jicama sprinkled with Tajin Fruit Seasoning

3 DUCHESS OF EARL

1 SERVING

INGREDIENTS

Lavender sugar, see note
½ jigger Earl Grey tea, cooled
½ jigger lavender syrup, see note
Champagne

DIRECTIONS

Moisten the rim of a Champagne glass with water and dip in lavender sugar to coat. Add Earl Grey tea and lavender syrup. Top with Champagne.

note: To make lavender sugar, combine 2 parts sugar and 1 part culinary lavender. To make lavender syrup, combine 1 part water and 1 part sugar in a pan. Add several sprigs of lavender and bring to a boil. Let cool. Strain to remove the lavender.

FIVE PAIRINGS FOR DUCHESS OF EARL

1 Miniature lavender scones and lemon shortbread cookies

2 A tiered serving platter displaying colorful glass

3 Delicate silver serving spoons in place of cocktail stirrers

4 Mismatched teacups filled with dried fruit

5 Lemons wrapped in cheesecloth and tied with lace

4 THE CHARLESTON

1 SERVING

INGREDIENTS

Handful of blueberries
½ jigger citrus-flavored vodka
Ice
Lemonade
Champagne

DIRECTIONS

Wrap all but two blueberries in cheesecloth and squeeze or mash with a fork to strain the juice into a cocktail shaker. Add the citrus vodka, shake with ice, and pour into a Champagne glass. Fill with 2 parts lemonade to 3 parts Champagne. Toss a few whole blueberries in for added punch.

FIVE PAIRINGS FOR THE CHARLESTON

1 Profiteroles with ricotta mascarpone and blueberry glaze

2 Tissue décor in flirty fringe

3 Delicate saucers brimming with almonds (raw, cinnamon-tossed, candied)

4 Clear glass pitchers in every shape and size

5 Sandals and seashells

5 THE CAN-CAN KICK

1 SERVING

INGREDIENTS

Champagne
Splash Absinthe (licorice-flavored liqueur)
Sprig rosemary

DIRECTIONS

Fill glass with Champagne, add a splash of absinthe, and insert a sprig of rosemary.

FIVE PAIRINGS FOR THE CHARLESTON

1 Rosemary-spiced meatballs perched on frilly toothpicks

2 Bold striped napkins

3 Colorful peppers stuffed with stinky French cheese such as Morbier

4 An icy silver platter clustered with oysters and rock salt

5 Ruffles of any kind

6 SOUTHERN BELLE

1 SERVING

INGREDIENTS

1 jigger sweet tea vodka
1 teaspoon honey
Champagne
Lemon wedge

DIRECTIONS

Combine sweet tea vodka and honey in a separate container and stir to mix fully. Add to glass, top with Champagne and a squeeze of lemon. Garnish with a lemon wedge.

FIVE PAIRINGS FOR SOUTHERN BELLE

1 Cornbread canapés drizzled with local honey

2 Gingham

3 Hot-chicken wings prepared Nashville style

4 Fancy silver cups with down-home paper napkins

5 Mason jars and mint leaves

Champagne Glasses That Sparkle

While the classic flute is the most common glass for sparkling wines of all kinds, consider mixing it up with an alternative vessel for your bubbly.

FLUTE

It's classic and works well, especially for inexpensive bubbles served cold. If you know us, you know that this will cover 99 percent of our Champagne/Cava/Prosecco drinking needs. The narrow flute is also the best shape for keeping your bubbly, well, bubbly.

TRUMPET

Similar to the flute in performance, trumpet-shaped glasses are common among high-end crystal offerings. While we aren't sure whether a gorgeous crystal trumpet will make your Champagne taste better, it certainly will make it shine.

TULIP

The tulip glass is said to be the most consistently outstanding shape for the sparkling wine experience. It is tall and elegant, yet expands at the top to allow the drinker to swirl and experience the aromatics.

COUPE

While the story goes that this glass was modeled after Marie Antoinette's left breast, it was actually designed for a popular nineteenth-century dessert Champagne sweetened with a dose of syrup. The shape of this glass makes it prone to spills and quick bubble dissipation. Fancy wine people dissuade its usage, but we think it's the most fun and nostalgic of all sparkler glasses.

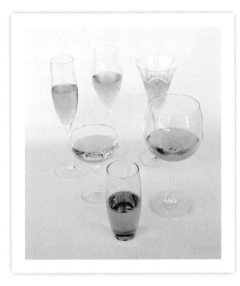

STEMLESS

Similar to the flute in shape, the stemless is great for casual sparkling wine consumption, like at outdoor parties and poolside events. The liquid will warm more quickly with a glass held directly in your hand, so consider keeping the chit-chat to a minimum.

BURGUNDY GLASS

If you are lucky enough to be sampling spectacular, high-quality Champagne, pour a bit into a red wine glass with a large bowl and long stem. It will ensure that you experience all that the vintage has to offer in taste and aroma. Also, you're fancy.

Cheers!

A Cup of Coffee Cake

The most popular recipe on our site—actually our most popular post ever—is this coffee cake in a cup. With a handful of ingredients you likely already have on hand, you can bake this treat in just a few microwave minutes. It's the perfect afternoon snack to make and share with the kiddo, or share with no one but yourself at midnight.

INGREDIENTS

2 tablespoons butter, divided
2 tablespoons sugar
1 egg, lightly beaten and divided
2 tablespoons sour cream
2 drops vanilla extract
¼ cup (30 g) + 2 tablespoons flour, divided
⅛ teaspoon baking powder
1 tablespoon brown sugar
1 teaspoon cinnamon

DIRECTIONS

FOR THE CAKE

1   In a mug, microwave 1 tablespoon of butter to soften (approximately 10 seconds).
2   Stir in the sugar until the mixture is fluffy and creamy, about 30 seconds.
3   Add ½ of the egg, the sour cream, and the vanilla.
4   Stir in ¼ cup (30 g) of flour and the baking powder.
5   Add crumb topping (see recipe below).
6   Microwave the cup, starting at 1 minute and adding 10 seconds at a time until the cake is done to your liking. Let it cool for a minute before digging in.

FOR TOPPING

In a separate ramekin or bowl, mix 1 tablespoon butter, 2 tablespoons flour, the brown sugar, and the cinnamon. Smush it all together with your fingers to combine.

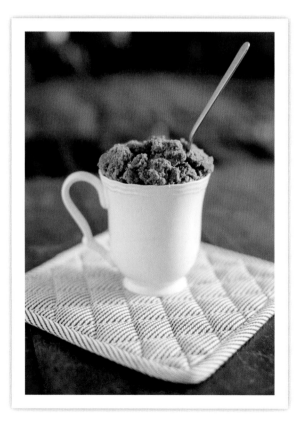

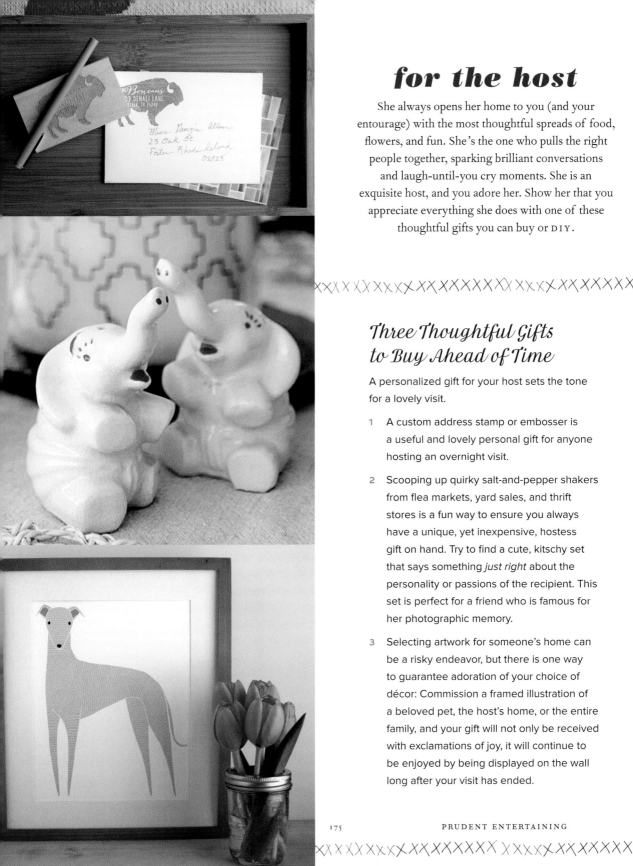

for the host

She always opens her home to you (and your entourage) with the most thoughtful spreads of food, flowers, and fun. She's the one who pulls the right people together, sparking brilliant conversations and laugh-until-you cry moments. She is an exquisite host, and you adore her. Show her that you appreciate everything she does with one of these thoughtful gifts you can buy or DIY.

Three Thoughtful Gifts to Buy Ahead of Time

A personalized gift for your host sets the tone for a lovely visit.

1   A custom address stamp or embosser is a useful and lovely personal gift for anyone hosting an overnight visit.

2   Scooping up quirky salt-and-pepper shakers from flea markets, yard sales, and thrift stores is a fun way to ensure you always have a unique, yet inexpensive, hostess gift on hand. Try to find a cute, kitschy set that says something *just right* about the personality or passions of the recipient. This set is perfect for a friend who is famous for her photographic memory.

3   Selecting artwork for someone's home can be a risky endeavor, but there is one way to guarantee adoration of your choice of décor: Commission a framed illustration of a beloved pet, the host's home, or the entire family, and your gift will not only be received with exclamations of joy, it will continue to be enjoyed by being displayed on the wall long after your visit has ended.

Three Faux-Thoughtful Gifts to Grab on Your Way to the Party

Run into your local grocery store and pull together a last-minute gift that seems more thoughtful than it actually was.

1   Spice it up with a fancy salt, a jar of vanilla beans, or some saffron with a bow.

2   Pick one perfect pineapple, known as a symbol of hospitality.

3   For a real treat, create a s'mores kit by bundling together graham crackers, marshmallows, chocolate bars, and skewers, then wrap them in a paper grocery bag.

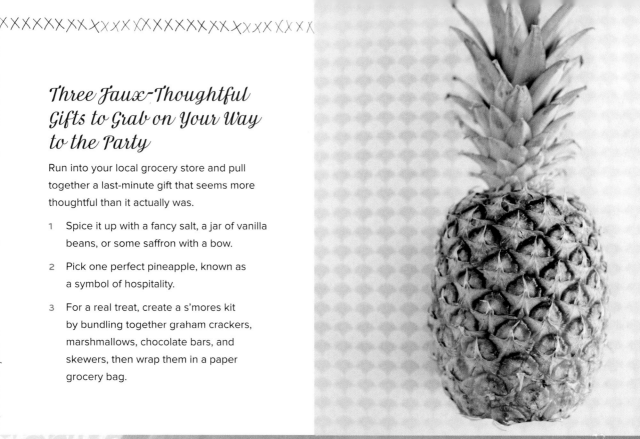

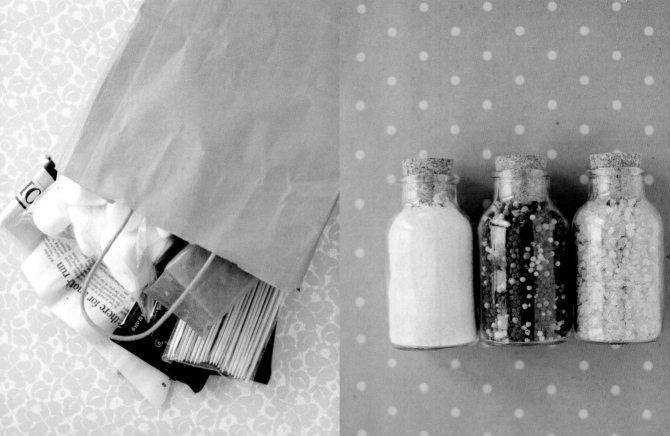

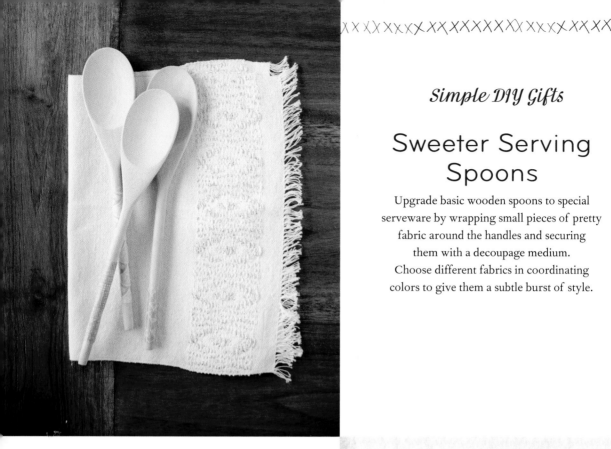

Sweeter Serving Spoons

Upgrade basic wooden spoons to special serveware by wrapping small pieces of pretty fabric around the handles and securing them with a decoupage medium. Choose different fabrics in coordinating colors to give them a subtle burst of style.

Iron-On Stationery

The easiest of all appliqué, the store-bought iron-on patch gets a life beyond the denim jacket on some lovely luxe semi-DIY stationery.

MATERIALS

Iron-on patches or transfers
Notecards with envelopes
Press cloth (a piece of white cotton sheet works great)
Iron and ironing board

INSTRUCTIONS

1. Position the iron-on patch on the front side of a notecard.
2. Carefully place the press cloth over the patch.
3. Iron the patch according to manufacturer's instructions. Lift off the cloth and let cool.
4. Write a lovely note and send your sweet card to a friend.

Calligraphy by Lauren Essl of blueeyebrowneye.com.

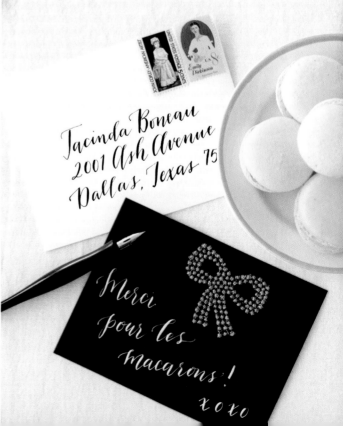

Neighborhood Map Tray

We love to keep these decoupage trays on hand. They will be so convenient when our husbands finally decide they want to serve us breakfast in bed. Until then, they are awesome for holding mail, smoothie supplies, and giving your clutter some eye-catching containment. Tear into last year's road atlas and create a custom map tray of your city for a new neighbor. Add more local treats to the gift for added wow factor. It's a thoughtful, useful, and beautiful gift.

MATERIALS

Unfinished wood serving tray

Latex paint

Paintbrush

Ruler

Map, atlas page, or any decorative paper

Craft knife

Cutting mat

4 oz. (112 g) decoupage medium, gloss or matte finish

Foam brush

Clear acrylic (or polyurethane) spray sealant

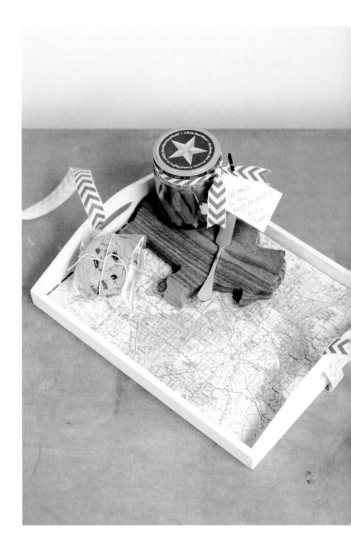

INSTRUCTIONS

1   Paint the wood tray in your desired color. If you're using a light color, you may need multiple coats. Let dry.

2   Measure the interior of the tray. (You can also place the map in the bottom of the tray and crease the paper where it meets the sides so you'll know how much to trim away. Very technical stuff.)

3   Trim the map to size using the ruler, craft knife, and cutting mat.

4   Apply an even coat of decoupage medium to the entire bottom of the tray.

5   Starting at one short end, place the map in the tray, pressing and smoothing away any wrinkles or bubbles as you move toward the opposite end. Let dry.

6   Apply two layers of decoupage medium to the map, letting it dry thoroughly between each coat.

7   Apply a coat of spray sealant to the entire tray; let dry.

Beginner's Guide to
Hand Appliqué

Appliqué can turn a blank canvas into a work of art. It's a great way to use the beautiful scraps of your favorite fabrics, and the design options are endless. Machine embroidery and machine sewing are quick and lovely for finishing appliqué projects, but hand-stitched appliqué has charm beyond compare.

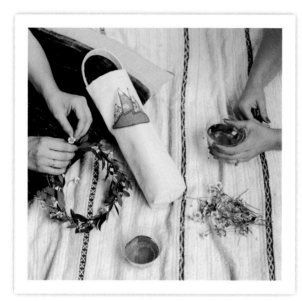

MATERIALS

Four 4" (10-cm) squares of fabric, three with different
patterns and one in solid green
Iron and ironing board
Double-sided interfacing (we used Therm O Web Heat n Bond® Lite
iron-on adhesive, which has a paper backing on one side)
Light box or window
Hand Appliqué Mountain template (see page 222)
Pencil
Scissors
Wine tote
Embroidery needle
1 skein brown embroidery floss

INSTRUCTIONS

1   Iron your appliqué fabrics.

2   Cut pieces of interfacing slightly smaller than your fabrics. Iron the interfacing to the wrong side of the fabrics.

3   If you want a larger appliqué, use a photocopier to enlarge the template to your preferred size. Using a light box or a window, trace each section of the template onto the wrong side of the fabric pieces. (Each wrong side should have the interfacing's paper side facing up.)

4   Carefully cut out each fabric section you traced.

5   Starting with the "grass," peel away the paper backing and iron it to your item. Repeat this step with the remaining pieces.

6   Thread your needle with embroidery floss and sew around the edge of each piece of fabric. We used blanket stitch (see page 120), but you may also use satin stitch (see page 121).

7   Give your handmade appliqué with pride.

See prettyprudent.com for tote-sewing instructions.

Fig Jam

Nothing makes a better gift than a homemade treat. We adore the traditional gift of homemade
jams and jellies because you can make them in a big batch and have them last all year. If you
have a garden that produces fruit, your gift is all the more special. My garden boasts a fig tree,
which makes for sweet jam, perfect for wine-and-cheese parties and pretty hostess gifts.

8 cups (2 L) of jam, or enough for 8 half-pint canning jars

INGREDIENTS

4 cups (620 g) figs (my Bedford figs are from a one-
  hundred-year-old cutting from my landlord's family
  farm, but any soft-skinned fig variety will work)
½ cup (120 ml) lemon juice
6 cups (1.2 kg) sugar
¼ teaspoon ground cloves
¼ teaspoon cinnamon
⅛ teaspoon allspice
¾ teaspoon butter
3-oz- (84-g-) packet liquid pectin

DIRECTIONS

1 Bring a large pot of water to a boil (or follow the
   instructions on your hot water canner). Prepare
   canning jars and lids by simmering in hot water.

2 Wash figs, remove stems and bases, and chop. (I like
   to chop half of the figs very finely and the other half
   more roughly, leaving a few bigger pieces for a pretty
   texture.)

3 In an 8-quart (7.5-liter) or larger saucepan, combine
   figs, lemon juice, ½ cup (120 ml) water, sugar, spices,
   and butter (to reduce foaming).

4 Turn heat to high and bring mixture to a steady rolling
   boil. Let it boil for at least 5 minutes, until no amount
   of stirring will reduce the boil.

5 Add liquid pectin and boil for an additional minute.
   Remove from heat.

6 Skim foam from the top of the mixture.

7 Transfer to canning jars using a sterilized ladle and
   funnel to avoid spilling on the jar rims. Leave ¼"
   (6 mm) of headspace at the top of each jar.

8 Wipe rims of jars with a clean cloth; attach lids and
   screw on bands. Process jars by boiling in a hot water
   bath for 10 minutes (longer at higher altitudes). Remove
   to cool on a towel-lined surface away from any curious
   little hands. Any popping or hissing sounds during the
   24-hour cooling period are normal.

9 After 24 hours, check the seal on each jar; the lids
   should not pop up or down when touched. Discard
   any jars that have not sealed properly.

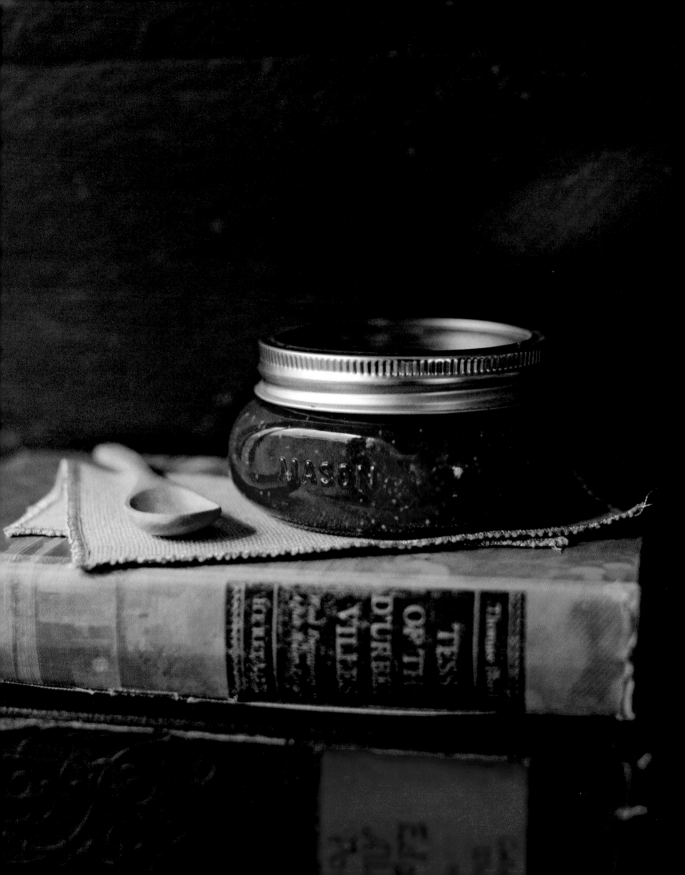

that's a wrap

Any gift can have a handmade touch when wrapped in pretty paper
and tied up with the perfect seasonal accent. Winter, spring, summer,
or fall, here's the gift-wrapping to make the girls swoon.

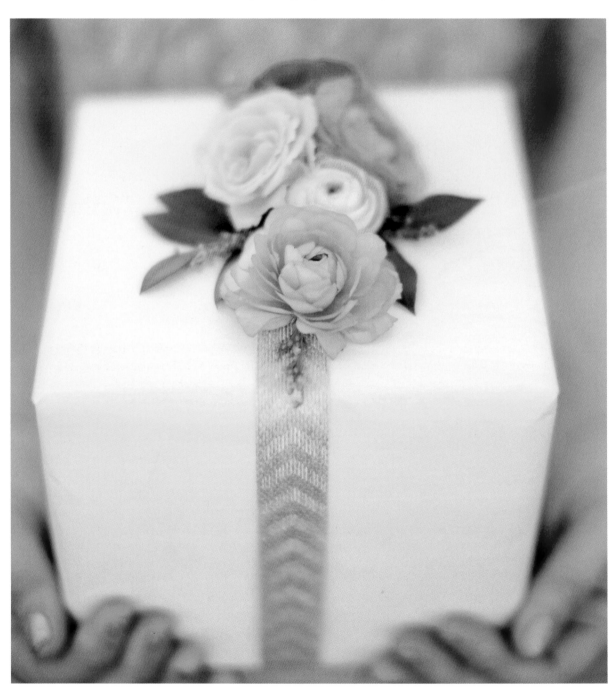

Fresh Flower Corsage Wrapping

Spring showers of the gifting sort call for pretty wrapping to be displayed on the party table. Why not add a fresh gift topper in the form of a flower corsage that the honoree can unwrap and then wear throughout the big day?

MATERIALS

Wrapped gift

Natural fiber ribbon, like burlap (synthetic ribbon will melt)

Fresh flowers (we love the look of ranunculus in coordinating shades of pink, coral, rust, and yellow)

Greenery (to make your flowers pop)

Hot glue gun and glue sticks

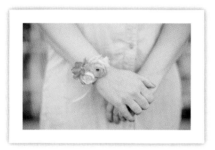

INSTRUCTIONS

1   Cut a length of ribbon long enough to wrap around the gift once. (It should also be long enough to tie around a wrist.)

2   Cut fresh flowers at their bases and arrange them along the center of your ribbon. Add some greenery.

3   Attach each flower and leaf to the ribbon using hot glue.

4   Let cool before tying the ribbon around your gift.

5   Once the honoree has opened her gift, tie the floral ribbon, now a beautiful corsage, around her wrist.

Twig Bundle Gift Wrap

Step up your burlap game by adding a bundle of twigs with a colorful twist to your fall gifts. Not only will your homemade wrapping kindle conversation at the party, gathering your materials is a great excuse to get outside and commune with nature before the cold touches down. (See photo on page 1.)

MATERIALS

Twigs

Craft paint, 8 different fall colors (we used burnt orange, pale yellow, peach, poppy, soft pink, leaf green, blue, and white)

Paintbrush

Kraft paper or a brown paper shopping bag

Scissors

Tape

Burlap

Hot glue gun and glue stick

Twine

INSTRUCTIONS

1   Gather 5 to 10 twigs. Make sure they are sturdy and dry.

2   Paint stripes on the twigs using multiple colors of paint, as shown or as desired.

3   While the paint is drying, wrap your gift in Kraft paper or a recycled shopping bag.

4   Cut a piece of burlap long enough to wrap around the gift once but much more narrow than the width of the box. Secure the burlap ends on the backside using the hot glue gun.

5   Secure your bungle of twigs by wrapping them a few times with a length of twine; tie a knot and trim the ends. Place the bundle on the front of the gift. Wrap a second length of twine around the gift and your beautiful twigs and tie them together with a pretty bow.

Fair Isle–Inspired Gift Wrap

We love pom-poms and always will: they're soft, fuzzy, and forever adorable. Create a colorful pattern with washi tape, then top your box with a re-usable pom-pom to create a gift that reads more "adorable Fair Isle hat" than "ugly Christmas sweater." If you want to pack an ugly sweater inside, well, that's up to you.

MATERIALS

White wrapping paper

Scissors

Tape

3 rolls of washi tape that resemble a Fair Isle sweater
  (we used patterned tape in red and two shades of gray)

2 pieces cardboard, 3" (7.5 cm) square

Yarn

Yarn needle

Hot glue gun and glue stick

INSTRUCTIONS

1   Wrap your gift in white wrapping paper.

2   Adhere lengths of washi tape (we used 9) around the entire gift, each one adjacent to the next.

3   To make the pom-pom, start by cutting two 3"- (7.5-cm-) diameter donut shapes out of cardboard.

4   Place both cardboard donuts together, edges even. Thread the yarn onto the yarn needle. Insert the needle through the center and up around both pieces of cardboard.

5   Continue wrapping the yarn around the cardboard donuts, as shown.

6   Wrap the yarn until the cardboard is completely covered. (The more yarn you use, the fuller your pom-pom will be.) Snip off the needle and the yarn attached to the skein.

7   Carefully cut the yarn around the edge so that the blades of your scissors go between the two pieces of cardboard.

8   Cut a 12" (30.5-cm) piece of yarn from the skein. Thread it between the two pieces of cardboard and bring the ends together; pull tight.

9   Tie the yarn in a knot, securing it.

10 Remove the pom-pom from the cardboard. If necessary, trim the pom-pom to make it rounder.

11 Adhere the pom-pom to the gift using the hot glue gun.

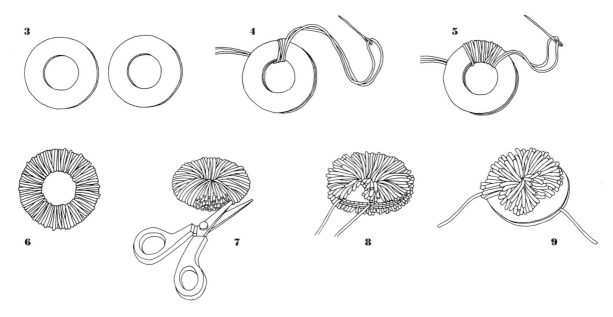

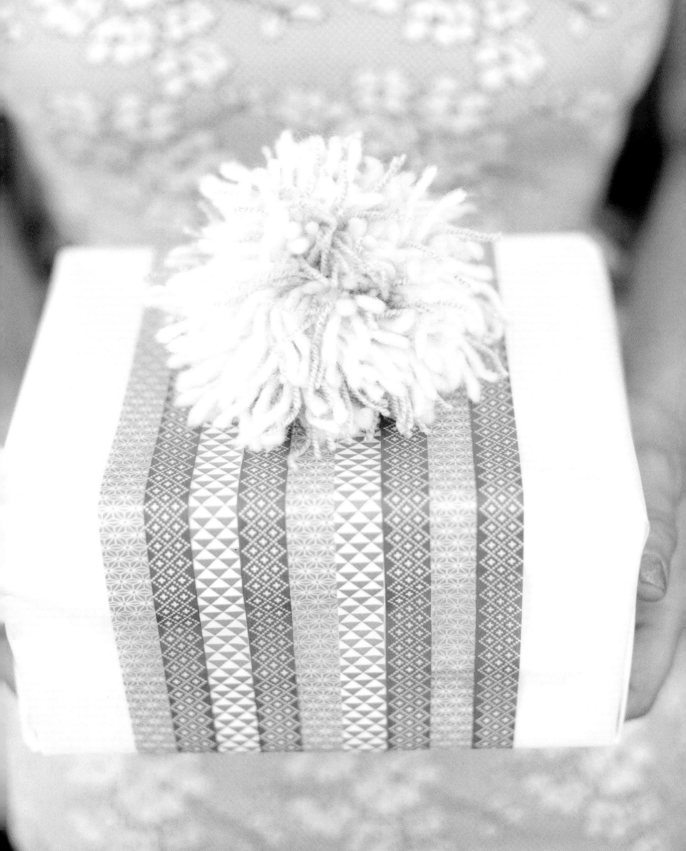

Knaughty Gift Wrap

Add a decorative element to your summer gifts with an attractive knot known as the double Carrick bend. Normally used for joining two sailing lines to create a strong knot that can withstand major force, it's perfect for summer wedding presents and gifts to someone you love.

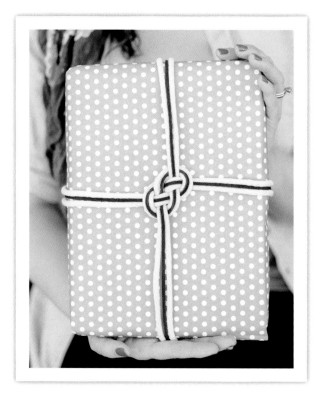

MATERIALS

Wrapped gift
Cotton rope, see note
Suede cord, see note
Hot glue gun and glue sticks

note: To determine how much rope and cord you need, measure your gift in all dimensions (width, length, and depth). Add these values and multiply the total by 5 for your amount of rope and by 2½ for your amount of cord.

INSTRUCTIONS

1 Cut the rope in half. Now fold each piece in half. Fold it in half again and place it on your work surface as shown.

2 Arrange the 2 folded pieces into 2 loops with the tails crossed, as shown.

3 Leave the loop on the right as is. Pick up the rope on the left at the fold. Leading with this folded end, weave the rope over and under multiple times through the loop on the right, exactly as shown. (It's really simple once you get the hang of it.)

4 Double-check the positioning of your rope. Pull the ends enough to make a loose knot.

5 Cut the suede cord in half. Set 1 piece aside. Beginning on the right, weave 1 piece through the knot, following the path of the original rope loop from step 2. You should come out on the same side you started. Repeat these steps to weave the second piece of suede on the left. Pull all 12 loose ends to tighten the knot.

6 Secure the knot to the front of the gift using the hot glue gun.

7 Pull all the loose ends around to the back of the gift. Trim and secure them in place using the hot glue gun.

8 Try *knot* to cry when the recipient rips the gift open.

1

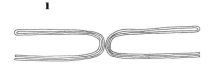

2

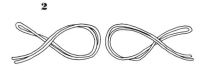

3

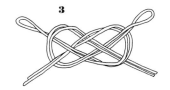

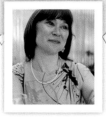

A Good Guest Always...

BY LAURA HOUSE, BROOKLYN-BASED WRITER AND EDITOR WHO EXPLORES THE ART OF HOSPITALITY AT GOODHOUSEGUEST.COM

SHOWS UP WITH A LITTLE TOKEN FOR THE HOST. Yes, it's old-fashioned, but if they open their home to you, let them know you appreciate all the effort they went to in sharing their space, food, and stash of wine with you.

UNPLUGS UPON ARRIVAL. Don't be the one with your face buried in your Instagram feed all night. Engage in live conversation with the real people in the room with you. Your status update can wait.

FENDS FOR THEMSELVES. Introduce yourself to other guests and find your way to the bar on your own. With dinging doorbells and buzzing oven timers calling, the early moments of a party are usually the busiest for hosts.

CALLS FIRST WHEN CHANGING UP THE PLAN. Need to bring along your brother who dropped into town last minute? Running more than thirty minutes late? Just give a call and let your host know so plans can be adjusted accordingly.

DOESN'T STEAL THE SHOW. Remember the guy you sat next to at that party last week who held you hostage with every last detail of his break-up? Don't be that guy. Share the road when it comes to conversation at a dinner party (or anywhere, really).

FOLLOWS A HOST'S LEAD. Some hosts genuinely appreciate (and expect) help in the kitchen. Others would rather not have you mess with their mountain-of-dishes order of things. Know how to read your host and go with the flow.

RESPECTS THE SURROUNDINGS. If staying with friends for an extended length of time, keep your space tidy, pick up around the house, and treat their home with the same level of respect you would your own. Homes—these places where we feel safe, vulnerable, and our most comfortable—are sacred spaces.

KNOWS WHEN TO SAY WHEN. Whether coming for dinner or bunking for the weekend, don't overstay your welcome. Don't be the one mixing another round of drinks at midnight when your hosts are yawning and checking their watches.

EXPRESSES GRATITUDE. Drop a little note in the mail, ring your host the next day, or send an email to express sincere thanks. More than just polite, it's a deeper way to connect and let friends and family know how important spending time with them truly is.

RECIPROCATES THE INVITATION. Keep the good times and kindness flowing by extending the next invite. It doesn't need to be splashy, either: have friends over for tea, invite them for a picnic, or treat them to a simple dinner.

4

a prudent *family*

It's a fact: Heading a family of your own is a whole new trip. Our children humble us, yet inspire us to be brave. They exhaust us to the point that we realize we've grown old, then energize us until we feel young again. A day with a child is a blank chalkboard, ripe with opportunities to explore, pretend, play, and learn. Nighttime holds the possibility of snuggles, rest, communication, and quiet love. Then morning arrives, and it all starts over from scratch. Every day as a family is hope; every sunrise is another chance to do it right.

What a gift it is to see the world from a few feet off the ground again, even as you tower above—to understand the love and responsibility our daughters and sons crave, and then look to ourselves to fulfill those needs by doing our very best, in every way that we can. Being a parent holds the potential—at least sometimes, in some moments—to feel good about what you've given to another person. We know that feeling, and we've loved talking with you about it on our website. We're excited to share that warmth and joy with you here. We at Pretty Prudent think you can have it all—not just a charming house but a graceful home as beautiful inside as your childrens' hearts.

Play! Create spontaneous lemonade stands, frequent picnics, impromptu adventures, pretty places to store treasures, and quiet spaces they can call their own. Fill the lives of the little people around you with wonder, delight, and comfort.

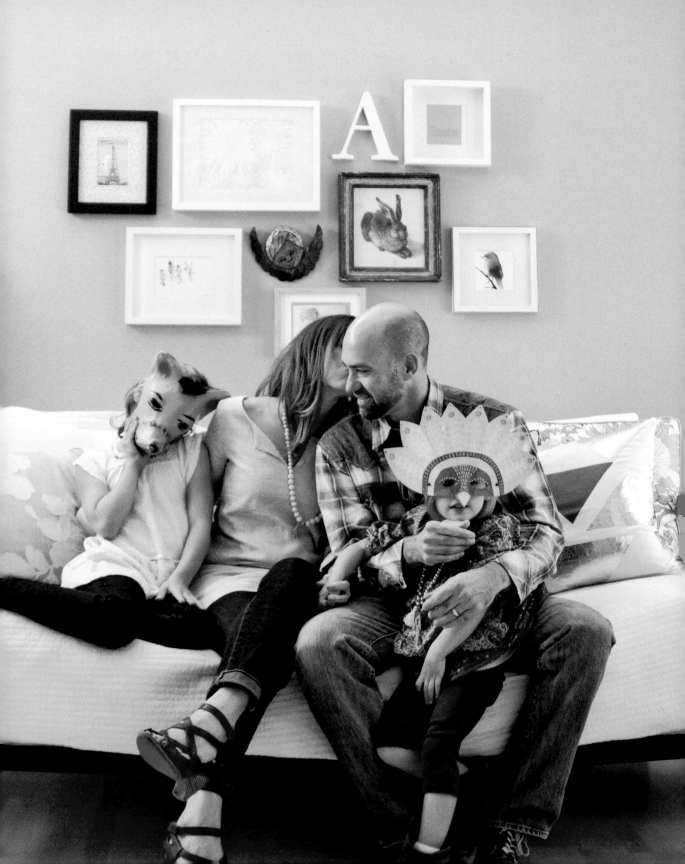

creating special spaces for kids

Everyone wants a little corner of the world to call their own. Some dads may dream of "man caves" and some moms may lust after craft studios, but kids everywhere are happy with the tiniest corner, closet, or windowsill to call their own. Here we share our own kids' special spaces and some of our favorite charming nooks put together by creative homemakers for their beautiful babes.

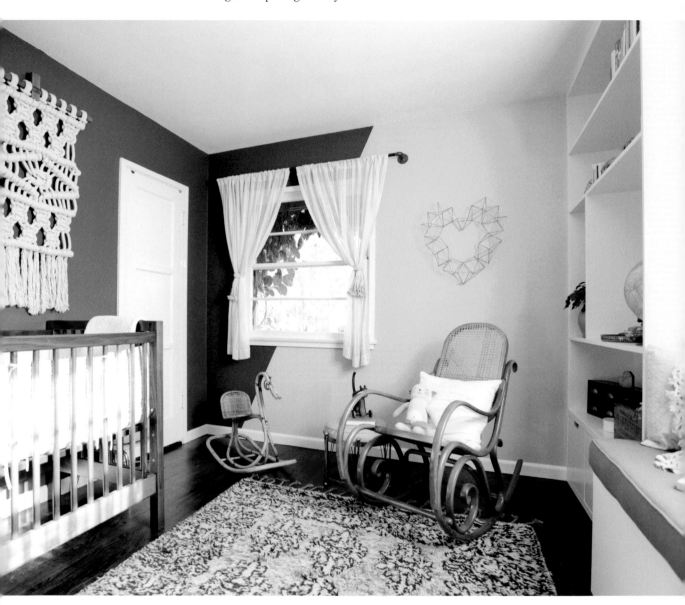

It's no surprise that this nursery, created by Bash, Please co-owner Kelly (bashplease. com) and her husband, Chris, for their daughter Lucy Roux, would exude style. Selectively decorated with rare, exclusive finds, the small space goes bold yet balanced with split room color in soothing gray and playful peach.

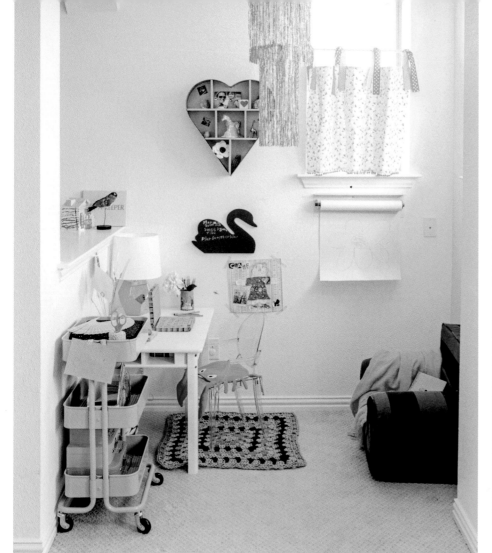
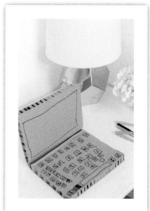
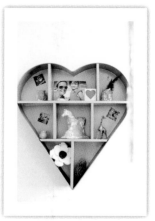

CLARE'S CORNER OFFICE

My daughters Clare and Quinn share a bedroom. My husband, Rick, and I agree that this is an important experience for these two young ladies, but I also feel that Clare, as the oldest and a rather serious girl, needs a small space to call her own. This separate corner of the family playroom makes the perfect oasis. I started by defining the space with one wall painted peach. We moved her desk and chair in, used a rolling storage cart to further establish the space, and finished up the area with a wall-mounted easel, a comfy seat, and a heart-shaped shelf filled with favorite photos and souvenirs. It's completed with our eye-catching Not-So-Granny Square Rug (see page 88 for instructions), a pretty peach throw, creative window treatments (see page 91 for ideas), and Clare's own shiny gold lamp, her favorite accent in her "home office." She is now open for business!

SCARLET'S SUNNY SEAT

Our small bungalow overflows with coziness; it's well suited for family time, snuggles, and togetherness. It's also well suited for feeling like there's no particular place set aside just for my darling daughter, Scarlet. This window nook is at counter height and would previously act as a holding place for packages, purses, and clutter, so we set about transforming it into a unique space for our voracious reader to perch. The cozy velvet seat, pocket pillow to hold her supplies (see page 102 for instructions), and light streaming in turned this odd little nook into a kids-only zone, completed with a stepstool and whimsical garland (see prettyprudent.com for instructions) to mark her space.

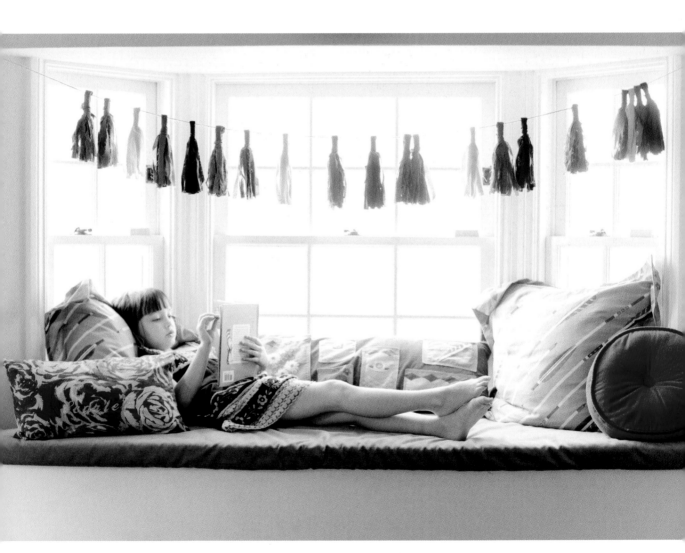

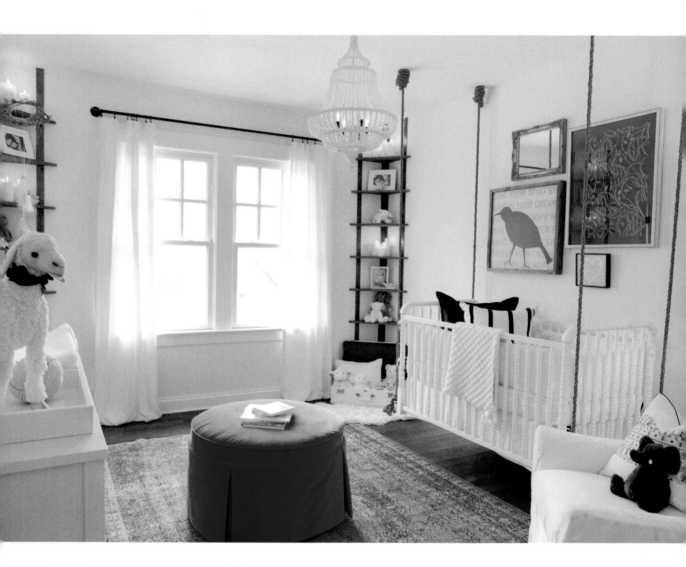

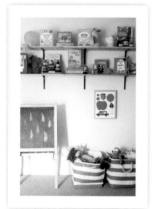
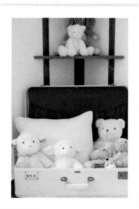

A FLOATING NURSERY

Beautiful light fills the lovely nursery that April Bermudez of April Dawn Designs (aprildawndesigns.me) created for a client's baby daughter. While most of the décor is calm and soothing in neutrals and shades of white, the bright pink kilim rug adds a pop of eye-catching color. The stunner in this space is clearly the floating crib. Have no fear, the crib is safely connected to the ceiling with strong rope tied in sailor knots to hooks in the ceiling beams, allowing baby to rest securely on waves of slight motion.

MORE SPECIAL SPACES FOR KIDS

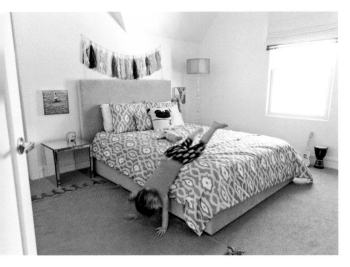

Adding an area rug—even over carpet—adds color and defines a play space.

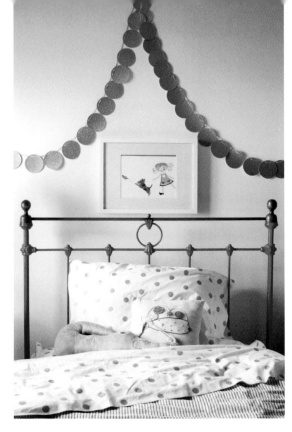

A vibrant coat of paint and a simple garland turn this bed into a royal place to rest.

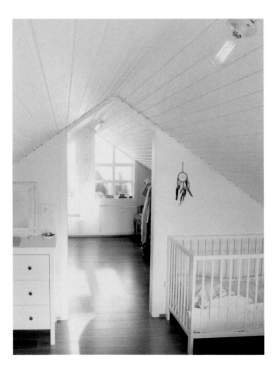

Monochromatic white and dramatic angles create a modern yet soothing nursery.

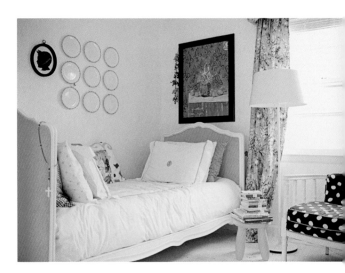

Oversize floral drapes and an undersized chair combined with a DIY day bed (created from two twin headboards) give this room an air of playful regency.

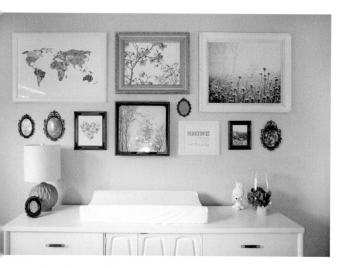

Replacing a traditional changing table with a painted mid-century dresser, complemented by a gallery wall of meaningful art pieces, creates a room that will grow with the child.

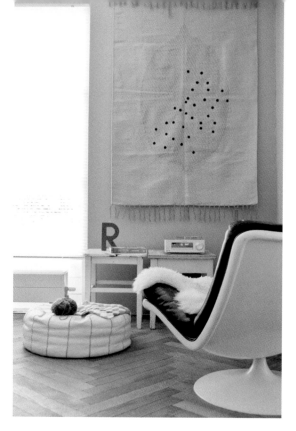

A fun, fruity rug becomes an unexpected piece of art when hung on the wall.

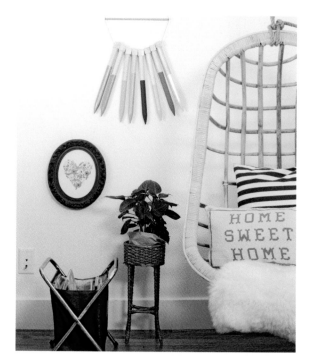

Kids love small cozy spaces to call their own like this hanging woven chair. Their isn't much more comforting than hanging out (literally) with a soft pillow and a favorite book.

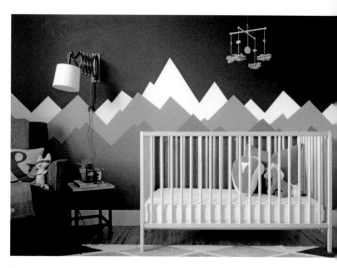

A simple yet bold landscape mural creates depth in this unexpectedly sophisticated—yet totally charming—nursery.

Stepped-up Step Stool

Helping little hands reach the sink doesn't have to be boring. Turn an inexpensive pre-fab
stool into a little piece of art with some pretty paper and decoupage medium. Try wrapping
paper, scrapbooking paper, or even recycled calendars and magazines.

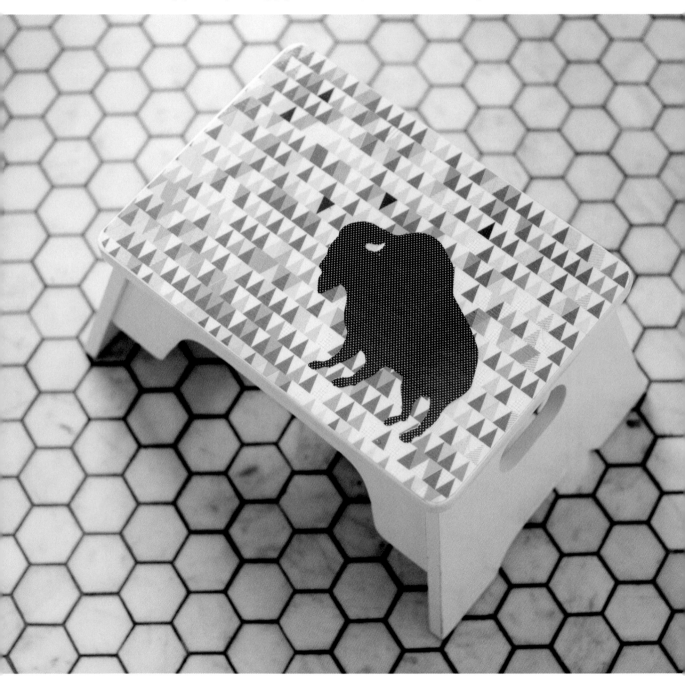

MATERIALS

Lightweight decorative paper, larger than the surface of the stool

Wood or plastic stool, painted or sealed
  (make sure it has a flat surface)

Pencil

Cutting mat

Craft knife

Soft bristle or foam brush

8 oz (240 ml) decoupage medium, gloss or matte finish

Stepped-up Step Stool Buffalo template (see page 222)

Lightweight decorative paper in a contrasting color (for the buffalo)

Clear acrylic (or polyurethane) spray sealant

INSTRUCTIONS

1   Place your decorative paper on your work surface wrong side up. Place the stool on top of the paper, upside down. Using a pencil, trace around the edge of the stool.

2   Place the paper on the cutting mat and use your craft knife to cut just inside your traced line. (Decoupage looks best when it has a small border around the outside edge.) If your stool has rounded corners, you can cut the paper more accurately by placing the stool upside down on the paper atop a cutting mat and cutting around the stool with your craft knife.

3   Using the brush, apply a thin coat of decoupage medium to the top of the stool. Immediately center the decorative paper on the stool. If you need to adjust your placement, gently slide the paper; don't lift or it will rip. Remove any wrinkles or bubbles by smoothing the paper from the center toward the outside edges with your hand.

4   Let the glue dry for 20–30 minutes. (Don't get impatient and apply your next coat before it's dry, or you'll get bubbles.)

5   Now apply a coat of decoupage medium to the top of your paper. Make sure it is the same thickness as the previous coat to avoid bubbling. Let dry completely.

6   Enlarge the template to fit the stool, print a copy, and cut it out. Place the template on the contrasting paper and trace around it using a pencil. Place the paper on the cutting mat and use a craft knife to carefully cut out the buffalo shape.

7   Apply another thin layer of decoupage medium to the top of the stool and position the buffalo. Let dry.

8   Apply another coat of decoupage medium to the top of the entire stool. Let dry completely.

9   To make your stool water-resistant, seal it with acrylic spray. This is an important step: Unsealed decoupage medium will not withstand the repeated exposure to water that is sure to happen in a bathroom.

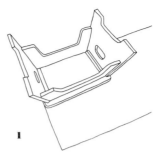

1

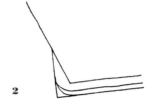

2

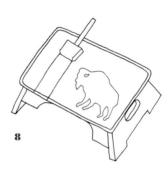

8

Binding Tape Crib Sheet

One of the first-ever tutorials on Pretty Prudent, then Prudent Baby, was a DIY crib sheet. While parents long to fill the new bundle's bed with linens worthy of a prince, the reality is that a newborn baby can only safely have a single fitted sheet—meaning no bumpers, no pillow, and no comforter. So that sheet should be spectacular. While there are many gorgeous fabrics with which to sew a crib sheet, they come in standard widths of 42–44" (107–112 cm), which is just a smidge too narrow to give the sheet a gift-worthy finished edge. This new tutorial adds a strip of binding around the bottom, giving the sheet the extra inches it needs to fit comfortably and look lovely both on and off of the bed. Here's how it's done.

INSTRUCTIONS

TO MAKE THE BINDING TAPE

1. Remove the fabric's selvages (the bound edge, which usually has writing on it). The easiest way to do this is to place the fabric flat on a cutting mat and use a straight edge and rotary cutter.

2. Fold over your fabric once or twice, parallel to the selvage edge. Make sure the layers are perfectly straight. Orient the folded fabric so the selvage runs horizontally. Place your ruler vertically on the fabric and cut 2½"- (6-cm-) wide strips. You'll need enough that when pieced together they're long enough to go around the edge of the sheet plus 12" (30.5 cm).

3. Place 1 strip on your work surface vertically and right side up. Place a second strip, horizontally and right side down, with the left short end overlapping the top of the first strip, as shown. Align the top and left edges of both strips.

4. Pin the strips together. Using the fabric marker, draw a line from the top right corner of the vertical strip to the bottom left corner of the horizontal strip.

5. Sew along this line. Trim away the corner fabric ¼" (6 mm) from the seam. Unfold the strip and iron the seam open.

6. Continue adding strips of fabric until your binding tape is long enough to go all the way around your sheet loosely plus an additional 12" (30.5 cm). Set it aside.

note: The strips of fabric for the binding tape are cut perpendicular to the selvage. This is called the cross-grain. Cross-grain has a little give. Cutting parallel to the selvage has almost no stretch, where cutting on the bias (the diagonal) gives you the most.

MATERIALS

6 yd (5.5 m) fabric, for binding tape
2 yd (1.8 m) fabric, for sheet
Ruler or straight edge (we used a 2½" [6-cm] quilting ruler, which makes it really easy)
Rotary cutter
Cutting mat
Straight pins
Air-erasable fabric marker
Sewing machine
Thread
5' (1.5 m) elastic, ⅜" (1 cm) wide

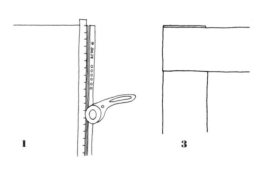

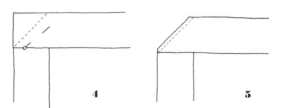

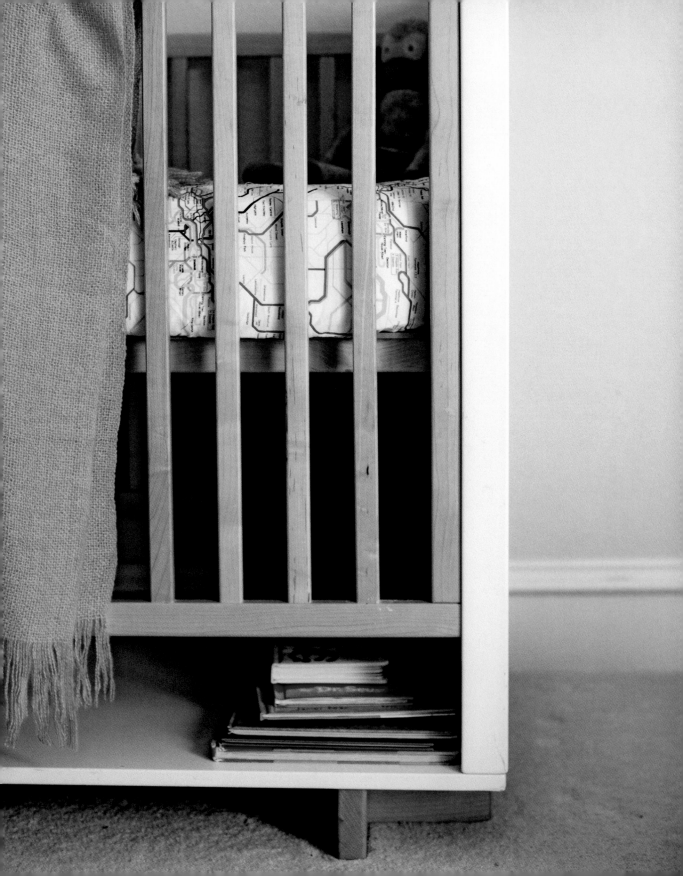

7   Cut a 44" × 68" (112 cm × 172 cm) piece of fabric for the sheet. Do not trim the selvage.

8   Place the fabric on your work surface horizontally and right side up. At each corner, cut away an 8" (20-cm) square of fabric. To make this process go faster, you can fold it in half, long sides together, and cut through two layers at a time on the open corners.

9   Open the fabric back up and place it right side up. At one corner, bring the two edges together, right sides facing.

10 Serge along the edges to make the corner of the sheet. If you don't have a serger, sew using a straight stitch, using a ⅜" (1-cm) seam allowance and then use a zigzag stitch along the edge. Repeat steps 3–4 to serge the remaining three corners of the sheet.

11 To add the binding tape, place the sheet right side up. Start in the middle of the left side. Place the binding tape right side down, left edges even. Fold down the top right corner of the binding tape, as shown, and pin. Continue to pin the binding tape to the edge of the sheet all the way around. When you reach the starting point, overlap the ends with an extra 2" (5-cm) length of binding tape. Sew or serge the binding tape to the sheet, using a ¼" (6-mm) seam allowance.

12 On the unsewn inside edge of the binding tape (the one farthest from the edge of the sheet) fold over ¼" (6 mm), wrong sides together, all the way around.

13 With the right inside edge of the binding tape folded, bring it around to the wrong side of the sheet to enclose the raw edge. (After you wrap it around, make sure the binding tape just barely covers the stitch line from step 11 on the wrong side.) Pin the binding tape in place.

14 With the sheet right side up, top stitch the binding tape on the fold where it meets the sheet, all the way around, leaving a 2"- (5-cm-) wide opening. (If you've pinned correctly, the top stitching will catch the edge of the binding tape on the wrong side of the sheet, securing both sides at the same time.) This is the casing that will house the elastic.

15 Pin one end of the elastic to your sheet near the opening in the casing. (This will prevent it from slipping inside while you work.) Attach a safety pin to the opposite end and insert it into the opening. Work it through the casing until you reach the starting point. Gather both the elastic ends, overlap them, and sew them together.

16 Sew the opening in the casing closed.

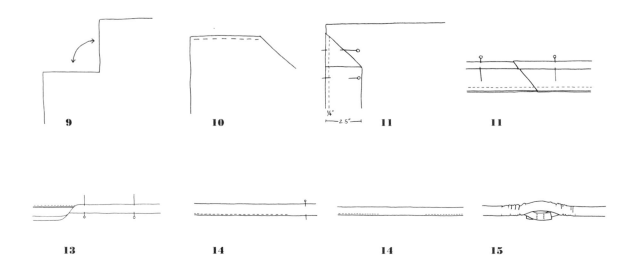

9   10   ¼" ⊢2.5"⊣ 11   11

13   14   14   15

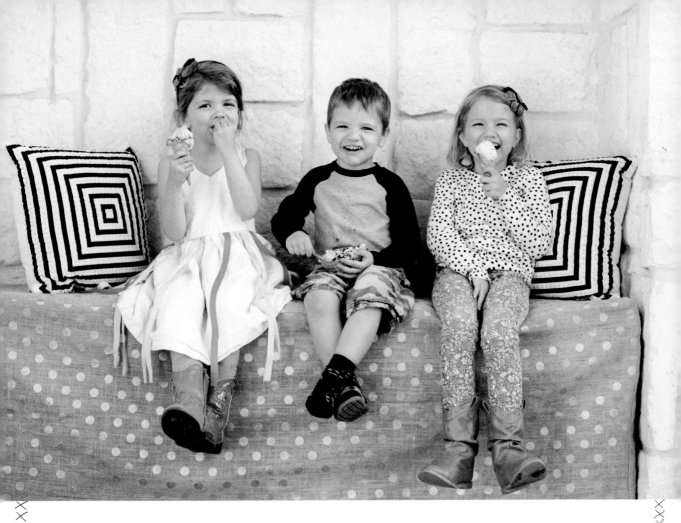

Ten Kid-Friendly Upholstery Fabric Tips

1. Micro suede is incredibly stain-resistant and easy to clean, even in white.

2. There are many suggested methods for removing ink from leather, but a Mr. Clean Magic Eraser sponge stands as our champion. Test an inconspicuous spot first, of course.

3. Dark fabrics can be as unforgiving as light fabrics.

4. Bold patterns are great for hiding spills, and babies are attracted to high-contrast color combinations.

5. Use washable slipcovers, especially on throw pillows.

6. Designate some furniture as a place to relax, put up your feet, and not worry about marker stains and snacks.

7. Designate some furniture as off-limits for wild child behavior.

8. Use a throw blanket to protect the arms, back, or seat of a high-traffic piece.

9. Use a throw blanket to hide a permanent stain.

10. Use a throw blanket to cuddle under with your kid. There will always be stains to clean, but there won't always be babies to cuddle.

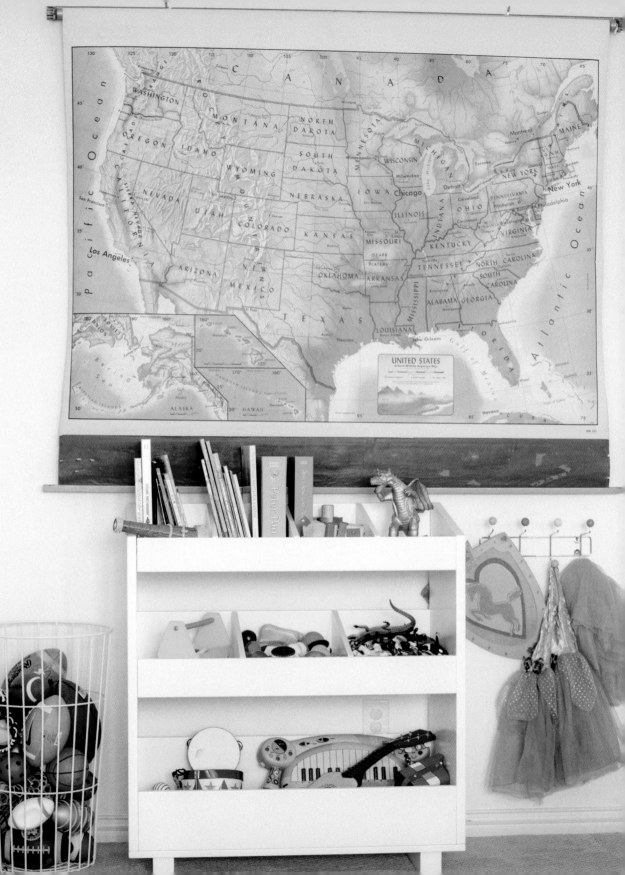

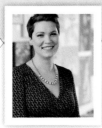

Playroom/Toy Organization Tips

BY DANIELLE KURTZ, CREATIVE DIRECTOR,
LAND OF NOD (LANDOFNOD.COM).

1　Organize toys in bins and baskets by type—a bin for dolls, for action figures, for trains. It's an easy way for kids to understand where things belong so they can, hopefully, participate in cleaning up.

2　Tall bookcases are ideal for shared spaces. Use the top shelves for decorative objects and the lower shelves for books and toys.

3　Invest in toy boxes that have a life beyond the playroom. Look for a piece that can transition into a mudroom, entryway, or living room. Then when your kids outgrow the toys, you can use the box to store hats, mittens, sport equipment, or blankets.

4　Even if you have a separate playroom, keep an attractive basket in the living room to catch strays for quick cleanup. Choose one that fits seamlessly into your décor and has a lid to hide the mess.

5　While you may want toys out of sight, they still need to be accessible to the kids. Choose storage with easily removable lids and low profiles. Also, be sure the overall size is small enough that the kiddos can carry the bins even when they're brimming with blocks.

6　Look for a coffee table with drawers or cubbies. Stash the toys there to keep them close at hand but out of sight.

7　A teepee or small playhome makes a great play space and doubles as storage for dolls and stuffed animals. Also, you can hide in there if you need a moment of peace—we won't tell.

8　Choose furniture pieces with clean, slim profiles. Bulkier pieces will make a room seem cramped. Take this one step further by adding a bookcase or table in acrylic. It disappears in the space and gives the illusion of more room.

9　Some large toys, like an art easel, simply can't be disguised. But that doesn't mean you should surrender your style. Instead look for pieces that are beautiful and functional. Take cues from the colors and materials that you'd traditionally put in your living room. You don't have a yellow and blue plastic couch, do you?

10　At least once a year, take a random day off while the kids are at school and sort through *all* the toys. Purge toys with missing or broken pieces and donate ones they've outgrown or never use. Organize the rest. They'll never notice. You'll feel 20 pounds lighter. Win-win.

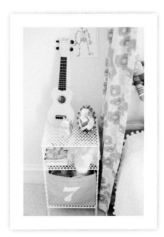

making family time

When your family is together, you always feel at home. Whether exploring
your neighborhood, goofing off inside, or doing kid-oriented activities, we find
there's something especially prudent in taking time to play together.

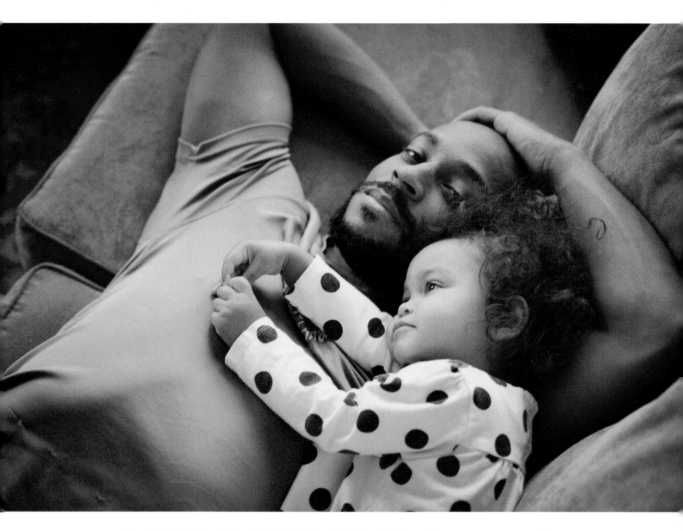

LOVE DON'T COST A THING.

Our favorite little ways to laugh together at home:

1 Ride around the house on office chairs.

2 Turn cardboard boxes into forts or "computers."

3 Throw the kids on the bed while singing made-up songs.

4 Take off our socks and have a stinky puppet show.

5 Invent hopscotch courses in the driveway.

6 Talk in a robot voice. *Meep. Morp.*

7 Roll the kids in the rug to make baby burritos.

8 Wear a rubber horse head and proceed with your day.

9 Use the couch as a balance beam for indoor Olympics.

10 Tickle fight.

Crinkle Critter Fox

Four out of four prudent babies approve of this crinkle toy, which gets its irresistible crunchy sound from a disposable wipe bag. The reward of watching your little one enjoy a handmade toy is the best feeling. Make a few extra for tiny friends while you're at it. They are sure to be a baby hit.

MATERIALS

Crinkle Critter Fox template (see page 222)
Scissors
Wool felt in orange, white, and brown
Plastic bag from disposable baby wipes
1 skein orange embroidery floss
1 skein black embroidery floss
Embroidery needle
Brown satin ribbon, for the feet
Orange satin ribbon, for the ears

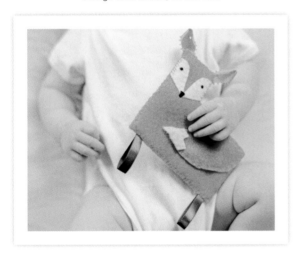

INSTRUCTIONS

1   Enlarge the template to your desired size, print a copy, and cut it out.

2   Place 2 pieces of orange felt together, edges even, with the plastic bag sandwiched between them.

3   Place the template on top and pin in place. Cut through all the layers. (You may cut the plastic bag separately to save the blades of your scissors.)

4   Use the template and scissors to cut out the fox's face and tail pieces from the white and brown felt. Arrange these on the front layer of orange felt.

5   Hand-sew the face and tail pieces to only the front layer of the fox using the orange embroidery floss and needle.

6   Hand-sew the eyes and nose to only the front layer of the fox using the black embroidery floss and needle. Make sure the stitches are very secure.

7   Reassemble the fox with the plastic sandwiched between the pieces of felt. Trim the plastic bag, if necessary, to make sure it's not showing.

8   Cut two 2" (5-cm) pieces of orange ribbon and two 3" (7.5-cm) pieces of brown ribbon. Fold each piece of orange ribbon in half and pin them between the layers of felt to make the fox's ears. Then fold each piece of brown ribbon in half and pin them between the layers of felt to make the fox's feet.

9   If you are machine stitching, sew around the outside edges using a zigzag stitch. If you are hand-sewing, use a whip stitch or blanket stitch to sew around the outside edges.

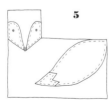
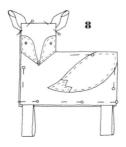
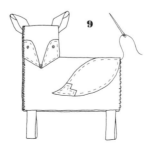

A PRUDENT FAMILY

Robin's Egg Cascarones

These hollowed out eggshells stuffed with confetti are a popular Mexican tradition in the spring. We gave them a robin's egg twist and some homemade confetti, then let the kids crack them all over the yard.

MATERIALS

Straight pins

Polystyrene (Styrofoam) block (any foam will do; we used some from a shipping box)

Eggs

Wooden skewers

Bowl

White vinegar

Food coloring

Paper in blue, Kraft, and gold

Hole punches in two different diameters

Funnel

Tissue paper in a coordinating color to the eggs

Scissors

White glue

Brown acrylic paint

Toothbrush

INSTRUCTIONS

1. To make a drying rack for the eggs, insert rows of straight pins into a polystyrene block. (This isn't absolutely necessary, just very helpful.)

2. Tap the large end of 1 uncooked egg to make a hole. Remove some of the shell and use a skewer to widen the opening.

3. Drain the egg out of the shell and into a bowl. (Use the eggs to make a quiche or some other delicious egg dish. We obviously don't support the wasting of perfectly good eggs.)

4. Rinse the eggshell until clean. Then set it on one of the pins in your drying rack to drain and dry. Repeat steps 2–4 to prepare more eggshells.

5. Color your eggs however you like. To make blue eggs like ours, mix together ½ cup (120 ml) of boiling water, 1 teaspoon vinegar, 12 drops of blue food coloring, and 4 drops of green food coloring. Let them sit for as long as needed to achieve the desired color. Place the eggshells back on the drying rack.

6. While the eggs dry, make your confetti using the paper and hole punches.

7. Use a funnel to fill each dry egg with confetti.

8. Cut tissue paper into squares just large enough to cover the opening on the eggs. Use the glue to adhere a tissue square to a hole to seal the confetti inside. Let dry. Repeat this step for the remaining eggs.

9. Thin the paint with a few drops of water. Dip the toothbrush into the paint and flick it with your finger toward the eggshells to create speckles.

10. Let dry and then get crackin'.

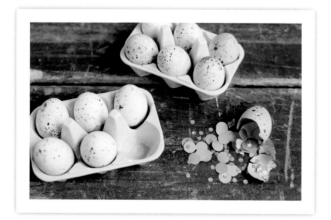

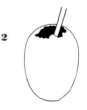

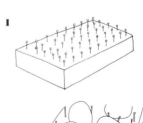

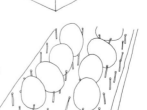

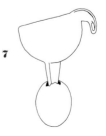

IN SPRING WE'RE SMITTEN WITH...

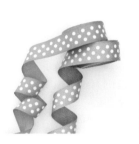 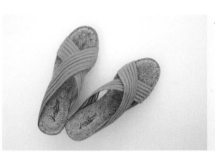 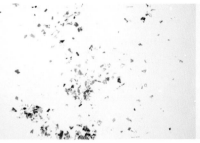

1	Rainbows	3	Peonies	6	Corsages	8	Macarons
2	Tea	4	Confetti	7	Cork	9	Cardigans
	parties	5	Kites		Wedges	10	Polka dots

IN SUMMER WE'RE SWEET ON...

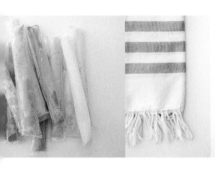 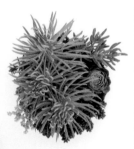 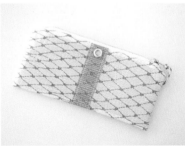 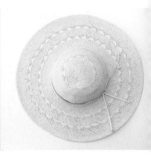

1	Popsicles	3	Straw baskets	6	Pedicures	9	Floppy
2	Beach	4	Stripes	7	Succulents		hats
	glass	5	Linen	8	Paper straws	10	Neon

A PRUDENT FAMILY

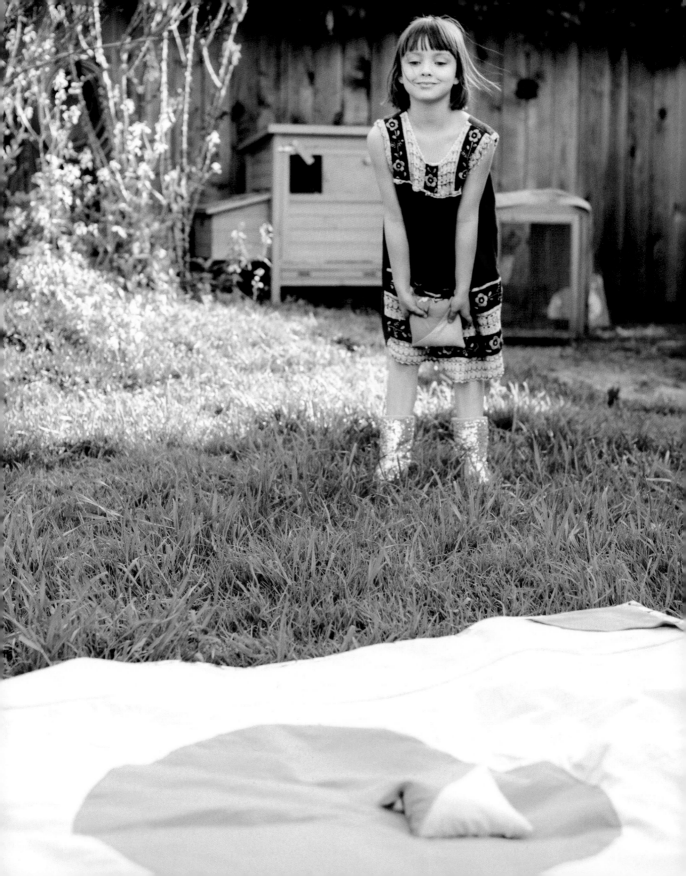

Playtime Picnic Blanket

This picnic blanket does double-duty. The circle in the center is a serving tray of sorts, while the beanbags keep the corners weighted to avoid flyaways. Then, when the feast is over, clear off the crumbs and get ready for a game of toss. Stand back and see who can get the beanbags into the circle—winner gets to pick the first popsicle.

MATERIALS

FOR THE PICNIC BLANKET

1 piece linen or cotton fabric, 41" × 60" (104 cm × 152 cm)

2 pieces linen or cotton fabric, each 10½" × 60" (26.5 cm × 152 cm)

4 pieces contrasting color linen or cotton fabric,
each 18" (46 cm) square

1 piece contrasting color linen or cotton fabric, 30" (76 cm) square

60"- (152-cm-) square piece rip-stop nylon

60"- (152-cm-) square piece batting

30"- (76-cm-) square piece double-sided interfacing
(we used Therm O Web Heat n Bond® Lite iron-on adhesive,
which has a paper backing on one side)

20'6" (6.2 m) double-fold bias tape, 1" (2.5 cm) wide

FOR THE BEAN BAGS

2 squares solid color linen or cotton fabric,
each 6½" (16.5 cm) square

2 squares contrasting solid color linen or cotton
fabric, each 6½" (16.5 cm) square

4 squares coordinating patterned linen or cotton
fabric, each 6½" (16.5 cm) square

Tape measure

Rotary cutter

Cutting mat

Iron and ironing board

Straight pins

Quilting ruler

Air-erasable fabric marker

String

Scissors

Sewing machine

Thread

Funnel

2 pounds (896 g) dry beans or rice

Hand-sewing needle

INSTRUCTIONS

TO MAKE THE PICNIC BLANKET

1 Iron the fabric pieces for the blanket. Place the 41" × 60" (104 cm × 152 cm) piece on your work surface right side up. Position one 10½" × 60" (26.5 cm × 152 cm) piece, right side down, on top, aligning the 60" (152 cm) sides. Pin then sew the 60" (152-cm) side using a straight stitch.

2 Iron the seam open. Repeat step 1 to sew the remaining 10½" × 60" (26.5 cm × 152 cm) piece to the opposite 60" (152-cm) side of the blanket. You should now have a 60" (152-cm) square. This is the top of the picnic blanket.

3 Iron the 30" (76-cm) square of contrasting fabric. To cut it into a circle, start by folding it into perfectly even quarters.

4 Place the quartered fabric on your work surface with the folded corner (the center of the whole piece) on the bottom left. Position the ruler on the diagonal from the bottom left to the top right corner across the fabric. Measure and mark 15" (38 cm) from the folded corner using the fabric marker.

5 Tie a string around the base of the fabric marker. At the opposite end of the same string either hold or pin it to the folded corner. Place the fabric marker at the 15" (38-cm) mark. While holding the string taut, swipe the marker across the fabric to the right and left of the mark to draw an arc. Cut along the line through all the layers.

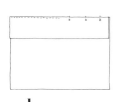

1

2

3

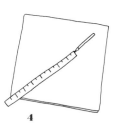

4

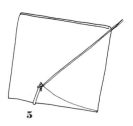

5

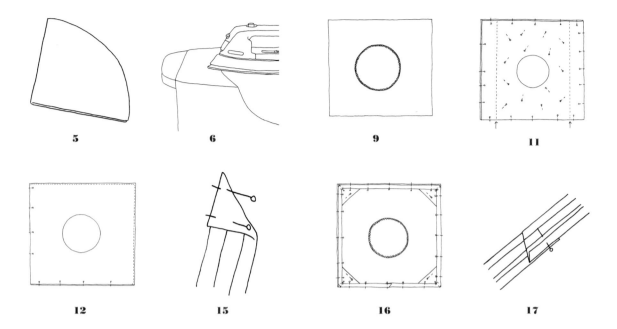

5   6   9   11

12   15   16   17

6   Open the fabric up to reveal a circle. Iron out the creases.

7   Place the circle on your work surface wrong side up. Position the square of double-sided interfacing on top and iron. Trim the interfacing so the edges are even with the fabric circle.

8   Remove the paper backing from the interfacing side of the fabric circle. Place it, fabric side up, in the center of the picnic blanket top. Iron it in place.

9   Sew around the edge of the circle using a satin stitch or tight zigzag stitch.

10   Place the piece of rip-stop nylon on your work surface wrong side up (if it has a wrong side). Place the batting on top of the nylon, edges even. Place the picnic blanket top, right side up, on top of the batting, edges even. Starting in the center of the blanket, pin the three layers together, working toward the edges.

11   Sew along the two original 60" (152-cm) seam lines (made in steps 1 and 2) using a straight stitch. (This is known as "stitching in the ditch.") As you sew, keep the layers flat to avoid bunching. If you have a walking foot for your sewing machine, use it to help avoid puckering.

12   Pin around the edges of the blanket. Sew using a straight stitch, rounding slightly at the corners rather than pivoting, using a ¼" (6-mm) seam allowance. Trim away the corners and notch the rounded edges at ½"- (12-mm-) intervals to reduce bulk.

13   Fold each 18" (46 cm) square of contrasting fabric in half along the diagonal, wrong sides together. Iron each flat to make four triangles.

14   Pin 1 triangle to each corner of the picnic blanket top, raw edges even.

15   To add bias tape around the outside edge of the blanket, start in the middle of one side. (The blanket should be right side up.) Open the bias tape and pin it right side down, raw edges even. (If you're using store-bought bias tape, place the more narrow folded edge closest to the blanket edge.) Fold down the top right corner of the bias tape into a triangle and pin it in place, as shown.

16   Pin the bias tape through all layers around the edges of the blanket, right sides together, raw edges even. Gently curve the bias tape at the corners.

17   When you reach the starting point, pin the end of the bias tape on top of the folded triangle (from step 15), overlapping by a few inches.

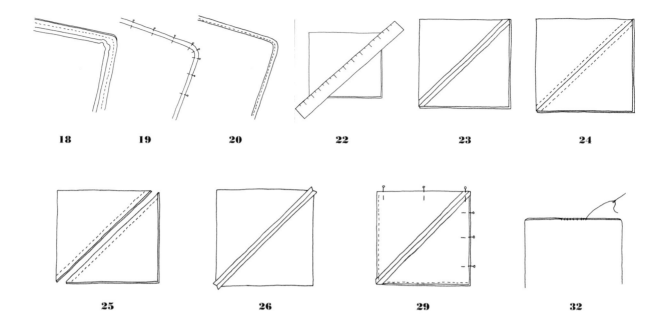

18   **19**   **20**   **22**   **23**   **24**

25   **26**   **29**   **32**

18 Sew on the narrow fold line of the bias tape using a straight stitch, all the way around the blanket.

19 Fold over the outside edge of the bias tape then bring it around to the wrong side of the picnic blanket, enclosing the raw edge of the blanket. Pin in place. (Make sure you are completely covering the previous stitch line with the bias tape.)

20 With the blanket right side up, top stitch the far edge of the bias tape (the bias tape fold, where it meets the blanket) all the way around. (If you've pinned correctly, the top stitching will catch the edge of the bias tape on the wrong side of the blanket, securing both sides at the same time.)

21 Now your blanket is complete. Time to make your bean bags!

TO MAKE THE BEAN BAGS

22 To make the tops of your beanbags, place 2 squares in different solid colors, right sides together, edges even. (Place the lighter fabric on top so you can see your markings more easily.) Draw a diagonal line between two corners using the ruler and fabric marker.

23 Draw two lines, each ¼" (6 mm) away from and parallel to the original line.

24 Sew along the two drawn lines from step 2 using a straight stitch.

25 Cut along the center line drawn in step 1.

26 Unfold the two sets of triangles and iron the seams open.

27 Trim away the excess seam fabric at the corners. Set aside.

28 Repeat steps 22–27 to make two more bean bag tops from the fabrics in solid colors.

29 Place 1 bean bag top and 1 square from the pattern fabric right sides together, edges even. Pin then sew with a straight stitch, using a ⅜" (1-cm) seam allowance and leaving a 1½" (4-cm) opening for turning. Back stitch at the beginning and end.

30 Trim the corners. Turn right side out through the opening and iron flat.

31 Using a funnel, fill the bag with beans to the desired fullness.

32 Use the needle and thread to hand-stitch the opening closed. Repeat steps 29 to 32 to make the remaining 3 bean bags.

33 Play!

Felt Swiss Cross
Hot Water Bottle Cover

Sometimes your family members just need a little compassion to overcome a back-to-school bug
or the inevitable "man cold." When you need to take TLC to a new level, whip up an easy felt cover for
a generic rubber water bottle and snuggle up. It's sure to warm their tootsies and your heart.

MATERIALS

Felt Swiss Cross Hot Water Bottle Cover template (page 222)
Rubber hot water bottle
½ yd (45 cm) winter-white wool felt
4" (10 cm) square red wool felt
Air-erasable fabric marker
Scissors
Straight pins
Cotton embroidery floss, off-white and red
Embroidery needle
Sewing machine
Thread

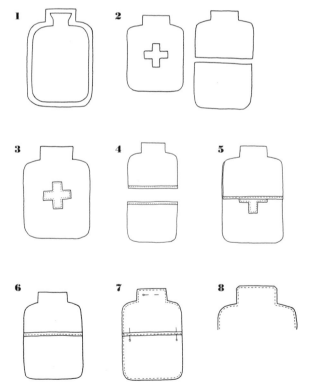

INSTRUCTIONS

1   Enlarge bottle templates A, B, and C to a size that is
    1" (2.5 cm) larger than will comfortably fit your water
    bottle and make any necessary adjustments to the shape.
    Enlarge the cross template to fit the bottle. Print out
    copies and cut out all the pieces.

2   Fold the white felt in half. Place the templates for the
    bottle on the felt, aligning the fold with the dotted lines.
    Trace around them using the fabric marker. Remove the
    templates and cut along the traced lines through both
    layers of fabric. Unfold the pieces. Place the template
    for the cross on the red felt. Trace around it using the
    fabric marker. Remove the template and cut it out.

3   Position the red cross in the center of the front piece
    (A) of white felt. Hand-sew the cross in place using a
    running stitch and off-white thread.

4   Position the back, top piece (B) of white felt wrong
    side up. Fold up the bottom edge ½" (12 mm) and pin
    in place. Hand-sew this hem using a running stitch and
    red thread. Position the back, bottom piece (C) of white
    felt wrong side up. Fold down the top edge ½" (12 mm)
    and pin in place. Hand-sew this hem using a running
    stitch and red thread.

5   Place the front piece (A) on your work surface right
    side up. Place the back, top piece (B) right side down
    on top, as shown.

6   Place the back, bottom piece (C) right side down on
    top, as shown.

7   Pin the three layers together and machine stitch around
    the entire edge with a ¼" (6-mm) seam allowance.

8   Trim the two corners at the top. Turn the cover right
    side out and insert the water bottle through the opening.

9   Give it to a friend. You can always make another.

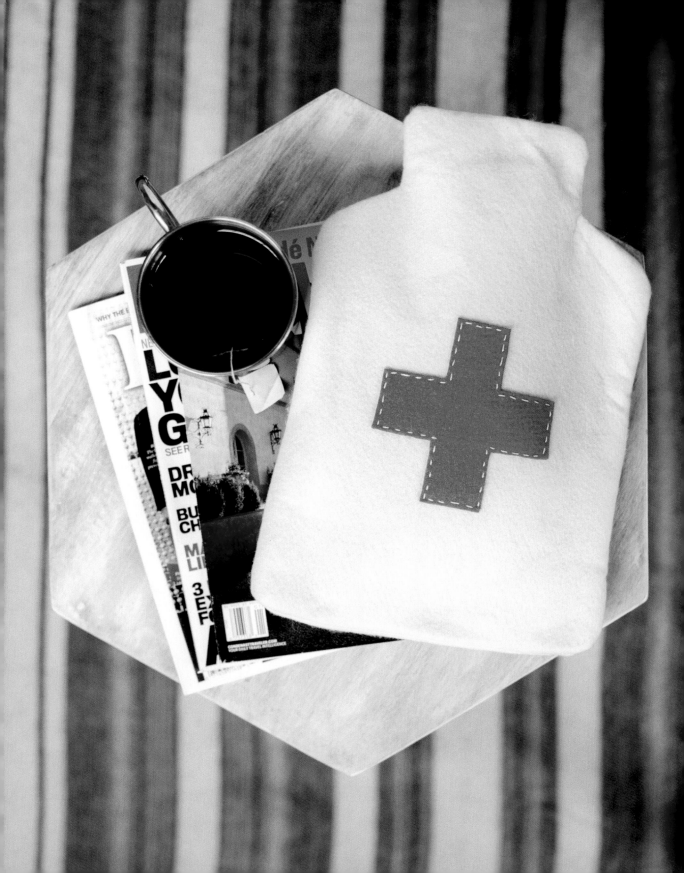

No-Sew Felt Tree Skirt

A Christmas tree without a skirt is like a child without pants; there's nothing wrong with it, it just looks kind of naked. Now you can cover that trunk easily and adorably with just felt and glue. No-sew pants not recommended. (For instructions, visit prettyprudent.com)

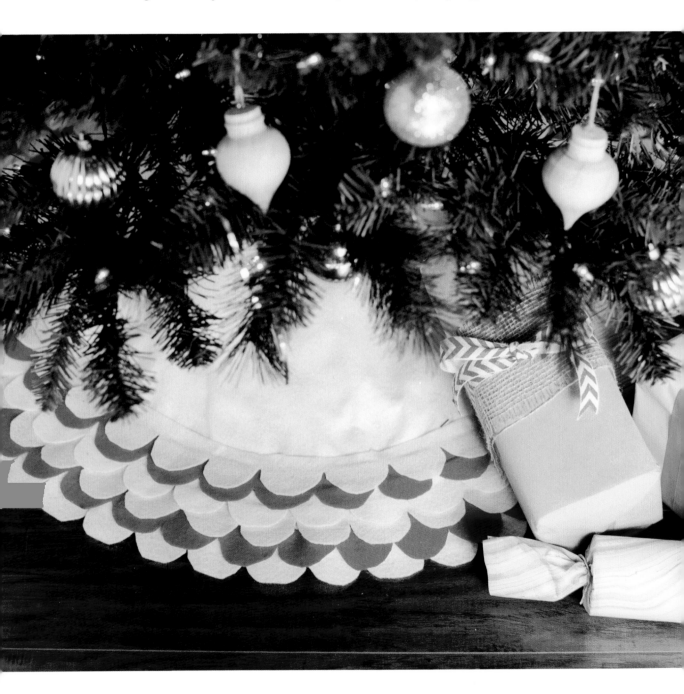

IN FALL WE
FLIP OVER...

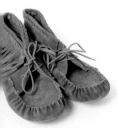 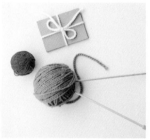 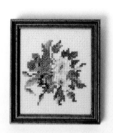 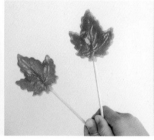 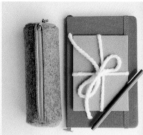

1 Moccasins
2 Yarn
3 Needlepoint

4 Tights
5 Hot
   Toddies

6 Maple everything
7 Elbow patches
8 Kraft paper

9 Fresh-baked
   bread
10 Wool felt

IN WINTER WE'RE
WILD ABOUT...

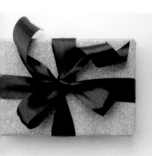 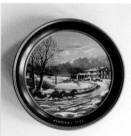 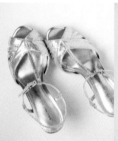 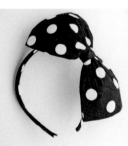 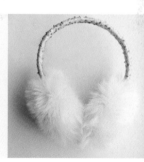

1 Glitter
2 Vintage
   cookie tins

3 Party shoes
4 Doilies
5 Bow headbands

6 Marshmallows
7 Earmuffs
8 Velvet ribbon

9 Pom-poms
10 Holly

A PRUDENT FAMILY

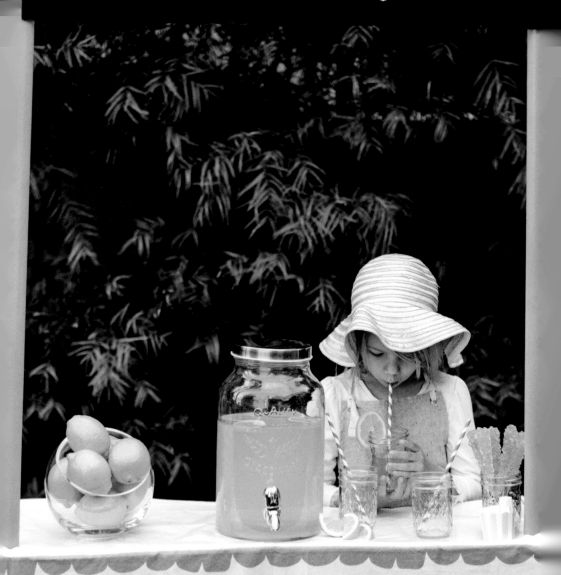

Cardboard Lemonade Stand

So your little entrepreneur wants to start slinging treats on the corner. You'd love to offer your venture capital, but how best to invest? We say give it a bit of your time and build our cardboard sale stand, then watch them use it again and again. The big payoff? This is one project that fits in just about any closet or budget, yet guarantees returns. Pretty sweet.

MATERIALS

FOR THE STAND

Cardboard sheets or cardboard boxes
Box cutter
Duct tape
Spray paint
2 dowels, 66" (168 cm) long, ¼" (6 mm) diameter
2 cup hooks
4 jump rings
Chalkboard paint
Chalk or chalk marker

FOR THE SLIPCOVER

13" × 37" (33 cm × 94 cm) piece of oilcloth
29½" × 65" (75 cm × 165 cm) piece of cotton fabric
Ruler
Rotary cutter
Cutting mat
Scissors
Quilting clips or binder clips
Sewing machine
Thread
Craft knife

INSTRUCTIONS

TO MAKE THE STAND

1   Cut the cardboard to the following dimensions:
    Piece A (Front): 28" × 36" (71 cm × 91 cm) with the corrugation parallel to the 28" (71-cm) side
    Piece B (Top): 12" × 36" (30.5 cm × 91 cm) with the corrugation parallel to the 12" (30.5-cm) side
    Piece C (Sides): four 12" × 28" (30.5 cm × 71 cm) with the corrugation parallel to the 28" (72-cm) side
    Piece D (Sign): 8" × 36" (20 cm × 91 cm)

2   Place pieces A and B on your work surface horizontally. (The 36"- [91-cm-] long sides should be on top and bottom.) Measure and mark 18" (46 cm) on every 36" (91-cm) side using a pencil. Use a straight edge to draw a line from the mark on the top edge to the mark on the bottom edge on each piece.

3   Score pieces A and B through just one layer of cardboard along the lines you drew in step 2 using the box cutter.

4   Tape all four outside edges of each piece of cardboard except for piece D.

5   Tape together two C pieces along the 28" (71-cm) sides. Place one strip of tape on the front side and one on the back side. (This will allow the pieces to bend.) Repeat this step to tape together the remaining two C pieces.

2

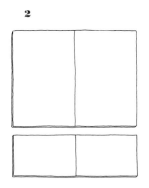

3

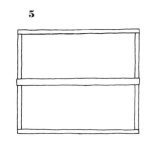

4

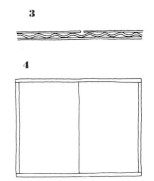

5   **6**

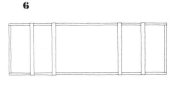

6   Stand piece A horizontally with the scored side facing out. (This will be the front of your lemonade stand.) Tape one set of C pieces to the right of the stand, 28" (71-cm) sides together. Tape the remaining set of C pieces to the left of the stand, 28" (71-cm) sides together.

7   Completely cover piece B with duct tape to make it water resistant. (This is the top of your lemonade stand.) Place piece B on top of the stand and tape each 12" (30.5-cm) side to the 12" (30.5-cm) tops of the adjacent C pieces. (The two C pieces on the ends wrap around to the back, as shown.)

8   To make the sign, start by spray painting the dowels; let dry. Then screw 1 hook into the top of each dowel, as shown.

9   Paint piece D (the sign) with chalkboard paint; let dry.

10 Cut a small "X" in each top corner of the sign using the box cutter. Insert 2 jump rings into each hole.

11 Make a slipcover following the instructions at right.

12 On the top piece of cardboard (piece B), cut a small "X" 1" (2.5 cm) from each of the front corners. (This is where the dowels will go.) Then place the slipcover on top, aligning the "X" marks.

13 Insert the dowels. Write on the sign with chalk or a chalk marker and hang.

TO MAKE THE SLIPCOVER:

1   Place the oilcloth on your work surface wrong side up. On one long side, fold over ½" (12 mm). Clip in place, then sew with a straight stitch using a ¼" (6-mm) seam allowance.

2   Iron the cotton piece flat and place on your work surface wrong side up. On both short sides, fold over ½" (12 mm). Iron, clip in place, then sew with a straight stitch using a ¼" (6-mm) seam allowance. On one long side, fold over ½" (12 mm). Iron, clip in place, then sew with a straight stitch using a ¼" (6-mm) seam allowance. Serge or use a zigzag stitch to secure the unfinished long side.

3   Orient this piece vertically and right side up with the serged (or zigzag-stitched) side on the left. Position the oilcloth horizontally and right side down, aligning the hemmed side of the oilcloth with the short side of the cotton. Clip in place.

4   Sew the short side of the oilcloth to the serged (or zigzag-stitched) long side of the cotton, using a ½" (12-mm) seam allowance and stopping ½" (12 mm) before you reach the corner.

5   Turn the project over so that the wrong side of the cotton is facing up. Bunch up the excess fabric in the corner and clip in place.

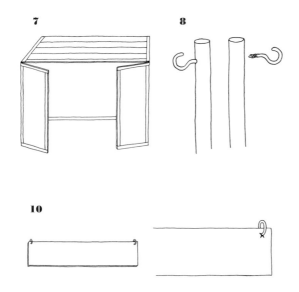

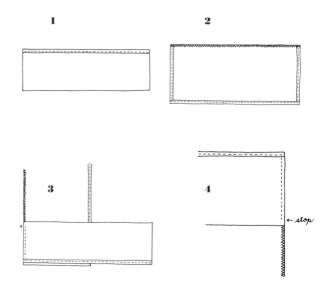

6   Turn the project back over, oilcloth side up. Align the long unfinished edge of the oilcloth with the serged (or zigzag-stitched) side of the cotton. (You'll have to fold the cotton, as shown, to get the pieces flat.) Clip in place, then begin sewing where you left off (½" [12 mm] from the corner). Continue sewing the long side, using a ½" (12-mm) seam allowance and stopping ½" (12 mm) from the corner, as before. Bunch the fabric, then proceed sewing the remaining short side.

7   On the top of the slipcover, cut a small "X" 1" (2.5 cm) from each of the front corners, as shown. (This is where the dowels will go.) Cover your lemonade stand and get to selling!

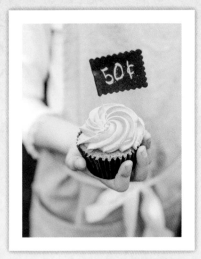

Bake Sale Tips

Sprinkles, sprinkles, and more sprinkles.

It's all about the packaging. Slide individual cookies into wax-paper bags and seal with washi tape; tie loaves of breakfast bread with pretty burlap bows.

Make bestsellers new again with fun twists. Try cutting classic rice crispy treats with fun cookie cutter shapes, or perch sandwich cookies on lollipop sticks.

Fancy cupcakes catch the little ones' eyes; add cute toppers for extra punch.

Label everything with prices so no time is wasted asking, or consider taking donations instead of pricing items. People will surprise you with their generosity.

Offer a "healthier" option such as apple slices with caramel dip.

Be sure to offer guaranteed nut-free and gluten-free options for guests with allergies.

Adding drink options to the menu will quench your customers' thirst after gobbling up your goodies.

Bags of little treats packaged together are always great for families looking to split their haul.

Consider adding a blank gift tag to each item for guests to fill in. They'll think of their friends while purchasing and spread your home-baked love around the neighborhood.

A PRUDENT FAMILY

5

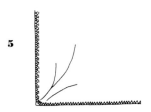

6

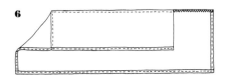

7

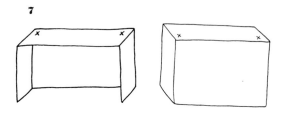

templates

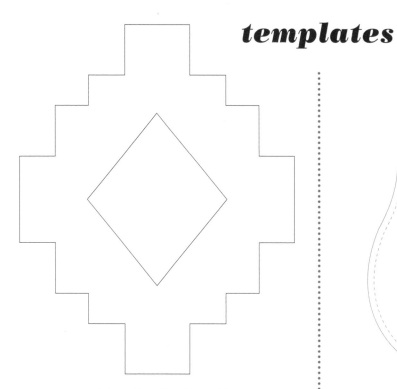

Outdoor Floor Stencil (page 82)

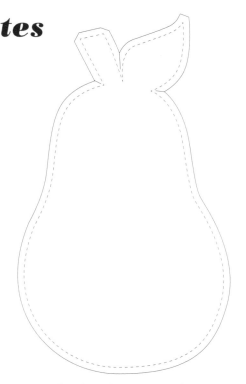

Pear Pillow Template (page 101)

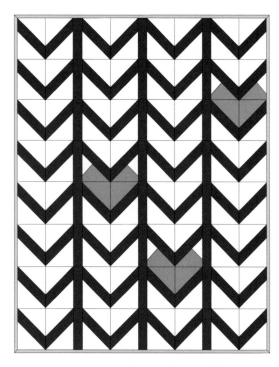

Herringbone and Heart Quilt (page 107)

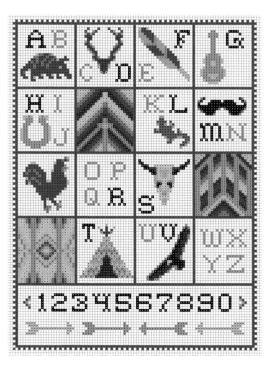

Hot Cross Stitch 1 Pattern (page 117)

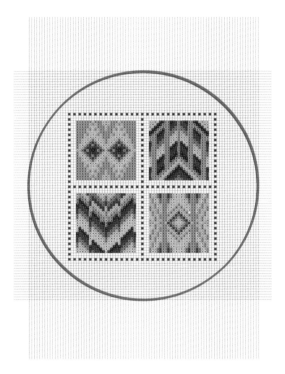

Hot Cross Stitch 2 Pattern (page 117)

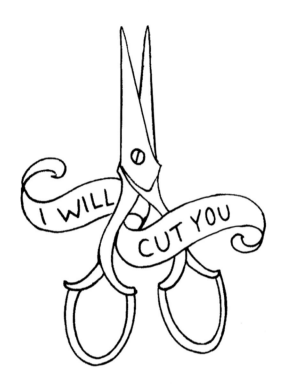

I Will Cut You Embroidery Pattern (page 118)

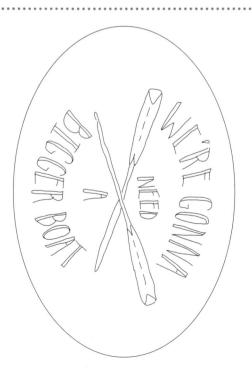

Bigger Boat Wood Burning Template (page 122)

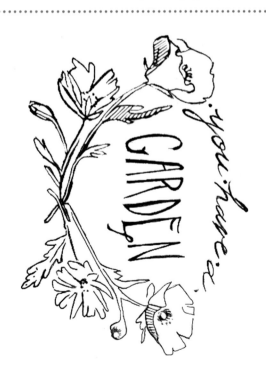

You Have a Garden Wood Burning Template (page 122)

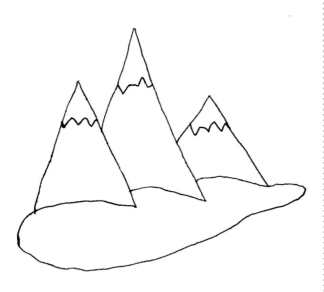

Hand Applique Mountain Template (page 179)

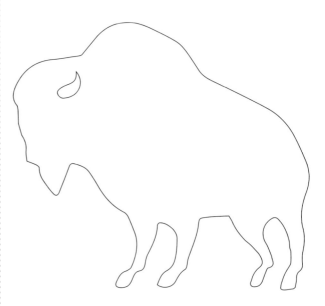

Buffalo Template (page 196)

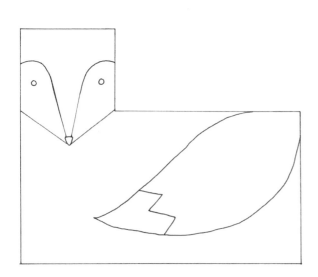

Fox Crinkle Toy Template (page 205)

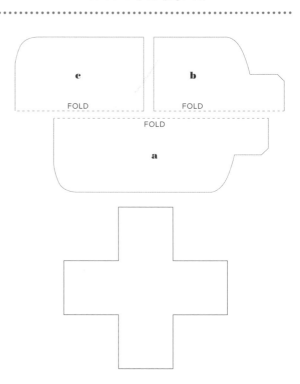

Swiss Cross Hot Water Bottle Template (page 212)

contributors

The Alder Family

Lisa Alexakis (sewmodern.com)

Amy Anderson (modpodgerocks.com)

Erin Basset (erinbasset.com)

Sonya Lee Benham
(artpusher.com, parlordiary.com)

Nina & Daryl Berg

Mona Berman (monarossberman.com)

April Bermudez (aprildawndesigns.me)

Meg Biram (megbiram.com)

Brad Blake & Alan Gove

Stacie Bloomfield (gingiber.com)

Marielle Boneau

Phyllis Boneau

Amanda Brown (SpruceAustin.com)

Lindsay Buchman

Lisa Call (olivejuiceletters.com)

Hannah Canvasser
(hannahcanvasser.com)

Raya Carlisle (ainsleycarlisle.com)

Sophia Deininger (sophiadeininger.com)

Lauren Essl (blueeyebrowneye.com)

Fabricworm (fabricworm.com)

Noel Fahden (onekingslane.com)

Frederick Holmes & Company
(frederickholmesandcompany.com/)

Sara & Rocky Garza
(saraandrocky.com, ourcozycasa.com)

Sam & Lesley Graham
(magnolialeatherworks.com,
lesleywgraham.com)

Francisco Guerra

Kelly & Chris Harris (bashplease.com)

Justine Hernandez
(apairofpowerfulspectacles@gmail.com)

Lewis Hess (atlastattoo.com/lewis-hess)

Laura House (goodhouseguest.com)

Suzan Howard

Annabel Inganni & Brendan Sowersby
(wolfum.com, 100xbtr.com)

Melissa Irish-Miller
(melissaraephotography.com)

Ingrid Jansen
(woodwoolstool.blogspot.com)

The Jayaseelan Family

Ýr Káradóttir & Anthony Bacigalupo
(reykjaviktrading.com)

Elka Karl

Danielle Keene (sheilamae.com)

Lauren Kelp (laurenkelp.com)

Tricia Kerr

Emmi Kohout

Danielle Kurtz (landofnod.com)

Lamps Plus (lampsplus.com)

The Land of Nod (landofnod.com)

Whitney May (onekingslane.com)

Annie McElwain (ainsleycarlisle.com)

Whitney McGregor (whiminteriors.com)

Michaels Arts and Crafts (michaels.com)

Jackie Miller
(instagram.com/jackbean_)

One Kings Lane (onekingslane.com)

Kelly Peak (peakphotog.com)

Greta Pechter (glasswingfloral.com)

Julia Perry (blessherhearth.com)

Sherry & John Petersik
(younghouselove.com)

Pat Piasecki (patpiasecki.com)

Amanda Saccoccio

Erin Schlosser (erinschlosser.com)

Gina Seaman

Simplicity (simplicity.com)

Lanier Skalniak

Misty Spencer (objectsliving.com)

Andrea & Steve Stanford
(spoonflower.com)

Kirby Stuart (dietcokestraightup.com)

Kelly Christine Sutton
(Kelly-Christine.com)

Manja Swanson (LampsPlus.com)

Joslyn Taylor (simplelovelyblog.com)

Kevin Truong (kevintruong.com)

Elke Van der Steen (elkvan@gmail.com)

Christine & Steven Visneau
(veecaravan.com)

Hilary & David Walker
(ourstylestories.com,
www.hilaryrosewalker.com)

Erin Weir

Heather Williams
(twigandtwinedesign.com)

Amber & Nick Wills (willscasa.com)

The Wilson Family

Gina Witcher

Colleen Zarate (colleenzarate.com)

photo credits

All illustrations including cover art © Sonya Lee Benham
All photographs © Ainsley / Carlisle except:
p. 4 © Kelly Christine Sutton; p. 7 © William Brinson; p. 8 © Kelly Christine Sutton; p. 12-13 (all) © Hilary Walker, Our Style Stories; p. 14 (all) © Nicole LaMotte, One Kings Lane; p. 15 (all) © Chad Crawford Photography; p. 16 (all) © Pat Piasecki; p. 17 (all) © Hilary Walker, Our Style Stories; p. 18 (all) © Anthony Bacigalupo, anthonybacigalupo.com; p. 19 (all) © Half Orange Photography; p. 20 (all) © Hilary Walker, Our Style Stories; p. 23 © Colleen Zarate, colleenzarate.com; p. 24 © Hilary Walker, Our Style Stories; p. 25 (top left quadrant): top left © 100xbtr, top right © Pretty Prudent, bottom left © Lamps Plus, bottom right © Pretty Prudent; (top right quadrant): top left, top right, and bottom left © Lamps Plus, bottom right © The Land of Nod; (bottom left quadrant): top left © Pretty Prudent, top right © Anthropologie.com, bottom left © Pretty Prudent, bottom right © Lamps Plus; (bottom right quadrant): top left © Pretty Prudent, top right © Schoolhouse Electric & Supply Co., bottom left and bottom right © Anthropologie.com; p. 26 (top left quadrant): top left © Pretty Prudent, top right © Rifle Paper Company, bottom left © Pretty Prudent, bottom right © The Land of Nod; (top right quadrant): top left and top right © The Land of Nod, bottom left © 100xbtr, bottom right © The Land of Nod; (bottom left quadrant): top left © Wolfum, top right © Reykjavík Trading Co., bottom left © Schoolhouse Electric & Supply Co., bottom right © Lamps Plus; (bottom right quadrant): top left © The Land of Nod, top right © Schoolhouse Electric & Supply Co., bottom left © The Land of Nod, bottom right © Anthropologie.com; p. 28 © Pretty Prudent; p. 29 (all) © Pretty Prudent; p. 30 © Colleen Zarate, colleenzarate.com; p. 31 (top) © Dalliance Design Inc.; p. 31 (bottom) © Adza Aubry, photobyadza.com, courtesy of Elka Karl; p. 32 © Colleen Zarate, colleenzarate.com; p. 34 © Ethan Luck; p. 35 © Pretty Prudent; p. 36 © Jacyln Campanaro; p. 37 (top) © Jacyln Campanaro; p. 39 © Lamps Plus; p. 41 © Adza Aubry, photobyadza.com, courtesy of Elka Karl; p. 44 © Nicole LaMotte, One Kings Lane; p. 47 © Pretty Prudent; p. 50 © Pretty Prudent; p. 52 (headshot) © Cole Collective; p. 52 (top right, bottom right) © Kimberly Jones; p. 53 (toy chest, "before" stool, and "before" rocking chair) © Pretty Prudent; p. 68 © Katie Oblinger; p. 69-70 © Pretty Prudent; p. 77 (all) © Pretty Prudent; p. 82 © Pretty Prudent; p. 86 © Katie Bower, bowerpowerblog.com; p. 95 (right) © Pretty Prudent; p. 113 © Nicole LaMotte, One Kings Lane; p. 126 © Mike Choi; p. 128 (middle) © Greta Petcher; p. 128 (bottom) © Francisco Guerra; p. 131 © Greta Petcher; p. 136 © Pretty Prudent; p. 166 (right) © Pretty Prudent; p. 167 © Pretty Prudent; p 173 © Pretty Prudent; p. 175 (top) © Pretty Prudent; p. 175 (bottom) © Stacie Bloomfield, gingiber.com; p. 187 © Todd Beeby; p. 189 © Kelly Christine Sutton; p. 190 © Shade Degges Photography; p. 193 (all) © April Dawn Designs; p. 194 (top left) © Kelly Christine Sutton; p. 194 (top right) © Lesley Graham; p. 194 (bottom left) © Anthony Bacigalupo, anthonybacigalupo.com; p. 194 (bottom right) © Whitney McGregor / Heidi Geldhauser; p. 195 (top left) © Lisa Mezzanotte, Elisabeth Arin Photography; p. 195 (top right) © Ingrid Jansen, woodwoolstool.blogspot.com; p. 195 (bottom left and bottom right) © Amber Wills; p. 203 (all) © The Land of Nod; p. 204 ©Melissa Irish-Miller; p. 207 (all) © Pretty Prudent; p. 215 (all) © Pretty Prudent
Back cover author photo © Ainsley / Carlisle

SONYA BENHAM, ILLUSTRATIONS
PARLORDIARY.COM

ANNIE MCELWAIN & RAYA CARLISLE,
PHOTOGRAPHY
AINSLEYCARLISLE.COM

COLLEEN ZARATE, PRODUCER
COLLEENZARATE.COM

acknowledgments

When we began the adventure of writing *Pretty Prudent Home*, we had no idea what a long, strange trip it would be. From our first draft of a table of contents (in 2009!), to elaborate photo shoots last year, to final copy edits just a few months ago, so many gracious, kindhearted people have contributed their time, energy, and creativity to this endeavor. We would first like to thank our husbands, Rick and Carleton, for their tolerance of our all-hours brainstorming phone calls, weekend-long writing sprees across the North American continent, and frenzied bouts of creative mania in the form of sewing, painting, and occasional screaming. We love each of you more than we love each other.

We would like to thank our kids for being adorable and always ready to craft, cuddle, and give constructive criticism ("These cookies would be much better with MORE SPRINKLES") and inspiring us to start the website (then called Prudent Baby) that would change our lives and career paths forever. Clare, Quinn, Gordon, and Scarlet, thank you for exhilarating us, exhausting us, and always reminding us that our homes and hearts are wherever you are.

This book simply would not have been possible without the endless attention, enthusiasm, and vision of our website's managing editor, Colleen Zarate. When she emailed us to ask for a job, we immediately admired her moxie, and each year since we have only learned to love and cherish her in new and deeper ways. A more gifted editor or thoughtful friend simply could not be found.

Artist Sonya Lee Benham worked tirelessly and cheerfully on more than 1,000 illustrations for this book with nary a complaint, despite almost constant henpecking from us two perfectionists. Her skill as an artist is surpassed only by her patience and humor; who else would take the time to draw additional (highly inappropriate) illustrations just to make us laugh? Thank you, Sonya (wink, wink).

We always admire a fellow lady duo, so we were honored to invite photographers Annie McElwain and Raya Carlisle to partner with us on the beautiful photography in this book. The lightness and brightness of their photography is outshined only by their personalities. If you are going to attempt making a dizzying number of photographs in a fleeting few days, you might as well have fun, and together, we certainly did.

Our deepest gratitude to Erin Weir for letting us use her home as the backdrop to many of the images in this book. We apologize for the mess we left, but we hope you enjoyed the cake and Champagne cocktails. We owe you a billion bottles of bubbly and our infinite thanks.

We are indebted to our publisher, ABRAMS, and both of our editors, Dervla Kelly for taking on our vision, and Rebecca Kaplan for helping craft that vision into the book you see here. We also owe infinite praise to tech editor Genevieve Sterbenz for every paper model made, absurdly detailed question answered, and late-night panicked email replied to with calm reassurance. Designer Sarah Gifford took our extremely detailed (perhaps slightly confusing?) creative direction and turned each page of our book into a reflection of our vision, and for that we are eternally grateful. Thank you all for bringing our book to life with your attention and warmth.

To our agent, Alison Fargis, and the team at Stonesong Press, we share with you our deepest gratitude for your guidance, attention, and tutelage since that first proposal in 2009. Your coaching helped raise this book as it sprouted, developed, and thrived over the past six years. We hope this baby makes you proud.

And finally, to our community of prudent mamas, dads, and readers: You are the reason we get up each morning and scramble to the site and our social media forums, excited to start our day with your encouragement and enthusiasm. Sharing our children's childhoods and our creative endeavors with you over these past six years has been our pleasure and our privilege; we hope we have done right by you with this book and look forward (prudently) to our future together. From the bottom of our hearts: Thank you.